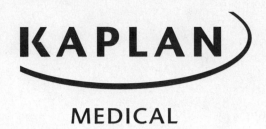

MEDICAL

USMLE® STEP 2 CK
Lecture Notes 2016 | Internal Medicine

Published by Kaplan Medical, a division of Kaplan, Inc.
750 Third Avenue
New York, NY 10017

Printed in the United States of America
10 9 8 7 6 5 4 3 2 1

Course ISBN: 978-1-62523-665-4 | Item Number: BL4017L

Retail Kit ISBN: 978-1-5062-0087-3
This item comes as a set and should not be broken out and sold separately.

Kaplan Publishing print books are available at special quantity discounts to use for sales promotions, employee premiums, or educational purposes. For more information or topurchase books, please call the Simon & Schuster special sales department at 866-506-1949.

EDITOR

Charles Faselis, M.D.
Chairman of Medicine
VA Medical Center
Washington, DC

Professor of Medicine
George Washington University School of Medicine
Washington, DC

CONTRIBUTORS

Joseph J. Lieber, M.D.
Associate Director of Medicine
Elmhurst Hospital Center

Associate Professor of Medicine
Associate Program Director in Medicine for Elmhurst Site
Ichan School of Medicine at Mount Sinai
New York, NY

Frank P. Noto, M.D.
Assistant Professor of Internal Medicine
Icahn School of Medicine at Mt. Sinai
New York, NY

Site Director, Internal Medicine Clerkship and Sub-Internship
Mount Sinai School of Medicine
New York, NY

Hospitalist
Elmhurst Hospital Center
Queens, NY

Contents

CANCER SCREENING

> A 39-year-old woman comes to the clinic very concerned about her risk of developing cancer. Her father was diagnosed with colon cancer at age 43, and her mother was diagnosed with breast cancer at age 52. She is sexually active with multiple partners and has not seen a physician since a motor vehicle accident 15 years ago. She denies any symptoms at this time, and her physical examination is normal. She asks what is recommended for a woman her age.

Screening tests are done on seemingly healthy people to identify those at increased risk of disease. Even if a diagnostic test is available, however, that does not necessarily mean it should be used to screen for a particular disease.

- Several harmful effects may potentially result from screening tests.
- Any adverse outcome that occurs (large bowel perforation secondary to a colonoscopy) is iatrogenic.
- Screening may be expensive, unpleasant, and/or inconvenient.
- Screening may also lead to harmful treatment.

Finally, there may be a stigma associated with incorrectly labeling a patient as "sick."

For all diseases for which screening is recommended, effective intervention must exist, and the course of events after a positive test result must be acceptable to the patient. Most important, the screening test must be valid, i.e., it must have been shown in trials to decrease overall mortality in the screened population. For a screening test to be recommended for regular use, it has to be extensively studied to ensure that all of the above requirements are met.

The 3 malignancies for which regular screening is recommended are **cancers of the colon, breast**, and **cervix**.

Colon Cancer

In the patient with no significant family history of colon cancer, screening should begin at age 50. The preferred screening modality for colon cancer is colonoscopy every 10 years. Other choices include annual fecal occult blood testing and sigmoidoscopy with barium enema every 5 years.

In the patient with a single first-degree relative diagnosed with colorectal cancer before age 60 or multiple first-degree relatives with colon cancer at any age, colonoscopy should begin at age 40 or 10 years before the age at which the youngest affected relative was diagnosed, *whichever age occurs earlier*. In these high-risk patients, colonoscopy should be repeated every 5 years. The U.S. Preventive Services Task Force (USPSTF) does not recommend routine screening in patients age >75.

Breast Cancer

The tests used to screen for breast cancer are mammography and manual breast exam. Mammography with or without clinical breast exam is recommended every 1–2 years from age 50–74. The American Cancer Society no longer recommends monthly self breast examination alone as a screening tool. Patients with very strong family histories of breast cancer (defined as multiple first-degree relatives) should consider prophylactic tamoxifen, discussing risks and benefits with a physician. Tamoxifen prevents breast cancer in high-risk individuals.

Cervical Cancer

The screening test of choice for the early detection of cervical cancer is the Papanicolaou smear (the "Pap" test). In average risk women, screening with Pap smear should be started at age 21, **regardless of onset of sexual activity**. It should be performed every 3 years until age 65. As an alternative, women age 30–65 who wish to lengthen the screening interval can do co-testing with Pap and HPV testing every 5 years. In higher risk women, e.g., HIV, more frequent screening or screening beyond age 65 may be required.

TRAVEL MEDICINE

A 44-year-old executive comes to the clinic before traveling to Thailand for business. He has no significant past medical history and is here only because his company will not let him travel until he is seen by a physician. The patient appears agitated and demands the physician's recommendation immediately.

It is important to set up a pretravel counseling session approximately 4 to 6 weeks before the patient's departure.

Hepatitis A infection is travelers' most common vaccine-preventable disease. Hepatitis A infection is possible wherever fecal contamination of food or drinking water may occur. Infection rates are particularly high in nonindustrial countries. If a patient is leaving within 2 weeks of being seen, both the vaccine and immune serum globulin are recommended. A booster shot given 6 months after the initial vaccination confers immunity for approximately 10 years.

All travelers to less-developed countries should get hep A vaccine.

Hepatitis B vaccination is recommended for patients who work closely with indigenous populations. Additionally, patients who plan to engage in sexual intercourse with the local populace, to receive medical or dental care, or to remain abroad for >6 months should be vaccinated.

Malaria: Mefloquine is the agent of choice for malaria prophylaxis. It is given once per week; it may cause adverse neuropsychiatric effects such as hallucinations, depression, suicidal ideations, and unusual behavior. Doxycycline is an acceptable alternative to mefloquine, although photosensitivity can be problematic. For pregnant patients requiring chemoprophylaxis for malaria, chloroquine is the preferred regimen.

Rabies vaccination is recommended for patients traveling to areas where rabies is common among domesticated animals (India, Asia, Mexico). Chloroquine can blunt the response to the *intradermal* form of rabies vaccine. Therefore, in patients who require malaria prophylaxis, in addition to rabies prophylaxis the *intramuscular* form of the vaccine should be administered. Rabies vaccination is not considered a routine vaccination for most travelers.

Typhoid vaccination is recommended for patients who are traveling to developing countries and will have prolonged exposure to contaminated food and water. Typhoid vaccination comes in 2 forms, an oral live attenuated form and a capsular polysaccharide vaccine given parenterally. The live attenuated form (1) needs to be refrigerated, and (2) is contraindicated in patients who are HIV positive. The polysaccharide vaccine is given intramuscularly as a single injection. Side effects include irritation at the injection site. Fever and headache are rare adverse reactions to the vaccine. The polysaccharide vaccine is the preferred form for almost all subjects as it is well-tolerated and convenient (no need for refrigeration). It is safe for HIV patients.

Polio: Adults who are traveling to developing countries and have never received a polio vaccine should receive 3 doses of the inactivated polio vaccine. Patients who have been previously immunized should receive a one-time booster. The live attenuated polio vaccine is no longer recommended because of the risk of vaccine-associated disease.

Patients traveling to areas where **meningococcal meningitis** is endemic or epidemic (Nepal, sub-Saharan Africa, northern India) should be immunized with the polysaccharide vaccine. Additionally, Saudi Arabia requires immunization for pilgrims to Mecca. Patients with functional or actual asplenia and patients with terminal complement deficiencies should also receive the vaccine. Meningococcal vaccine is now routinely administered at age 11.

To prevent **traveler's diarrhea**, patients should be advised to avoid raw and street vendor salads, unwashed fruit, and tap/ice water. Patients who experience mild loose stools without fever or blood can safely take loperamide. Treatment with a fluoroquinolone or azithromycin is reserved for patients with moderate to severe symptoms.

IMMUNIZATIONS

> A 52-year-old man comes to the clinic for a health maintenance evaluation. His recent colonoscopy showed no evidence of carcinoma. Recent serum fasting glucose, serum cholesterol, and blood pressure measurements are all within normal limits. The patient has a history of smoking, continues to smoke 2 packs per day, and was diagnosed with COPD 3 years ago.

Note

Patients must get pneumovax, meningococcal, and Haemophilus vaccines 2 weeks before a splenectomy.

Immunization is the best method available to prevent serious infectious disease. Between 50,000 and 70,000 adults die every year from preventable infectious diseases (influenza, invasive pneumococcal disease, and hepatitis B). Surveys have shown that among patients who have an indication for any vaccination, very few actually receive it (pneumococcal vaccination 20%, influenza 40%, hepatitis B 10%). It is for this reason that the American College of Physicians recommends that every patient's immunization status should be reviewed at age 50. Risk factors that would indicate specific vaccinations should be evaluated at that time.

Most patients received a primary immunization against tetanus and diphtheria as children. Adults who were never vaccinated should receive a total of 3 doses, the first 2 of which are given 1 to 2 months apart, with the third dose given 6 to 12 months later. The principle is that adults require a total of 3 vaccinations against tetanus and diphtheria. A booster vaccination should be given every 10 years for life. One of the boosters should use Tdap instead of Td booster. If the wound is dirty, revaccinate after 5 years.

Influenza Vaccine

Recommended annually for all adults regardless of age. Patients who have a history of cardiopulmonary disease, diabetes mellitus, or hemoglobinopathy, or are age 50+ residents of chronic care facilities derive the greatest benefit from an annual influenza vaccination. Pregnant women who will be in their second or third trimester during the influenza season should also receive the vaccine.

Pneumococcal Vaccine

Indicated for all adults age ≥65. Additionally, patients with a history of sickle-cell disease or splenectomy, those who have a history of cardiopulmonary disease, alcoholism, or cirrhosis, and Alaskan natives and certain Native American populations should receive the vaccine regardless of age. Immunocompromised patients (patients with hematologic malignancies, chronic renal failure, or nephrotic syndrome; HIV-positive patients; or patients receiving immunosuppressive medications) should also receive the vaccine at any age. Revaccination should be performed in healthy patients who received their initial vaccination age <65 and were age <60 at the time of primary vaccination. Patients with a high risk of fatal infection (CKD, asplenic patients, immunocompromised patients) should be revaccinated once after 5 years. No one gets >1 booster shot per lifetime.

Hepatitis B Vaccine

Recommended when there is a history of IV drug abuse, male homosexuality, household or sexual contact with hepatitis B carriers, or frequent exposure to blood or blood products. Additionally, patients with a history of chronic liver disease should receive the vaccine. Immunity is confirmed serologically. Also recommended for all children through age 18, those with STIs, those who are sexually active but not monogamous, workers with occupational exposure to blood, and prison inmates.

Hepatitis A Vaccine

The vaccine against hepatitis A protects against the virus in >95% of cases. There are 2 types of vaccine; both types stimulate active immunity against a future infection.

- One contains inactivated hepatitis A virus
- One contains a live but attenuated virus

For the best protection, the vaccine should be given in 2 doses; a booster should follow up the initial dose 6-12 months later. Protection against hepatitis A begins approximately 2-4 weeks after the initial vaccination. Those who miss the follow-up booster dose should receive only the remaining booster dose.

In the United States, the vaccine is strongly recommended for all children age 12-23 months in an attempt to eradicate the virus nationwide. There are also recommendations that the following populations should be vaccinated:

- All children age >1 year
- People whose sexual activity puts them at risk
- People with chronic liver disease
- People who are being treated with clotting factor concentrates
- People who are living in communities where an outbreak is present

Hepatitis A is the most common vaccine-preventable virus acquired during travel, so people travelling to places where the virus is common (Indian subcontinent, Africa, Central America, South America, the far East, and Eastern Europe) should be vaccinated.

Varicella Vaccine

A live attenuated vaccine recommended for use in all adults who lack a history of childhood infection with varicella virus. Being a live attenuated vaccine, varicella vaccine should not be given to immunocompromised patients, HIV-positive patients when symptomatic or <200 CD4 cells, or pregnant women.

Patients age ≥60 are recommended to receive the varicella zoster (shingles) vaccine, which has been shown to reduce the risk of zoster and its associated pain (post-herpetic neuralgia). It is indicated regardless of whether there is a history of shingles, as it is possible to have a second herpes zoster infection.

Measles, Mumps, Rubella (MMR) Vaccine

A live attenuated vaccine usually given in childhood. Healthy adults born after 1956 should receive one dose of the vaccine. Pregnant women and immunocompromised patients should not be vaccinated. HIV-positive patients who are asymptomatic may receive the vaccine.

Meningococcal Vaccine

Recommended for everyone at age 11 visit. Also recommended for young adults living in dormitories or barracks, people exposed to outbreaks, those with asplenia or terminal complement deficiencies, those who travel to endemic regions (traveling to Mecca), and those exposed to *Neisseria menigitidis*.

Human Papillomavirus (HPV) Vaccine

Recommended for women age 9-26, regardless of sexual activity. Do not use in pregnancy. Regimen is in 3 doses: 0, 2, and 6 months.

Herpes Zoster Vaccine

The zoster vaccine is a live vaccine that has been shown to reduce the incidence of shingles by 50%. It has also been shown to reduce the number of cases of post-herpetic neuralgia, as well as the severity and duration of pain/discomfort associated with shingles. The vaccine is, basically, a larger-than-normal dose of the chicken pox vaccine, as both shingles and chickenpox are caused by the same virus, varicella zoster (VZV).

The shingles vaccine (Zostavax) is recommended for adults age ≥60, whether they have already had shingles or not. The shingles vaccine is a live vaccine given as a single injection. Some people report a chickenpox-like rash after receiving it. The vaccine should NOT be given to:

- Those with a weakened immune system due to HIV/AIDS or another disease that affects the immune system
- Those who are receiving immune system-suppressing drugs or treatments, such as steroids, adalimumab (Humira), infliximab (Remicade), etanercept (Enbrel), radiation or chemotherapy
- Those who have neoplasia, which affects the bone marrow or lymphatic system, such as leukemia or lymphoma

SMOKING CESSATION

A 25-year-old man comes to the clinic for evaluation of a stuffy nose and fever. Over the course of the interview the patient states that he smokes 3 packs of cigarettes per day and has been doing so for the last 7 years.

Smoking is responsible for 1 in every 5 deaths in the United States. Smoking cessation is the most preventable cause of disease. Physicians can take the following steps to assist:

ASK about smoking at every visit.

ADVISE all smokers to quit at every visit.

ATTEMPT to identify those smokers willing to quit.

ASSIST the patient by setting a quit date (usually within 2 weeks) and using nicotine patches/gum, the oral antidepressant bupropion or varenicline as supportive therapy. Varenicline and bupropion are more effective than patches.

ARRANGE follow-up. Provide positive reinforcement if the quit attempt was successful. If the quit attempt was not successful, then determine why the patient smoked and elicit a recommitment to smoking cessation. Most patients will require several attempts before being successful.

Monotherapy treatment for smoking cessation includes nicotine replacement therapy (transdermal nicotine patches, gum, lozenges, inhalers), bupropion, and varenicline. Bupropion lowers the seizure threshold so do not use in cases of alcohol abuse. With varenicline, screen first for depression since it causes increased rate of suicidal thoughts.

Place a follow-up call 1-2 weeks after quit date. The use of pharmacotherapy doubles the effect of any tobacco cessation intervention.

Note

Varenicline should not be used in patients with a history of psychiatric disease.

OSTEOPOROSIS

All women age >65 should be given DEXA bone density scan. Screening should begin at age 60 if there is low body weight or increased risk of fractures. A bone density test uses x-rays to measure how many grams of calcium and other bone minerals are packed into a segment of bone. The bones that are tested are in the spine, hip and forearm. Bone density test results are reported in 2 numbers: T-score and Z-score.

The **T-score** is the bone density compared with what is normally expected in a healthy young adult of the same sex. The T-score is the number of units—standard deviations—that bone density is above or below the average. T-score >2.5 SD indicates the likelihood of osteoporosis and increased risk of fracture. The diagnosis of osteoporosis by DEXA scan also means that treatment should be initiated with bisphosponates, oral daily calcium supplementation, and vitamin D.

The **Z-score** is the number of standard deviations above or below what is normally expected for someone of the same age, sex, weight, and ethnic or racial origin. Z-score ≤-2 may suggest that something other than aging is causing abnormal bone loss (consider drugs causing osteoporosis such as corticosteroids). The goal in this case is to identify the underlying problem.

ABDOMINAL AORTIC ANEURYSM

U/S should be done once in men age >65 who have ever smoked. There are no screening recommendations for male nonsmokers and women, regardless of smoking history.

HYPERTENSION, DIABETES MELLITUS, AND HYPERCHOLESTEROLEMIA

> A 45-year-old man comes to the physician anxious about his health. Five years ago his mother was diagnosed with diabetes and high cholesterol. He is worried about his health and risk for heart disease. Physical examination is within normal limits.

Cholesterol screening should commence at age 35 in men who have no risk factors. In both men and women with risk factors for coronary artery disease, screening should be done routinely after age 20. Management should not be determined by an isolated reading because cholesterol levels may fluctuate between measurements. Repeat in 5 years in low-risk individuals.

Screening for diabetes mellitus should be considered only for patients with hypertension (>135/80 mm Hg). Diabetes mellitus is diagnosed when:

- 2 fasting glucose measurements are >125 mg/dL, HbA1c > 6.5%, or
- random glucose >200 mg/dL accompanied by symptoms

There is insufficient evidence for or against routine screening. The strongest indication is for those with hypertension and hyperlipidemia.

Screening is recommended for elevated blood pressure in those age >18, at every visit. Screening is not recommended for carotid artery stenosis with duplex.

ALCOHOL ABUSE

> A 55-year-old man comes to the office for evaluation of a sore throat. The patient admits that he was recently fired from his job and is having marital problems at home. The patient has no significant past medical history, and physical examination is within normal limits. He attests to drinking 3 shots of whiskey every day after work.

Physicians should screen for alcohol abuse by using the CAGE questionnaire:

Have you ever felt the need to:	Cut down on your drinking?
Have you ever felt:	Annoyed by criticism of your drinking?
Have you ever felt:	Guilty about your drinking?
Have you ever taken a morning:	Eye opener?

A positive screen is 2 "yes" answers. One "yes" should raise the possibility of alcohol abuse.

PREVENTION OF VIOLENCE AND INJURY

A 27-year-old woman presents to the emergency department complaining of right-arm pain. When asked how she sustained the injury, she states that she fell down the steps in front of her house. The patient appears anxious and nervous. On physical examination there are various 2 cm wide lacerations on her buttocks.

Injuries are the most common cause of death in those age <65. The role of the physician is to advise patients about safety practices that can prevent injury, e.g., using seat belts, wearing bicycle helmets, and not driving after drinking alcohol.

Identifying women who are at increased risk of physical or sexual abuse is an essential role for physicians. Simply asking women if they have been hit, kicked, or physically hurt can increase identification by >10%.

DISEASES OF THE PITUITARY GLAND

The pituitary is surrounded by the sphenoid bone and covered by the sellar diaphragm, an extension from the dura mater. It lies in the sella turcica near the hypothalamus underneath the optic chiasm.

The pituitary is divided into 2 lobes—the adenohypophysis or anterior lobe, which constitutes 80% of the pituitary, and the neurohypophysis or posterior lobe, which is the storage site for hormones produced by the neurosecretory neurons (supraoptic and paraventricular nuclei) within the hypothalamus. The 2 hormones stored in the posterior lobe are ADH (antidiuretic hormone or vasopressin) and oxytocin.

There is a very close relationship between the hypothalamus and the pituitary. The hypothalamus regulates the release of hormones from the anterior pituitary by different hypothalamic releasing and inhibiting hormones (hypothalamic–pituitary axis).

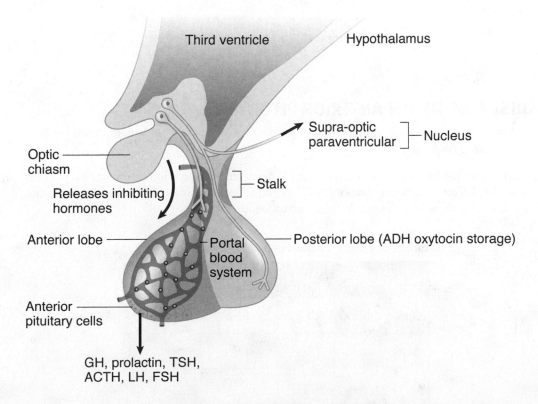

Figure 2-1. Pituitary Gland

As a sample summary, the hypothalamus secretes releasing factors for each respective pituitary stimulatory hormone. Each pituitary hormone stimulates release of the active hormone from the final target gland. The active hormones then inhibit release of releasing factors and stimulatory hormones from the hypothalamus and pituitary gland, respectively. This is feedback inhibition, and it leads to a steady state of both respective hormones involved in the axis.

Clinically, disease states involving overproduction of target hormones lead to suppressed levels of pituitary hormones, while those involving underproduction of target hormones lead to increased levels. We use this physiology to screen and diagnose these diseases.

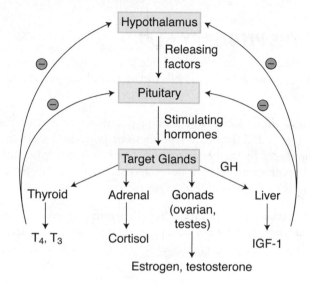

Figure 2-2. Summary of Action

DISEASES OF THE ANTERIOR PITUITARY

Syndromes causing excess production of hormones usually arise from benign tumors only of a single cell type.

Microadenomas are defined as tumors <1 cm in diameter. Macroadenomas are tumors >1 cm in diameter. Larger tumors can occasionally compress the optic chiasm and can cause visual deficits. Microadenomas are more common than macroadenomas.

Table 2-1. Pituitary Adenomas by Function

Prolactin	50–60%
Growth hormone (GH)	15–20%
ACTH	10–15%
Gonadotroph	10–15%

Hyperprolactinemia

A 32-year-old woman comes to your office because she has noticed milk-like discharge from her breasts the past 4 weeks. She also states that she has not menstruated in 2 months. The examination reveals galactorrhea but is otherwise normal.

Definition. Excess prolactin secretion is a common clinical problem in women and causes the syndrome of galactorrhea-amenorrhea. The amenorrhea appears to be caused by inhibition of hypothalamic release of gonadotropin-releasing hormone (GnRH) with a decrease in luteinizing hormone (LH) and follicle-stimulating hormone (FSH) secretion. Prolactin inhibits the LH surge that causes ovulation. The LH/FSH-producing cells are not destroyed, just suppressed. Although hyperprolactinemia is also seen in men, gynecomastia and especially galactorrhea are very rare. The most common presenting symptom in men is erectile dysfunction and decreased libido.

Etiology. Hyperprolactinemia can be seen in natural physiologic states such as pregnancy, early nursing, hypoglycemia, seizure, exercise, stress, sleep, cirrhosis, nipple stimulation, and chronic renal failure (due to PRL clearance).

Autonomous production of prolactin occurs with pituitary adenomas; these so-called pro-lactinomas are the most common functioning pituitary adenomas, accounting for 60% of all pituitary tumors. They are usually microadenomas when they occur in women and macroadenomas in men, usually presenting with visual field deficits, etc. Macroadenomas can obstruct the pituitary stalk, increasing prolactin release by blocking dopamine transport from hypothalamus (stalk effect). Other examples are tumors, such as craniopharyngioma, meningioma, and dysgerminoma; empty sella; and trauma.

Hyperprolactinemia can also occur with decreased inhibitory action of dopamine. This occurs with the use of drugs that block dopamine synthesis (phenothiazines, metoclopramide) and dopamine-depleting agents (α-methyldopa, reserpine). Tricyclic antidepressants, narcotics, cocaine, SSRIs, and risperidone can also cause increased prolactin.

Stimuli that overcome the normal dopamine inhibition can also lead to hyperprolactinemia. An example of this is primary hypothyroidism (resulting in an increase in thyrotropin-releasing hormone [TRH]) and subsequently an increase in prolactin release.

Always check TSH in patients with elevated prolactin.

Clinical. Hyperprolactinemia presents with galactorrhea, menstrual abnormalities amenorrhea/oligomenorrhea, osteopenia and osteoporosis in long-standing cases, infertility, and gynecomastia in women; men present with hypogonadism, erectile dysfunction, decreased libido, gynecomostia, and infertility. Men typically do not develop galactorrhea. Women are detected earlier because of menstrual symptoms. Hence, microadenomas are more common in women.

Diagnosis. Always exclude states such as pregnancy, lactation, hypothyroidism and medications before starting the work-up of hyperprolactinemia. Prolactinomas may co-secrete growth hormone (GH).

Prolactin levels >100 ng/mL suggest probable pituitary adenoma. Prolactin level should be commensurate with tumor size, with prolactin levels of 100 ng/mL correlating with tumor approximately 1 cm, of 200 ng/mL correlating with tumor approximately 2 cm, etc.

Note

Cabergoline is used more often than bromocriptine because of a better side-effect profile. It should be considered the preferred medical treatment for galactorrhea.

Note

A basal, fasting, morning PRL level >100 to 200 mg/L (normal <20 mg/L) in a nonpregnant woman indicates a need for an MRI of the pituitary.

Management. For prolactinomas, initially treat with cabergoline or bromocriptine (a dopamine agonist), which reduce prolactin levels in almost all hyperprolactinemic patients. Dopamine normally inhibits prolactin release. Surgery is reserved only for adenomas not responsive to cabergoline or bromocriptine, or if the tumor is associated with significant compressive neurologic effects. Surgery is more effective for microadenomas than macroadenomas. Only 30% of macroadenomas can be successfully resected (long-term recurrence >50% in macroadenoma). About 90% of patients treated with cabergoline have a drop in prolactin to <10% of pretreatment levels. Radiation therapy is used if drug therapy and surgery are ineffective in reducing tumor size and prolactin levels.

Acromegaly

Definition. Acromegaly is a syndrome of excessive secretion of growth hormone. In children this is called gigantism. Acromegaly is an insidious, chronic debilitating disease associated with bony and soft tissue overgrowth, and increased mortality.

Etiology. Acromegaly is caused by pituitary adenomas, usually a macroadenoma in 75% of the cases that produce growth hormone. Rarely ectopic tumors can produce GH or growth hormone releasing hormone (GHRH) and cause this syndrome. Less than 1% are malignant. Growth hormone is produced by 20% of pituitary tumors.

Clinical Findings. Growth hormone excess occurs most frequently between the third and fifth decades of life.

- Various skeletal and soft tissue changes occur.
- Enlargement of the hands and feet, coarsening of facial features, and thickened skin folds occur. Shoe, hat, glove, and ring sizes increase.
- The nose and mandible (prognathism and separation of teeth) enlarge, sometimes causing underbite.
- The voice becomes deeper.
- There is increased sweating.
- Obstructive sleep apnea can also develop.
- Internal organs are enlarged, including heart, lung, spleen, liver, and kidneys.
- Interstitial edema, osteoarthritis, and entrapment neuropathy (carpal tunnel syndrome) are seen.
- Menstrual problems are common because prolactin is co-secreted by the GH-producing tumor.
- About 10-20% of patients develop cardiac anomalies such as hypertension, arrhythmias, hypertrophic cardiomyopathy, and accelerated atherosclerosis.

Metabolic changes include impaired glucose tolerance (80%) and diabetes (13–20%). Hypertension is seen in one third of patients. Headaches and visual field loss can also occur. Articular cartilage proliferates and causes severe joint disease.

Note

The most common cause of death in acromegaly is cardiovascular mortality.

Diagnosis. Patients with acromegaly have symptoms for an average of 9 years before the diagnosis is made. The best initial test is IGF-1 level. A significantly elevated IGF level compared to the average IGF-1 for age-matched equivalents is a positive screen for acromegaly.

Confirmatory testing involves the measurement of GH after 100 g of glucose is given orally; this test is positive if GH remains high (>5 ng/mL) and suggests acromegaly. Normally a glucose load should completely suppress levels of GH.

Measurement of insulin-like growth factor (IGF) or somatomedin correlates with disease activity.

Radiologic studies such as CT scanning and MRI are used to localize the tumor but should be done only after GH excess is documented biochemically. MRI is superior to CT scan. MRI will show a tumor in 90% of people with acromegaly.

Management. The objectives are to decrease GH levels to normal, stabilize or decrease tumor size, and preserve normal pituitary function. Transsphenoidal surgery provides a rapid response. Hypopituitarism can result in 10–20%. Primary treatment is surgery.

Somatostatin analogues are the drugs of choice. Octreotide and lanreotide reduce GH values in around 70% of patients and cause partial tumor regression in 20–50% of patients. Octreotide is the best medical therapy for acromegaly. The main side effect of concern with somatostatin analogues is cholestasis, leading to cholecystitis.

Dopamine agonists such as bromocriptine and cabergoline are used if surgery is not curative. 10% of patients respond to these drugs.

Pegvisomant is a growth hormone analogue that antagonizes endogenic GH by blocking peripheral GH binding to its receptor in the liver. Important to note, pegvisomant is a second-line agent.

Radiotherapy, used only if surgery and drug therapy do not work, results in slow resolution of disease and hypopituitarism in 20% of patients.

Complications. Complications of acromegaly can arise from pressure of the tumor on the surrounding structures or invasion of the tumor into the brain or sinuses. Other complications include cardiac failure (most common cause of death in acromegaly), diabetes mellitus, cord compression, and visual field defects.

Hypopituitarism

Definition. Hypopituitarism is partial or complete loss of anterior function that may result from any lesion that destroys the pituitary or hypothalamus or that interferes with the delivery of releasing and inhibiting factors to the anterior hypothalamus. GH and gonadotropins (FSH, LH) are typically lost early.

Etiology. Large pituitary tumors, or cysts, as well as hypothalamic tumors (craniopharyngiomas, meningiomas, gliomas) can lead to hypopituitarism. Pituitary adenomas are the most common cause of panhypopituitarism. The mass compresses the gland, causing pressure, trauma, and necrosis.

Pituitary apoplexy is a syndrome associated with acute hemorrhagic infarction of a preexisting pituitary adenoma, and manifests as severe headache, nausea or vomiting, and depression of consciousness. It is a medical and neurosurgical emergency.

Inflammatory diseases can lead to hypopituitarism: granulomatous diseases (sarcoidosis, tuberculosis [TB], syphilis), eosinophilic granuloma, and autoimmune lymphocytic hypophysitis (usually associated with other autoimmune diseases such as Hashimoto thyroiditis and gastric atrophy). Trauma, radiation, surgery, infections, and hypoxia may also damage both the pituitary and hypothalamus.

Vascular diseases such as *Sheehan postpartum necrosis* (initial sign being the inability to lactate) and infiltrative diseases including hemochromatosis and amyloidosis may induce this state as well.

Stroke can also damage these cells. Stroke can cause central diabetes insipidus due to damage of hypothalamus and/or posterior pituitary.

Clinical Findings. The following hormones will appear in the order in which they are lost in hypopituitarism.

- Gonadotropin deficiency (LH and FSH) can occur in women and lead to amenorrhea, genital atrophy, infertility, decreased libido, and loss of axillary and pubic hair.

- In men, decreased LH and FSH results in impotence, testicular atrophy, infertility, decreased libido, and loss of axillary and pubic hair.

- GH deficiency occurs next and is not clinically detectable in adults, though it may manifest as fine wrinkles and increased sensitivity to insulin (hypoglycemia). GH deficiency gives an asymptomatic increase in lipid levels and a decrease in muscle, bone, and heart mass. It also may accelerate atherosclerosis, and it increases visceral obesity.

- GH deficiency in children results in growth failure and short stature.

- Thyrotropin (TSH) deficiency results in hypothyroidism with fatigue, weakness, hyperlipidemia, cold intolerance, and puffy skin without goiter.

- Adrenocorticotropin (ACTH) deficiency occurs last and results in secondary adrenal insufficiency caused by pituitary disease.

- There is decreased cortisol, which results in fatigue, decreased appetite, weight loss, decreased skin and nipple pigment, and decreased response to stress (as well as fever, hypotension, and hyponatremia).

Electrolyte changes like hyperkalemia and salt loss are minimal in secondary adrenal insufficiency because aldosterone production is mainly dependent on the renin-angiotensin system. ACTH deficiency does not result in the salt wasting, hyperkalemia, and death that are associated with aldosterone deficiency.

Diagnosis. The first step in diagnosing pituitary insufficiency is to measure GH, TSH, LH, and IGF1. The most reliable stimulus for GH secretion is insulin-induced hypoglycemia. After injecting 0.1 µ/kg of regular insulin, blood glucose declines to <40 mg/dL; in normal conditions that will stimulate GH levels to >10 mg/L and exclude GH deficiency. Random GH and IGF levels are not sensitive enough to diagnose GH deficiency. This is why a provocative test is used.

Arginine infusion can also stimulate growth hormone release. Measure GH levels after infusing arginine. This is less dangerous because it does not lead to hypoglycemia.

To diagnose ACTH deficiency, basal cortisol levels may be preserved (the problem could be only in response to stress). Insulin tolerance test is diagnostic and involves giving 0.05–0.1 U/kg of regular insulin and measuring serum cortisol; plasma cortisol should increase to >19 mg/dL. Metyrapone tests for decreased ACTH production. Metyrapone blocks cortisol production, which should increase ACTH levels. A failure of ACTH levels to rise after giving metyrapone would indicate pituitary insufficiency. Cosyntropin (ACTH) stimulation may give abnormally low cortisol output if pituitary insufficiency has led to adrenal atrophy.

To diagnose gonadotropin deficiency in women, measure LH, FSH, and estrogen. In males, gonadotropin deficiency can be detected by measuring LH, FSH, and testosterone. To diagnose TSH deficiency, measure serum thyroxine (T_4), and free triiodothyronine (T_3), which are low, with a normal to low TSH.

Management. Management of hypopituitarism involves treating the underlying causes. Multiple hormones must be replaced, but the most important is cortisol replacement.

Empty Sella Syndrome (ESS)

ESS is in the differential diagnosis of enlarged sella caused by pituitary tumors. In ESS, the sella has no bony erosion. It is caused by herniation of the suprasellar subarachnoid space through an incomplete diaphragm sella. No pituitary gland is visible on CT or MRI. The syndrome can be primary (idiopathic) and is also associated with head trauma and radiation therapy. *Most patients with these syndromes are obese,* multiparous women with headaches; 30% will have hypertension; endocrine symptoms are absent. Therapy is reassurance.

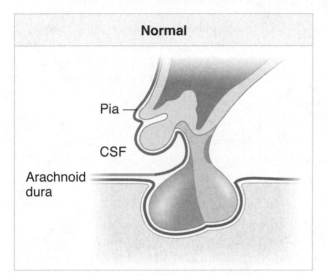 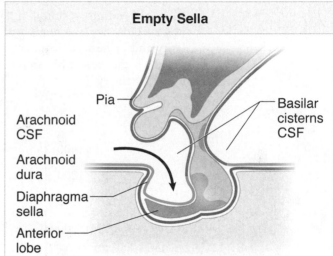

Figure 2-3. Empty Sella Syndrome

DISEASES OF THE POSTERIOR PITUITARY LOBE

Vasopressin or ADH and oxytocin are synthesized in neurons of the supraoptic and paraventricular nuclei in the hypothalamus, then transported to the posterior pituitary lobe to be released into the circulatory system. The syndrome associated with an excess secretion of ADH is called SIADH (syndrome of inappropriate secretion of ADH), and the syndrome associated with a deficiency of ADH is called diabetes insipidus (DI).

Central and Nephrogenic Diabetes Insipidus

Definition. Central diabetes insipidus (CDI) is a disorder of the neurohypophyseal system caused by a partial or total deficiency of vasopressin (ADH), which results in excessive, dilute urine and increased thirst associated with hypernatremia. Nephrogenic DI is caused by renal resistance to the action of vasopressin.

Etiology. DI frequently starts in childhood or early adult life and is more common in men than women. DI caused by ADH insufficiency is called central diabetes insipidus and DI caused by renal unresponsiveness to ADH is nephrogenic diabetes insipidus.

The causes of central DI include neoplastic or infiltrative lesions of the hypothalamus or pituitary (60% also have partial or complete loss of anterior pituitary function); in the hypothalamus these lesions can be secondary to adenomas, craniopharyngiomas, etc.; in the pituitary gland, adenomas, leukemias, or sarcoid histocytosis can lead to DI. Other causes of central DI include pituitary or hypothalamic surgery, radiotherapy, severe head injuries, anoxia, hypertension, and meningitis. Idiopathic DI starts in childhood. Encephalitis, TB, and syphilis may affect the pituitary as well.

Nephrogenic DI can be idiopathic or it can be secondary to hypercalcemia, hypokalemia, sickle cell disease, amyloidosis, myeloma, pyelonephritis, sarcoidosis, or Sjögren syndrome. Drugs (lithium, demeclocycline, colchicine) are among the most common causes of nephrogenic DI.

Clinical Findings. Clinical findings of DI include polyuria, excessive thirst, polydipsia (16–20 L/d), hypernatremia with high serum osmolarity and coexisting low urine osmolarity and urine specific gravity <1.010. Nocturia is expected. Hypertonicity is not usually present if the patient has an intact thirst mechanism and can increase water intake to keep up with urinary loss.

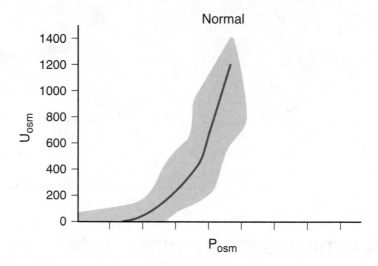

Figure 2-4. P_{osm} versus U_{osm} during Dehydration in Normal Subjects

Diagnosis. The water deprivation test compares U_{osm} after dehydration versus U_{osm} after vasopressin. In a normal person, the response to fluid restriction is to increase urine osmolality and decrease urine volume. In DI, the urine volume remains high despite volume depletion. ADH levels will be low in central DI and high in nephrogenic DI. If they fall to the right of the shaded area, the patient has DI (see Figure 2-4).

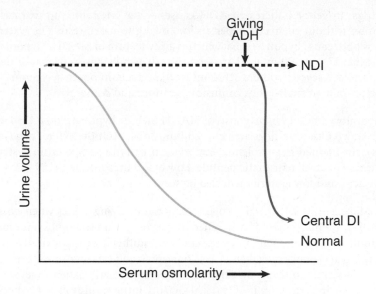

Figure 2-5. Water Restriction Test

Differential Diagnosis. The differential diagnosis of DI includes primary disorders of water intake (psychogenic polydipsia, drug-induced polydipsia from chlorpromazine, anticholinergic drugs, or thioridazine) and hypothalamic diseases.

Management. The management for central DI includes hormone replacement with vasopressin subcutaneously or desmopressin subcutaneously, orally, or intranasally. Some drugs can be used that stimulate the secretion of ADH or increase release (chlorpropamide, clofibrate, or carbamazepine).

For nephrogenic DI, HCTZ or amiloride may be used, which enhances the reabsorption of fluid from the proximal tubule. Chlorthalidone is effective as well. Abnormalities of calcium and potassium should be corrected as well.

Syndromes Associated with Vasopressin (ADH) Excess

Syndromes associated with ADH excess involve a mechanism of defense against hypovolemia or hypotension. This includes adrenal insufficiency, excessive fluid loss, fluid deprivation, and probably positive-pressure respiration.

Excessive release of ADH from the neurohypophysis is associated with drugs or diseases (SIADH).

Syndrome of Inappropriate Secretion of ADH (SIADH)

Etiology. The etiology of SIADH includes malignancies such as *small cell carcinomas,* carcinoma of the pancreas, and ectopic ADH secretion. Nonmalignant pulmonary diseases such as TB, pneumonia, and lung abscess can also lead to SIADH. CNS disorders including head injury, cerebral vascular accident, and encephalitis are other etiologies. Drugs such as chlorpropamide, clofibrate, vincristine, vinblastine, cyclophosphamide, and carbamazepine can induce SIADH.

Clinical Findings. In general, increased ADH causes water retention and extracellular fluid volume expansion without edema or hypertension, owing to natriuresis. The water retention and sodium loss both cause hyponatremia, which is a key feature in SIADH. Hyponatremia and concentrated urine (U_{osm} >300 mOsm) are seen, as well as no signs of edema or dehydration. When hyponatremia is severe (sodium <120 mOsm), or acute in onset, symptoms of cerebral edema become prominent (irritability, confusion, seizures, and coma).

Diagnosis. Laboratory findings in diagnosis of SIADH include hyponatremia <130 mEq/L, and P_{osm} <270 mOsm/kg. Other findings are urine sodium concentration >20 mEq/L (inappropriate natriuresis), maintained hypervolemia, suppression of renin–angiotensin system, and no equal concentration of atrial natriuretic peptide. Low blood urea nitrate (BUN), low creatinine, low serum uric acid, and low albumin will also be seen.

Management. Management of SIADH involves treating underlying causes when possible. Fluid restriction to 800–1,000 mL/d should be obtained to increase serum sodium. Demeclocycline can be used in chronic situations when fluid restrictions are difficult to maintain. Demeclocycline inhibits ADH action at the collecting duct (V2). Conivaptan and tolvaptan are V2 receptor blockers indicated for moderate to severe SIADH. For very symptomatic patients (severe confusion, convulsions, or coma), hypertonic saline (3%) 200–300 mL intravenously in 3–4 h should be used. The rate of correction should be between 0.5–1 mmol/L/h of serum Na.

DISEASES OF THE THYROID GLAND

Generalities. The normal function of the thyroid gland is directed toward the secretion of L-thyroxine (T_4) and L-3,5,5′-triiodothyronine (T_3), which influence a diversity of metabolic processes.

Diseases of the thyroid could be quantitative or qualitative alterations in hormone secretion, enlargement of thyroid (goiter), or both. Insufficient hormone secretion results in hypothyroidism; excess secretion results in hyperthyroidism. Focal enlargement of the thyroid can be associated with tumors (benign or malignant). Generalized enlargement can be associated with increased, normal, or decreased function of the gland depending on the underlying cause.

Laboratory Tests in Thyroid Disease. The most sensitive test in thyroid diseases is the TSH. If the TSH is normal, then the patient is euthyroid.

Total T_4 and T_3 do not always reflect actual thyroid function. For example, increased TBG levels are seen in pregnancy and the use of oral contraceptives. This will increase total T_4 but free or active T_4 level is normal. Decreased TBG levels are seen in nephrotic syndrome and the use of androgens. This will decrease total T_4 but free or active T_4 level is normal with the patient being euthyroid.

Clinical Pearl

Always check **free** T4 to assess thyroid function.

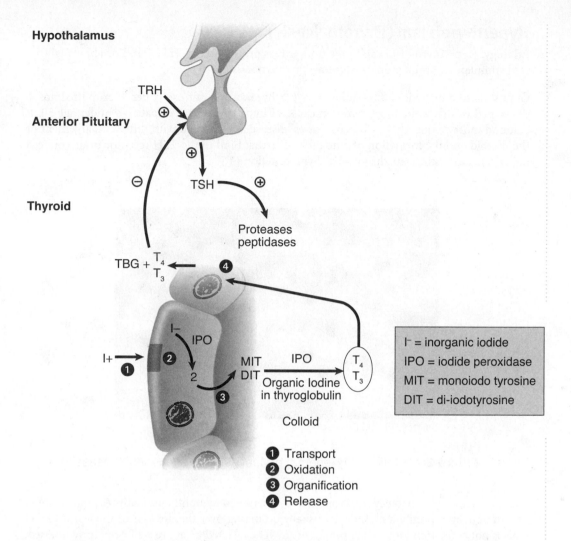

Hypothalamus

TRH

Anterior Pituitary ⊕

⊕

⊖ TSH ⊕

Thyroid

Proteases
peptidases

TBG + T_4
T_3 ④

④ Release

I⁻
IPO

I+
② ② IPO T_4
T_3
2 MIT
DIT
③ Organic Iodine
in thyroglobulin

Colloid

I⁻ = inorganic iodide
IPO = iodide peroxidase
MIT = monoiodo tyrosine
DIT = di-iodotyrosine

① Transport
② Oxidation
③ Organification
④ Release

Figure 2-6. Pathways for Synthesis and Secretion of Thyroid Hormones

RAIU (thyroid-reactive iodine uptake) varies directly with the functional state of the thyroid. After 24 hours, normal uptake is 5–30% of administered dose. RAIU is *increased* in Graves' disease or toxic nodule and *decreased* in thyroiditis or surreptitious ingestion of thyroid hormone.

Table 2-2. Evaluating Thyroid Function

Thyroid Hormones and TSH	RAI Uptake Scan	Diagnosis
↓ TSH; free ↑ T_4, ↑ T_3	↑ RAIU	
↓ TSH; free ↑ T_4, ↑ T_3	↓ RAIU	
↓ TSH; free ↓ T_4, ↓ T_3	↓ RAIU	

Note

The answers to Diagnosis column can be found on the next page

Other tests include antimicrosomal and antithyroglobulin antibodies, which are detected in Hashimoto thyroiditis. In Graves' disease, thyroid-stimulating immunoglobulin (TSI) is found. Serum thyroglobulin concentration can be used to assess the adequacy of treatment and follow-up of thyroid cancer.

Hyperthyroidism (Thyrotoxicosis)

Etiology. Hyperthyroidism can result from excess production of TSH (rare) or abnormal thyroid stimulators. Amiodarone can induce thyrotoxicosis.

Graves' disease or toxic diffuse goiter = hyperthyroidism + diffuse goiter + exophthalmos + dermopathy. This is the most common cause of hyperthyroidism in patients under age 50. It is found more frequently in women. Graves' disease is associated with diffuse enlargement of the thyroid and the formation of autoantibodies that bind to the TSH receptor in thyroid cell membranes and stimulate the gland to hyperfunction (TSI).

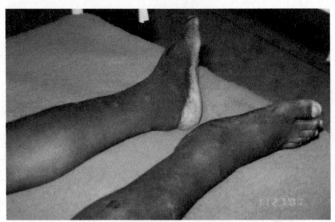

Courtesy of Tom D. Thacher, M.D.

Figure 2-7. Pretibial Myxedema, a Manifestation of Graves' Disease

Diagnosis Answers Table 2-2

De novo synthesis of hormone (primary hyperthyroidism)
Facticious hyperthyroidism or inflammation or destruction of the gland releasing preformed hormone into the circulation (subacute thyroiditis)
Secondary or tertiary hypothyroidism

Graves' disease, as previously mentioned, is accompanied by ophthalmopathy (exophthalmus) and dermopathy-pretibial myxedema, usually occurring over the dorsum of the legs and feet (this is not a manifestation of hypothyroidism). The affected areas are well demarcated, raised, and thickened, and may be pruritic and hyperpigmented. Graves' disease may be associated with other systemic autoimmune disorders such as pernicious anemia, myasthenia gravis, and diabetes mellitus. Eye disease is treated with steroids or radiation, skin disease with steroids.

Intrinsic thyroid autonomy can result from a hyperfunctioning adenoma (toxic). It can also be secondary to toxic multinodular goiter (Plummer disease), which is a nonautoimmune disease of the elderly associated commonly with arrhythmia and CHF and sometimes the consequence of simple goiter.

Transient hyperthyroidism results from subacute thyroiditis (painful) or lymphocytic thyroiditis (painless, postpartum).

Extrathyroid source of hormones include thyrotoxicosis factitia and ectopic thyroid tissue (struma ovarii, functioning follicular carcinoma).

Clinical Findings. In general, nervous symptoms predominate in the clinical picture of younger patients, whereas cardiovascular and myopathic symptoms are more common in older patients. Atrial fibrillation can occur from hyperthyroidism. Other clinical findings include emotional lability, inability to sleep, tremors, frequent bowel movements, excessive sweating, and heat intolerance. Weight loss (despite increased appetite) and loss of strength also are seen. Dyspnea, palpitations, angina, or cardiac failure may occur in older patients. The skin is warm and moist, and palmar erythema is present along with fine and silky hair in hyperthyroidism. Ocular signs include staring, infrequent blinking, and lid lag. Menstrual irregularity such as oligomenorrhea occurs. Osteoporosis and hypercalcemia can occur from increases in osteoclast activity.

Diagnosis. The diagnosis of hyperthyroidism is made on history and physical examination. Laboratory studies include suppressed TSH in primary hyperthyroidism and high TSH in secondary hyperthyroidism. Serum free T_4 and T_3 are elevated. RIAU is increased. Antithyroglobulin and antimicrosomal antibodies are elevated in Graves' disease and autoimmune thyroiditis.

Differential Diagnosis. The differential diagnosis of hyperthyroidism includes anxiety, neurosis, and mania, pheochromocytoma, acromegaly, and cardiac disease. Other causes of ophthalmoplegia and exophthalmus include myasthenia gravis and orbital tumors. It is very important to distinguish primary hyperthyroidism from thyroiditis.

Management. Immediate therapeutic approach to management of hyperthyroidism associated with Graves' and toxic nodular goiter is administration of propanolol (to control adrenergic symptoms), and antithyroid drugs such as propylthiouracil (PTU is safe in pregnancy) and methimazole. Methimazole is the drug of choice due to decreased hepatotoxicity compared to PTU. Both drugs can cause agranulocytosis. Ablative therapy can be accomplished with radioactive iodine. Subtotal thyroidectomy is only indicated in pregnancy (2nd trimester) and in children. After ablative therapy, the patient will become hypothyroid and hormone replacement treatment is indicated. Surgery is also used if the thyroid is so large that there are compressive symptoms.

Thyroid Storm

Thyroid storm is an extreme form of thyrotoxicosis. This is an endocrine emergency. It is precipitated by stress, infection, surgery, or trauma. It is manifested by extreme irritability, delirium, coma, tachycardia, restlessness, vomiting, jaundice, diarrhea, hypotension, dehydration, and high fever.

Treatment. The treatment of thyroid storm involves supportive therapy with saline and glucose hydration, glucocorticoids, and oxygen cooling blanket. Therapy for hyperthyroidism is also used and includes first, antithyroid agents. Next, iodine should be given to inhibit hormone release. This should be followed by adrenergic antagonists (e.g., β-adrenergic blockers). Finally, dexamethasone is given to inhibit hormone release, impair peripheral generation of T_3 from T_4, and provide adrenal support. Antithyroid drugs should be stopped several days (1–2 weeks) before and after the RAI treatment. The antithyroid medications, such as PTU, block the uptake of the radioactive iodine.

Hypothyroidism

Etiology. The etiology of hypothyroidism results from the thyroid in 95% of cases (primary). Primary hypothyroidism can occur secondary to chronic thyroiditis (Hashimoto disease); this is the most common cause of goitrous hypothyroidism and is associated with antimicrosomal antibodies. Postablative surgery or radioactive iodine, heritable biosynthetic defects, and iodine deficiency can lead to primary hypothyroidism. Drugs such as lithium and acetylsalicylic acid can elicit primary hypothyroidism. Amiodarone, interferon, and sulfonamides can cause hypothyroidism.

Suprathyroid causes of hypothyroidism include pituitary induced (secondary hypothyroidism) or hypothalamic induced (tertiary hypothyroidism).

Note

Thyroid stimulating immunoglobulin (TSI) is an auto-antibody against TSH receptors, specific to Graves' disease.

Clinical Findings. In the newborn, signs and symptoms of hypothyroidism include cretinism (in 1/5,000 neonates) and juvenile hypothyroidism. Persistent physiologic jaundice, hoarse cry, constipation, somnolence, and feeding problems are also seen. In later months, delayed milestones and dwarfism, coarse features, protruding tongue, broad flat nose, widely set eyes, sparse hair, dry skin, protuberant abdomen, potbelly with umbilical hernia, impaired mental development, retarded bone age, and delayed dentition are also seen.

Signs and symptoms of hypothyroidism in the adult in the early stages include lethargy, constipation, cold intolerance, stiffness and cramping of muscles, carpal tunnel syndrome, and menorrhagia. Later in the course of disease intellectual and motor activity slows, appetite decreases and weight increases, hair and skin become dry, voice gets deeper and hoarse, and deafness may occur. Slow deep tendon reflexes with prolonged relaxation phase are noted on examination. Cholesterol levels in the blood may be elevated. Ultimately, myxedema appears with an expressionless face, sparse hair, periorbital puffiness, large tongue, and pale, cool skin that feels rough and doughy. Hyponatremia and anemia also occur.

Diagnosis. Diagnosis of hypothyroidism is made by symptoms and physical findings. Laboratory tests are also used to confirm diagnosis (Table 2-3).

Table 2-3. Confirmation of Hypothyroid Diagnosis*

Primary Hypothyroidism	2° or 3° Hypothyroidism
↑ TSH	Normal or ↓ TSH
↓ T_4, ↓ FT_4	↓ T_4, ↓ FT_4
T_3 decreases in lesser extent	Accompanied by decreased secretion of other hormones

*Also seen: hypercholesterolemia, elevation of CPK, AST, hyponatremia, LDH; 12% associated to pernicious anemia

Management. The goal in management of hypothyroidism is to restore metabolic state gradually in the elderly and patients with coronary artery disease (CAD). Levothyroxine (T_4) should be administered with monitoring of TSH/T_3 levels (it takes 6 weeks to stabilize after dosing changes). If there is a strong suspicion of suprathyroid hypothyroidism of hypothalamic or pituitary origin, give hydrocortisone first, then replace thyroid hormone.

Myxedema coma results in patients who have severe long-standing hypothyroidism that is left untreated. They develop a hypothermic, stuporous state that is frequently fatal. It is associated with respiratory depression (CO_2 retention). Myxedema coma is precipitated by cold exposure, trauma, infections, and CNS depressants. Treatment includes very high doses of T_4 and T_3.

Thyroiditis

Thyroiditis includes disorders of different etiologies characterized by inflammation of the thyroid. They have different clinical courses, and each can be associated at one time or another with euthyroid, thyrotoxic, or hypothyroid state.

Subacute Thyroiditis. Subacute thyroiditis includes granulomatous, giant cell, or de Quervain thyroiditis. This can occur at any age, although most commonly in the fourth and fifth decades.

Clinical Pearl

- Hashimoto thyroiditis presents more commonly as **hypo**thyroidism.

- Subacute (de Quervain) thyroiditis presents more commonly as **hyper**thyroidism.

Subacute thyroiditis is probably of viral origin and follows upper respiratory infection symptoms including malaise, fever, pain over the thyroid, and pain referred to the lower jaw, ears, neck, or arms. The thyroid gland is enlarged and firm in this setting. Laboratory findings in subacute thyroiditis include elevated erythrocyte sedimentation rate (ESR), decreased radioactive iodine uptake, initial elevation in T_4 and T_3 (caused by leak of hormone from the gland), followed by hypothyroidism as the hormone is depleted.

The differential diagnosis of subacute thyroiditis includes mostly Graves' disease. Treatment is symptomatic with NSAIDs, prednisone, and propanolol. The disorder may smolder for months but eventually subsides with return to normal function.

Hashimoto Thyroiditis. Hashimoto thyroiditis is a chronic inflammatory process of the thyroid with lymphocytic infiltration of the gland, and is thought to be caused by autoimmune factors.

- **Etiology.** Hashimoto thyroiditis is a common disorder occurring most frequently in middle-aged women, and is the most common cause of sporadic goiter in children. Autoimmune factors are implicated as evidenced by lymphocytic infiltration, presence of increased immunoglobulin, and antibodies against components of thyroid tissue (antithyroglobulin Abs).

- **Clinical findings.** Clinical findings include a *goiter that is painless,* which is the main feature of this disease. The goiter is rubbery and not always symmetrical. Hypothyroidism occurs.

- **Diagnosis.** The diagnosis of Hashimoto thyroiditis is suggested by finding a firm, nontoxic goiter on examination. Laboratory values in the early stages are metabolically normal, then TSH increases, and T_4 and T_3 decrease. High titers of antithyroid antibodies, namely antimicrosomal antibodies, are present. Histologic confirmation is made by needle biopsy, but it is usually not needed. Antithyroperoxidase antibodies are found as well.

- **Management.** Hashimoto thyroiditis is managed by replacement with L-thyroxine.

Lymphocytic (Silent, Painless, or Postpartum) Thyroiditis. Lymphocytic thyroiditis is a self-limiting episode of thyrotoxicosis associated with chronic lymphocytic thyroiditis. It is more common in women of any age. The thyroid is nontender, firm, symmetrical, and slightly to moderately enlarged. T_4 and T_3 are elevated, RAIU is low, and ESR normal. If antithyroid antibodies are present, they are only in a low titer. Etiology and pathogenesis of lymphocytic thyroiditis is unclear. This disease may last for 2–5 months and be recurrent (as in postpartum thyroiditis). Treatment is symptomatic with propanolol.

Reidel Thyroiditis. Reidel thyroiditis results from intense fibrosis of the thyroid and surrounding structures (including mediastinal and retroperitoneal fibrosis).

Neoplasia of the Thyroid

Classification. Thyroid adenomas may be nonfunctioning or hyperfunctioning. They are slow growing over many years. Management for hyperfunctioning adenomas includes ablation with radioactive iodine. The types of thyroid adenomas are follicular (which is most common and highly differentiated, autonomous nodule), papillary, and Hürthle.

Types of thyroid carcinomas

Papillary Carcinoma. Papillary carcinoma is the most common thyroid cancer. It is associated with history of radiation exposure. 60–70% of all thyroid cancers are papillary. Women are affected by papillary carcinoma 2–3 times more than men. There is a bimodal frequency and peaks occur in the second and third decades and again later in life. This tumor is slow growing and spreads via lymphatics after many years. The treatment is surgery when the tumor is small and limited to a single area of the thyroid. TSH suppression therapy with levothyroxine is also used. With large tumors, radiation therapy is used with surgery.

Follicular Carcinoma. Follicular carcinoma accounts for 15–20% of all thyroid cancers. It is more common in the elderly and in women rather than men. This tumor is more malignant than papillary carcinoma. Follicular carcinoma spreads hematogenously with distant metastasis to the lung and bone. Treatment requires near total thyroidectomy with postoperative radio-iodine ablation.

Anaplastic Carcinoma. Anaplastic carcinoma accounts for 1–2% of all thyroid cancer. It occurs mostly in elderly patients. Women are affected more than men with this tumor. Anaplastic carcinoma is highly malignant with rapid and painful enlargement. Eighty percent of patients die within 1 year of diagnosis. This cancer spreads by direct extension.

Medullary Carcinoma. Medullary carcinoma accounts for 5% of all thyroid cancers. It occurs as a sporadic form or familial form. This tumor arises from parafollicular cells of the thyroid and is more malignant than follicular carcinoma. The tumor often produces calcitonin. Medullary carcinoma is the component of two types of MEN (multiple endocrine neoplasia). In type IIa (Sipple syndrome), pheochromocytoma, medullary thyroid carcinoma, and (in one-half of cases) parathyroid hyperplasia occur. In MEN type IIb, pheochromocytoma, medullary carcinoma, and neuromas occur. Medullary carcinoma may also occur in families without other associated endocrine dysfunctions. The only effective therapy is thyroidectomy. Calcitonin levels can also be increased from cancer of the lung, pancreas, breast, and colon. The only thyroid cancer with an elevated calcitonin level is medullary cancer.

When to suspect a thyroid carcinoma

Suspect a thyroid carcinoma when there is recent growth of thyroid or mass with no tenderness or hoarseness. Patients with a history of radiation therapy of the head, neck, or upper mediastinum in childhood average 30 years to develop thyroid cancer. The presence of a solitary nodule or the production of calcitonin are also clues to malignancy. Calcifications on x-rays such as psammoma bodies suggest papillary carcinoma; increased density is seen in medullary carcinoma. Do thyroid function tests first; cancer is never hyperfunctioning.

Diagnostic approach to solitary nonfunctioning nodule

Fine-needle aspiration (FNA) for cytology is the initial procedure of choice in the evaluation of most patients. Five percent of nonfunctioning thyroid nodules prove to be malignant; functioning nodules are very seldom malignant. The first test to do in a patient with a thyroid nodule is TSH; if this is normal, then proceed to FNA. U/S is useful to distinguish cysts from solid nodules.

PARATHYROID GLANDS

Generalities. The function of parathyroid hormone (PTH) is to maintain extracellular fluid calcium concentration. PTH acts directly on the bone and kidney, and indirectly on intestine (through its effects on synthesis of 1,25-dihydroxycholecalciferol [$1,25(OH)_2D_3$]) to increase serum calcium. It is closely regulated by the concentration of serum-ionized calcium. PTH increases osteoclast activity, which releases calcium. PTH also inhibits phosphate reabsorption in the kidney tubule. This also favors bone dissolution and calcium release from bones. PTH activates vitamin D, which increases the GI absorption of calcium.

Calcium Regulation—Overview. Calcium regulation involves 3 tissues, namely, the bone, kidney, and intestine. It involves 3 hormones: PTH (hypercalcemic), calcitonin (hypocalcemic), and activated vitamin D (hypercalcemic). See Figure 2-8.

Hypercalcemia

Hypercalcemia represents an increase in the total or free calcium level. About 98% of calcium is stored in bone. Calcium is absorbed from the proximal portion of the small intestine, particularly the duodenum. About 80% of an ingested calcium load in the diet is lost in the feces, unabsorbed. Of the 2% that is circulating in blood, free calcium is 50%, protein bound is 40%, with only 10% bound to citrate or phosphate buffers.

Etiology. The most common cause of hypercalcemia is primary hyperparathyroidism. Hyperparathyroidism, which is usually asymptomatic, comes to light because of routine office-based testing. The hypercalcemia of malignancy is due to a PTH-like protein produced by squamous cell carcinoma of the lung or metastatic disease to the bone. Granulomatous diseases such as sarcoidosis, tuberculosis, berylliosis, histoplasmosis, and coccidioidomycosis are all associated with hypercalcemia. Neutrophils in granulomas have their own 25-vitamin D hydroxylation, producing active 1,25 vitamin D. Rare causes include vitamin D intoxication, thiazide diuretics, lithium use, and Paget disease, as well as prolonged immobilization. Hyperthyroidism is associated with hypercalcemia because there is a partial effect of thyroid hormone on osteoclasts. Acidosis results in an increased amount of free calcium. This is because albumin buffers acidosis. Increased binding of hydrogen ions to albumin results in the displacement of calcium from albumin.

Familial hypocalciuric hypercalcemia (FHH) is a benign form of hypercalcemia. It presents with mild hypercalcemia, family history of hypercalcemia, urine calcium to creatinine ratio <0.01, and urine calcium <200 mg/day (hypocalciuria). Most cases are associated with loss of function mutations in the CaSR gene, which encodes a calcium sensing receptor (expressed in kidney and parathyroid tissue). The perceived lack of calcium levels by the parathyroid leads to high levels of parathyroid hormone. FHH is indicated by the presence of hypercalcemia at the same time with hypocalciuria. (**In all other causes of hypercalcemia, elevated calcium levels in the blood are correlated with elevated calcium urine levels, as a properly sensing kidney works to excrete calcium.**) No treatment is generally required, since patients are most commonly asymptomatic.

Clinical

- Neurologic: Hypercalcemia results in decreased mental activity such as lethargy and confusion.
- GI: Hypercalcemia results in decreased bowel activity such as constipation and anorexia but commonly gives nausea and vomiting as well. Pancreatitis occurs because of the precipitation of calcium in the pancreas. Severe pancreatitis, however, is associated with hypocalcemia because of binding of calcium to malabsorbed fat in the intestine. Ulcer disease is caused by hypercalcemia for unclear reasons.
- Renal: Hypercalcemia results in polyuria and polydipsia because of the induction of nephrogenic diabetes insipidus. Calcium also precipitates in the kidney, resulting in both kidney stones as well as nephrolithiasis.
- Cardiovascular: Hypertension occurs in 30–50% of patients with hypercalcemia. The EKG will show a short QT.

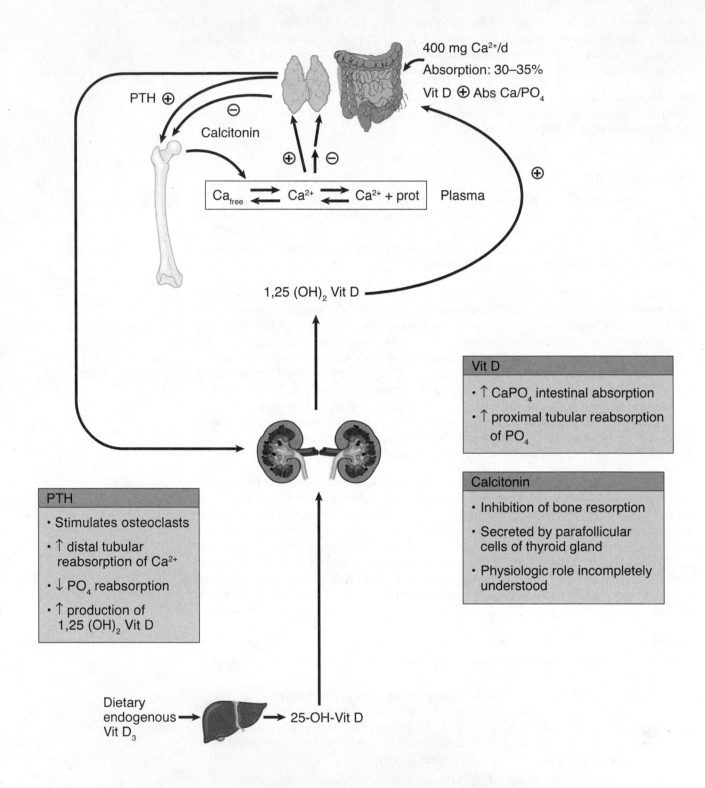

PTH ⊕

⊖

Calcitonin

400 mg Ca²⁺/d
Absorption: 30–35%
Vit D ⊕ Abs Ca/PO₄

⊕ ↑ ⊖

$Ca_{free} \rightleftarrows Ca^{2+} \rightleftarrows Ca^{2+} + prot$ Plasma

⊕

1,25 (OH)₂ Vit D

Vit D
- ↑ CaPO₄ intestinal absorption
- ↑ proximal tubular reabsorption of PO₄

PTH
- Stimulates osteoclasts
- ↑ distal tubular reabsorption of Ca²⁺
- ↓ PO₄ reabsorption
- ↑ production of 1,25 (OH)₂ Vit D

Calcitonin
- Inhibition of bone resorption
- Secreted by parafollicular cells of thyroid gland
- Physiologic role incompletely understood

Dietary endogenous Vit D₃ → → 25-OH-Vit D

Figure 2-8. Calcium Regulation

Treatment. Severe, life-threatening hypercalcemia is treated first with vigorous fluid replacement with normal saline or half-normal saline. This may be followed by the use of loop diuretics, such as furosemide, which promote calcium loss from the body. Loop diuretics are used **only after hydration in very severe cases**. IV bisphosphonates such as zoledronate and pamidronate inhibit osteoclasts and stimulate osteoblasts. The maximum effect of bisphosphonates takes 2–3 days. If fluid replacement and diuretics do not lower the calcium level quickly enough and you cannot wait the 2 days for the bisphosphonates to work, calcitonin can be used for a more rapid decrease in calcium level. Calcitonin inhibits osteoclasts.

Primary Hyperparathyroidism

Primary hyperparathyroidism represents 90% of mild hypercalcemias.

Etiology. It is most commonly due to one gland adenoma (80%), but hyperplasia of all 4 glands can lead to primary hyperparathyroidism (20%). Parathyroid cancer is a rare cause of this disease (<1%). Primary hyperparathyroidism can occur as part of MEN. In MEN type I, hyperparathyroidism, pituitary tumors (3 "Ps"), and pancreatic tumors are seen. In MEN type II, hyperparathyroidism, pheochromocytoma, and medullary carcinoma of the thyroid are seen.

Clinical Findings. One half of patients with hyperparathyroidism are asymptomatic. Osteitis fibrosa cystica with hyperparathyroidism occurs because of increased rate of osteoclastic bone resorption and results in bone pain, fractures, swelling, deformity, areas of demineralization, bone cysts, and brown tumors (punched-out lesions producing a salt-and-pepper-like appearance). Urinary tract manifestations of hypercalcemia include polyuria, polydipsia, stones, and nephrocalcinosis with renal failure. The polyuria and polydipsia are from nephrogenic diabetes insipidus. Neurologic manifestations include CNS problems, mild personality disturbance, severe psychiatric disorders, mental obtundation or coma, neuromuscular weakness, easy fatigability, and atrophy of muscles. GI manifestations include anorexia, weight loss, constipation, nausea, vomiting, thirst, abdominal pain with pancreatitis, and peptic ulcer disease. Cardiovascular findings include hypertension and arrhythmias (short QT).

Diagnosis. Diagnosis can be made by laboratory findings of serum calcium >10.5 mg/dL, with elevated PTH level. Urine calcium elevation is common, but because of the calcium-reabsorbing action of PTH, there may be normal levels in one-third of patients. Serum phosphate is usually low (<2.5 mg/dL). The differential diagnosis includes all other causes of hypercalcemia, especially hypercalcemia of malignancy. In every other cause of hypercalcemia the PTH level will be low. In primary hyperparathyroidism, PTH is always elevated.

Imaging studies such as CT, MRI, sonography, and nuclear scans are not used to diagnose hyperparathyroidism. A nuclear parathyroid scan (sestamibi) can be used to localize the adenoma. When combined with a neck sonogram, specificity rises significantly.

Management. Surgical removal of the parathyroid glands is effective. Medical treatment, used if surgery is contraindicated or if serum calcium ≤11.5 mg/dL and the patient is asymptomatic, includes bisphosphonates (pamidronate). The dietary calcium should be reduced to 400 mg/d. Oral hydration with 2–3 L of fluid is very effective. Phosphate supplementation with phospho-soda should be given. Estrogen may be indicated in hyperparathyroidism in postmenopausal women. Imaging studies may help localize the site of the affected gland prior to surgery.

Parathyroidectomy should be performed if there are symptoms of hypercalcemia, bone disease, renal disease, or if the patient is pregnant. Asymptomatic mild increases in calcium from hyperparathyroidism do not necessarily need to be treated.

Note

Calcitonin is an intermediary measure while waiting for IV bisphosphonate to act.

In primary hyperparathyroidism, surgery is indicated if any of the following are present:

- Symptomatic hypercalcemia
- Calcium >11.5 mg/dL
- Renal insufficiency
- Age <50 years
- Nephrolithiasis
- Osteoporosis

Emergency treatment for severe hypercalcemia includes IV normal saline to restore volume and rarely furosemide after hydration. Everyone gets IV bisphosphates such as pamidronate. Bisphosphonates are useful only temporarily for hyperparathyroidism and may take 2–3 days to reach maximum effect.

Hungry bones syndrome is hypocalcemia that occurs after surgical removal of a hyperactive parathyroid gland, due to increased osteoblast activity. It usually presents with rapidly decreasing calcium, phosphate, and magnesium 1–4 weeks post-parathyroidectomy.

Cinacalcet is a calcimimetic agent that has some effect in hyperparathyroidism by shutting off the parathyroids. This increases the sensitivity of calcium sensing (basolateral membrane potential) on the parathyroid. Cinacalcet is used as treatment of secondary hyperparathyroidism in hemodialysis patients. It is also indicated for the treatment of hypercalcemia in patients with parathyroid carcinoma and in moderate-to-severe primary hyperparathyroidism unamenable to surgery.

Hypocalcemia

Etiology. Hypocalcemia is most commonly caused by hypoparathyroidism, renal failure, hyperphosphatemia, and hypomagnesemia. Drugs such as loop diuretics, phenytoin, alendronate, and foscarnet will also lower calcium levels. Renal failure causes hypocalcemia because of the loss of activated 1,25-dihydroxy-vitamin D. This leads to decreased calcium absorption from the gut. In addition, hyperphosphatemia will cause the precipitation of calcium in tissues. Low magnesium levels from malnutrition of alcoholism prevent the release of parathyroid hormone from the parathyroid glands. Alkalosis decreases free calcium levels by causing increased binding of calcium to albumin. Pseudo hypocalcemia occurs with low albumin levels. The free calcium level remains normal, while the total calcium level decreases.

To correct for albumin, add 0.8 to calcium level for every 1 gram below 4 of albumin. Massive blood transfusion gives hypocalcemia because of binding of the calcium to the citrate in the transfused units of blood.

Clinical Findings. Hypocalcemia results in increased neural hyperexcitability such as seizures, tetany, circumoral numbness, and tingling of the extremities. Arrhythmias may develop because of a prolonged QT. Cataracts develop for unclear reasons.

Treatment of hypocalcemia is IV or oral calcium replacement, and vitamin D replacement as necessary.

Hypoparathyroidism

Etiology. The most common cause of hypoparathyroidism is surgical removal of the thyroid. Low PTH levels are also seen in hereditary hypoparathyroidism, acquired hypoparathyroidism (surgical removal), and hypomagnesemia. Magnesium deficiency prevents release of PTH from the gland. Hypomagnesemia occurs from decreased GI absorption or alcoholism. High PTH levels are seen in chronic renal failure, and decreased levels of active vitamin D, which is caused by decreased dietary intake or defective metabolism (secondary to anticonvulsant therapy or vitamin D-dependent rickets, type I). Ineffective vitamin D can also lead to high PTH levels; this is seen in intestinal malabsorption and vitamin D-dependent rickets, type II. Low or ineffective vitamin D is also associated with low calcium levels.

Clinical Findings. Clinical findings depend on the level of calcium, duration, acid-base disorder, and age at onset of disease.

Neuromuscular irritability is seen, such as tetany, laryngospasm, cramping, seizures, and impaired memory function. Chvostek sign may be positive (percussion of the facial nerve in front of the ear, which elicits a contraction of the facial muscles and upper lip). Trousseau sign may be positive (inflation of a blood pressure cuff on the arm to a pressure higher than the patient's systolic pressure for 3 min elicits flexion of the metacarpophalangeal joints and extension of the interphalangeal joints). Ocular findings such as cataracts and soft tissue calcifications can occur. The cardiovascular system may be affected, seen as QT prolongation, refractory CHF, and/or hypotension. Hypocalcemia frequently results in circumoral tingling as well as tingling of the hands and feet. Hyperventilation worsens symptoms of hypocalcemia because the alkalosis decreases free calcium levels.

Diagnosis. Diagnosis is suggested when the serum calcium is low; it is important to check an **albumin** and make the correction in calcium level. A low calcium may be due to low albumin; for a 1.0 g/dL drop in albumin, the total calcium will decrease by 0.8 mg/dL. It is better to measure ionized calcium. Depending on the etiology, PTH can be low (hypoparathyroidism) or high. Low calcium with high phosphorous can be due to renal failure, massive tissue destruction, hypoparathyroidism, and pseudohypoparathyroidism. Low calcium with low phosphorous is due to absent or ineffective vitamin D.

Management. In the acute stage of hypocalcemia, calcium gluconate can be given IV. Maintenance therapy includes oral calcium 2–4 g/d, vitamin D, and if there is hyperphosphatemia, diet restriction and phosphate binders ($CaCO_3$ or aluminum hydroxide).

DISORDERS OF CARBOHYDRATE METABOLISM

Diabetes Mellitus

Definition. A disorder of carbohydrate metabolism caused by relative or absolute deficiency of insulin, hyperglycemia, and end-organ complications, including nephropathy, retinopathy, neuropathy, and accelerated atherosclerosis. Diabetes affects approximately 6% of the population in the United States, and approaches 20% of patients over age 65.

Classification

- **Type 1 IDDM (insulin-dependent or juvenile onset)** accounts for 5–10% of diabetes worldwide, with males = females. The age of onset is usually age <30. Genetically, <10% of first-degree relatives are affected with a 50% occurrence in identical twins.

  There is an increased prevalence of autoantibodies to islet cells, glutamic acid decarboxylase (GAD), and other tissues with IDDM. Type 1 diabetes is associated with HLA-B8, HLA-B15, HLA-DR3, and HLA-DR4. Patients usually have a lean body build and are prone to ketosis owing to absent insulin production.

- **Type 2, or NIDDM (non-insulin-dependent or maturity onset)**, is the most common type of diabetes, accounting for 90% of cases, with males > females. Age of onset is usually age 40. Genetically >20% of first-degree relatives are affected with 90–100% occurrence in identical twins.

  No autoantibodies are associated with NIDDM. The body build of these patients is usually obese with >80% being >15% above ideal body weight. NIDDM patients are ketosis-resistant, and insulin levels may be high, normal, or low. About 90% of diabetes is type 2.

Pathophysiology. For IDDM, by the time the condition appears, most of the beta cells in the pancreas have been destroyed. The destructive process is most likely autoimmune in nature.

For NIDDM, there are 2 clear physiologic defects: abnormal insulin secretion and resistance to insulin action in target tissues.

Clinical Findings. Manifestations of symptomatic DM vary from patient to patient. Most often symptoms are associated with hyperglycemia, and polyuria, polydipsia, and polyphagia can be seen. The first event may be an acute metabolic decompensation, resulting in coma (ketoacidosis for IDDM and hyperosmolar coma for NIDDM). Occasionally the initial expression of DM is a degenerative complication like neuropathy.

Diagnosis. Symptomatic patients will have polyuria, polydipsia, ketonuria, and weight loss. Plasma glucose >200 mg/dL in these patients is sufficient for diagnosis with no further testing needed. A random glucose >200 mg/dL is diagnostic.

In asymptomatic patients, an elevated plasma or urine glucose during routine screening does not establish diagnosis but indicates a need for further evaluation. Patients who have DM will have a fasting plasma glucose ≥126 mg/dL on 2 occasions. The oral glucose tolerance test is rarely required. DM is diagnosed when plasma glucose ≥200 mg/dL at 2 h and on at least one of the earlier samples. HbA_{1c} >6.5% is diagnostic of diabetes.

Glycosylated hemoglobin A_{1c} (HbA_{1c}) is produced by nonenzymatic condensation of glucose molecules with free amino groups on the globin component of hemoglobin. It is used both for diagnosis and to follow compliance of the treatment and glucose control in diabetic patients. HbA_{1c} is high in diabetics with chronic hyperglycemia during the preceding 8–12 weeks.

Management. The objectives of diabetic therapy are to control symptoms, prevent acute complications, and limit long-term complications. Several steps should be considered, such as patient education, weight loss, low-fat diet, physical activity, and pharmacologic therapy with oral hypoglycemic drugs or insulin.

Weight reduction of as little as 4–7% body fat has an enormous effect on peripheral insulin sensitivity and on reduction of postprandial hyperglycemia. Exercise lowers glucose levels. Exercising muscle needs no insulin for glucose to enter. Resting muscle, in comparison, needs insulin for glucose entry. As many as 25% of diabetic patients can be kept off of medication with diet and exercise alone.

The effects of diet, exercise, and weight loss can last for many years. When diet and exercise do not keep the HbA1c <7%, medications are introduced.

Oral hypoglycemics should be prescribed for all type 2 diabetics. Metformin is the drug of choice and along with lifestyle intervention should be used in all newly diagnosed patients. One major advantage of metformin is that it does not cause hypoglycemia. Another is that it does not cause weight gain. (Metformin is contraindicated in those with renal insufficiency.)

- If a patient is initiated on metformin yet the diabetes does not become well-controlled, add a sulfonylurea.

- If a patient is already on sulfonylurea but the diabetes is not well-controlled, add metformin.

- If a patient is already taking both metformin and a sulfonylurea yet there is still poor glycemic control, then either switch to insulin or add a glitazone.

  – Glitazones can lead to fluid retention.

  – If one drug is not sufficient, a second or third oral agent may be combined to keep the patient off insulin.

- If metformin cannot be used, use a new glucagon-like peptide (GLP-1) agonist (exenatide or liraglutide). GLP-1 agonists are second-line agents that can be added to metformin or used individually if metformin cannot be used.

In all cases, metformin is clearly the "best initial therapy" for type 2 diabetes. After metformin, the choices are less clear.

- Sulfonylureas (glyburide, glipizide, glimepiride): increase weight, cause hypoglycemia; sulfa drugs

- Thiazolidinediones (rosiglitazone or pioglitazone): can worsen CHF

  – Thought to act by decreasing the resistance of tissues to insulin

  – Recent studies suggest pioglitazone may be linked to bladder cancer

  – Rosiglitazone only available through a special assessment program

- Incretin mimetics (exenatide, liraglutide): must be given by injection

  – Augment the naturally occurring hormones that are secreted from the GI tract in response to food; when food enters the intestine, incretins are released

  – Increase the release of insulin from the pancreas

  – Also called gastric inhibitory peptide or glucose-dependent insulinotropic peptide (both abbreviated as GIP); GIP increases insulin release and slows gastric motility

The other incretin is "glucagon-like peptide" or GLP. Though "glucagon-like," GLP does **not raise glucose levels** or mimic the effect on glucagon in terms of breaking down glycogen or increasing gluconeogenesis. The term "glucagon-like peptide" is very confusing because the effect of GLP is strictly to LOWER glucose levels. GLP also raises insulin levels and slows gastric motility. GLP is normally released from the small bowel but in the native form lasts only for 2 minutes.

The "incretin mimetic" drugs exenatide and liraglutide are direct analogues of GIP and GLP, except that their actions last much longer. The problem with these drugs is that they must be given by injection. They have an outstanding effect on slowing gastric motility and promoting weight loss, but because they are given by injection they are not used as one of the first 3 classes of medications to treat type 2 diabetes.

- Dipeptidyl peptidase IV (DPP-IV) inhibitors (sitagliptin, saxagliptin, linagliptin): natural hormones which prevent the metabolism of the incretins GIP and GLP

  – Increase insulin release from the pancreas and slow stomach emptying

  – Can be given orally

Only after therapy with multiple oral hypoglycemic fails should an insulin regimen be considered. When starting insulin, divide 50% into long-acting and 50% into pre-meal short-acting. This regimen is usually given as glargine insulin 1x/day injection along with 2–3×/day ultra-short-acting insulin such as lispro or aspart before meals. Glargine causes fewer episodes of hypoglycemia compared with NPH. Levemir is a newer, long-acting insulin, lasting 16–18 hours.

Table 2-4. Oral Hypoglycemic Drugs

Class	Generic Name	Brand Name	Doses/Day
Sulfonylureas	Glyburide, glipizide, glimepiride	Micronase, Diabeta, Amaryl	1–2
Biguanides	Metformin	Glucophage	2–3
Thiazolidinediones	Rosiglitazone, pioglitazone	—	1
Glucosidase inhibitors	Acarbose, miglitol	Precose	With every meal
Meglitinides	Repaglinide, nateglinide	—	—
DPP-IV inhibitors	Sitagliptin, saxagliptin, linagliptin	Januvia, Onglyza, Tradjenta	—
Subcutaneous agents			
GLP-1	Exenatide, liraglutide	Byetta, Victoza	2/day, 1/day

Table 2-5. Insulin Preparations

Type	Peak Action (Hours)	Duration of Action (Hours)
Ultra-short-acting		
• Insulin lispro	30–60 min	4–6
• Insulin aspart	20–30 min	3–5
Rapid		
• Regular	2–4	6–8
• Semilente	2–6	10–12
Intermediate		
• NPH	6–12	12–18
• Lente	6–12	12–18
Long-acting		
• Glargine	2	24
• Levemir	18–24	36

Complications of Diabetes Mellitus

Acute Complications. Diabetic ketoacidosis (DKA) is a result of severe insulin insufficiency. It occurs in type 1 diabetics and may be the presenting manifestation. Precipitating factors of DKA include insufficient or interrupted insulin therapy, infection, emotional stress, and excessive alcohol ingestion.

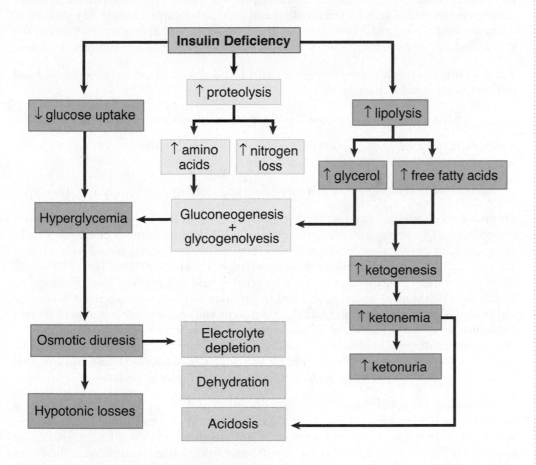

Figure 2-9. Pathophysiology of DKA

The main problems in DKA stem from acidosis with increased anion gap and dehydration. Clinical findings include anorexia, nausea or vomiting, abdominal pain, rapid breathing (Kussmaul respiration), "fruity" breath odor of acetone, signs of dehydration (dry skin and mucous membranes and poor skin turgor), and altered consciousness to coma. Acidosis can result in fatal rhythm disturbance.

Acutely, DKA is associated with hyperkalemia, which may be fatal. The total body level of potassium is depleted because of the urinary loss of potassium. As soon as the potassium level falls to ≤5 mEq/L, potassium replacement should be given.

The diagnosis of DKA can be made by finding elevated blood glucose, increased serum levels of acetoacetate, acetone, and hydroxybutyrate, metabolic acidosis (low serum bicarbonate and low blood pH), and increased anion gap (sodium − [bicarbonate + chloride]). DKA is managed with insulin, fluids, and electrolyte replacement. Normal saline should be given in high volume with insulin replacement. Bolus with 5–10 units of regular insulin.

Hyperosmolar nonketotic coma (HONK) is a syndrome that occurs predominantly in patients with type 2 diabetes and is characterized by severe hyperglycemia in the absence of significant ketosis. Precipitating factors include noncompliance with treatment plus the inability to drink sufficient water to keep up with urinary losses. This is common in elderly diabetics living in nursing homes. Infections, strokes, steroids, immunosuppressant agents, and diuretics are other precipitating factors. HONK can occur after therapeutic procedures such as peritoneal or hemo-dialysis, tube feeding of high-protein formulas, and high-carbohydrate infusion. The pathophys-iology involved is profound dehydration resulting from a sustained hyperglycemic diuresis. The clinical findings are weakness, polyuria, polydipsia, lethargy, confusion, convulsions, and coma.

The diagnosis of HONK is suggested by elevated blood glucose (typically ≥700 mg/dL) and extremely high serum osmolality

$$\text{Serum osmolality in mOsm/L} = 2[\text{sodium}] + [\text{glucose}/18] + [\text{BUN}/2.8]$$

A high BUN (prerenal azotemia) and mild metabolic acidosis (bicarbonate ~20 mEq/L) is also seen without ketosis.

Management of HONK involves high-volume fluid and electrolyte replacement, and insulin.

Chronic Complications. Chronic complications of diabetes involve the micro- and mac-rovasculature. The retina is affected, and diabetes is the leading cause of blindness; simple, background, or proliferative (microaneurysms, hemorrhages, exudates, retinal edema) dam-age can occur. Nephropathy affects 30–40% of type 1 and 20–30% of type 2 diabetics. Hyperproliferation, proteinuria, and end-stage renal disease can develop. The pathology can be diffuse, which is more common, and lead to widening of glomerular basement membrane and mesangial thickening. Nodular pathology can occur and results in hyalinization of afferent glomerular arterioles (Kimmelstiel-Wilson syndrome). Management of nephropathy involves strict control of diabetes, angiotensin-converting enzyme inhibitors, and dialysis or renal trans-plantation. All diabetics should be screened for proteinuria annually. Overt proteinuria is >300 mg/day. Microalbuminuria is >30 mg/day. Both are treated with ACE inhibitors.

Cardiovascular Complications. The number-one cause of death in patients with diabetes is cardiovascular disease. About 75% of all deaths in diabetes are from myocardial infarction, con-gestive failure, or stroke. For every 1% reduction in hemoglobin A1c, there is a 14% reduction in the risk of myocardial infarction. For every 10-point reduction in blood pressure, there is an additional 12% reduction in the risk of myocardial infarction. Coronary artery bypass should be performed in a diabetic patient even if there is only two-vessel coronary disease.

Diabetes is considered the equivalent of coronary disease in terms of management of hyperlip-idemia. Target LDL in a diabetic patient is <100 mg/dL.

- If LDL >100 mg/dL, lifestyle modifications such as diet and exercise should be initiated.
- Also, if LDL >100 mg/dL, drug therapy with a statin should be considered.

Renal Complications. Screening for proteinuria should occur annually for every diabetic patient. Trace proteinuria is detectable on a standard dipstick when the level >300 mg per 24 hours. Microalbuminuria is defined as a level 30–300 mg. All those with proteinuria should receive therapy with an ACE inhibitor or angiotensin receptor blocker. Diabetes is the most common cause of end stage renal disease in the United States.

Eye Complications. Screening for retinopathy should occur in every type 2 diabetic patient at diagnosis then annually. In type 1 diabetes, the first screening should take place 5 years after diagnosis, then annually thereafter. Proliferative retinopathy is defined as the presence of vitreous hemorrhages or neovascularization; it is treated with laser photocoagulation. Nonproliferative or background retinopathy can only be prevented with tight control of glucose levels.

Gastroparesis. Treated with metoclopramide or erythromycin.

Erectile Dysfunction. This occurs in as many as 50% of patients after 10 years of diabetes. Treatment is sildenafil.

Foot Exam. Podiatric examination should occur annually. Neuropathy leads to increased injury from trauma. Diabetes is responsible for 50% of all nontraumatic amputations in the United States.

Neuropathy. Neuropathy is another complication and has various types. Peripheral neuropathy is the most common and is symmetrical, with symptoms of numbness, paresthesia, and pain being prevalent; physical examination reveals absent reflexes and loss of vibratory sense. Mononeuropathy can also occur and affects a single nerve or nerve trunk (mononeuritis multiplex) and is vascular in origin; patients will have sudden foot drop, wrist drop, or paralysis of CN III, IV, or VI. Autonomic neuropathy can also occur and is usually devastating for the patient; patients will have orthostatic hypotension and syncope as main manifestations. Gastrointestinally, patient may have difficulty swallowing, delayed gastric emptying (gastroparesis), constipation, or diarrhea. Bladder dysfunction or paralysis can lead to urinary retention. Impotence and retrograde ejaculation are seen in men with this type of neuropathy.

Management of neuropathy depends on type. For peripheral neuropathy, analgesics, gabapentin, pregabalin, amitriptyline, and carbamazepine are used. Gabapentin and pregabalin are the best. For gastroparesis, metoclopramide or erythromycin can be used.

Additional Concepts. The "honeymoon" period (in IDDM patients) is an initial episode of ketoacidosis followed by a symptom-free interval during which no treatment is required. Presumably stress-induced epinephrine release blocks insulin secretion, causing the syndrome. In normal individuals insulin reserve is such that hormone release is adequate even in the face of stress.

The Somogyi effect is rebound hyperglycemia in the morning because of counterregulatory hormone release after an episode of hypoglycemia in the middle of the night.

The Dawn phenomenon is an early morning rise in plasma glucose secondary to a rise in counter-regulatory hormones cortisol, epinephrine, and GH requiring increased amounts of insulin to maintain euglycemia.

Hypoglycemia

Glucose is the primary energy source of the brain. Symptoms of hypoglycemia are divided into 2 groups and can occur because of excessive secretion of epinephrine, leading to sweating, tremor, tachycardia, anxiety, and hunger. Hypoglycemia can also occur because of dysfunction of the CNS, leading to dizziness, headache, clouding vision, blunted mental activity, loss of fine motor skills, confusion, abnormal behavior, convulsions, and loss of consciousness. There is no uniform correlation between a given level of blood sugar and symptoms. Major symptoms in normal persons may not be seen until blood sugar is 20 mg/dL.

Classification. Postprandial hypoglycemia (reactive) can be secondary to alimentary hyperinsulinism (after gastrectomy, gastrojejunostomy, pyloroplasty, or vagotomy), idiopathic, and galactosemia.

Fasting hypoglycemia can result from conditions in which there is an underproduction of glucose, such as hormone deficiencies (panhypopituitarism, adrenal insufficiency), enzyme defects, substrate deficiency (severe malnutrition, late pregnancy), acquired liver disease, or drugs (alcohol, propanolol, salicylates). Fasting hypoglycemia can also occur in conditions related to overutilization of glucose such as hyperinsulinism. Hyperinsulinism can occur secondary to insulinoma, exogenous insulin, sulfonylureas, drugs (quinine), endotoxic shock, and immune disease with insulin receptor antibodies. Overutilization of glucose can also occur in states in which there are appropriate insulin levels, such as extrapancreatic tumors and rare enzyme deficiencies.

Insulinoma (pancreatic B-cell tumor) can cause hypoglycemia. Ninety percent of these tumors are single and benign. Clinical findings include symptoms of subacute or chronic hypoglycemia such as blurred vision, headache, feelings of detachment, slurred speech, and weakness. Symptoms occur in the early morning or late afternoon or after fasting or exercise.

Diagnosis. This is made by finding a serum insulin level ≥8 mg/mL in the presence of blood glucose <40 mg/dL (i.e., inappropriately high serum insulin level when glucose is low), noted either spontaneously or during a prolonged fast (72 hours). CT scan, U/S, and arteriography may also be useful in detecting the tumor(s). Management of insulinoma is by surgery, diet, and medical therapy.

Factitious hyperinsulinism is caused by self-administration of insulin or ingestion of Equal or oral sulfonylureas. It is common and exceeds the incidence of insulinomas. Most often, these patients are associated with the health professions or have access to these drugs by a diabetic member of the family. A triad of hypoglycemia, high immunoreactivity, insulin, and suppressed plasma C peptide is pathognomonic of exogenous insulin administration.

Ethanol-induced hypoglycemia can also occur with prolonged starvation, when glycogen reserves become depleted in 18–24 hours and hepatic glucose output depends completely on gluconeogenesis. Ethanol at a concentration of 45 mg/dL can induce hypoglycemia by blocking gluconeogenesis.

Table 2-6. Differential Diagnosis of Insulinoma and Factitious Hyperinsulinism

Test	Insulinoma	Exogenous Insulin	Sulfonylureas
Plasma insulin	High (usually <200 µU/mL)	Very high (usually >1,000 µU/mL)	High
Proinsulin	Increased	Normal or low	Normal
C peptide (insulin connective peptide) 1:1	Increased	Normal or low	Increased
Insulin antibodies	Absent	+/– Present	Absent
Plasma or urine sulfonylurea	Absent	Absent	Present

DISEASES OF THE ADRENAL GLAND

Generalities. The adrenal gland is divided into 2 areas, the cortex and medulla. The cortex is divided into 3 areas, the outer zone (glomerulosa), which is the site of aldosterone synthesis; the central zone (fasciculata), which is the site of cortisol synthesis; and the inner zone (reticularis), which is the site of androgen biosynthesis. The disorders of hyperfunction of the gland are associated with the following specific hormones: increased cortisol is seen in Cushing syndrome; increased aldosterone in hyperaldosteronism; and increased adrenal androgens with virilization in women.

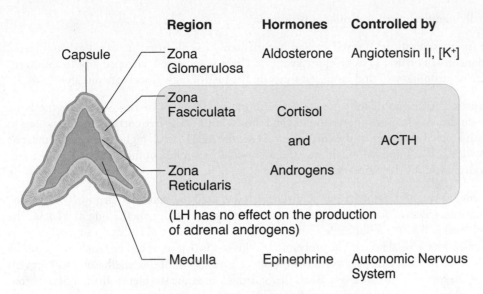

Region	Hormones	Controlled by
Zona Glomerulosa	Aldosterone	Angiotensin II, [K⁺]

Figure 2-10. Adrenal Cortex Regions

Hyperfunctioning of the Gland

Cushing syndrome

Definition. A group of clinical abnormalities caused by prolonged exposure to increased amounts of cortisol or related corticosteroids.

Etiology. Exogenous, iatrogenic causes are the most common overall causes of Cushing syndrome and can be secondary to prolonged use of glucocorticoids.

The etiology of Cushing syndrome includes adrenal hyperplasia. This can be secondary to pituitary ACTH production, which occurs in pituitary-hypothalamic dysfunction, and pituitary ACTH-producing adenomas (microadenoma, e.g., Cushing disease). ACTH-producing pituitary adenomas cause about 60–80% of Cushing cases. Adrenal hyperplasia can also be secondary to ACTH or corticotropin-releasing hormone (CRH), produced by nonendocrine tumors (bronchogenic carcinoma, carcinoma of the thymus, pancreatic carcinoma, and bronchial adenoma). Adrenal neoplasia, such as adenoma or carcinoma, and adrenal nodular hyperplasia account for about 30% of Cushing cases. Excessive cortisol production by an autonomous adrenal results in a low ACTH level. About 15% of Cushing cases are from ACTH from a source that cannot be located.

Clinical Findings. The clinical findings of Cushing syndrome include deposition of adipose tissue in characteristic sites such as upper fat, moon facies; interscapular buffalo hump; and mesenteric bed, truncal obesity. Other clinical findings include *hypertension*, muscle weakness, and fatigability related to mobilization of peripheral supportive tissue; osteoporosis caused by increased bone catabolism; cutaneous striae; and easy bruisability. Women may have acne, hirsutism, and oligomenorrhea or amenorrhea resulting from the increased adrenal androgen secretion. Emotional changes range from irritability or emotional lability to severe depression or confusion; even psychosis can occur as well. Glucose intolerance is common in Cushing disease, with 20% of patients having diabetes.

Cushing and glucocorticoid use are also associated with hypokalemia and leukocytosis. Hypokalemia occurs because of the mineralocorticoid effect of the steroids.

Clinically significant hypokalemia is uncommon.

Other manifestations are delayed wound healing, renal calculi from increased calcium levels, and glaucoma. Polyuria is from hyperglycemia. There is increased susceptibility to infections because neutrophils exhibit diminished function because of high glucocorticoid levels.

Diagnosis. The diagnostic tests used to establish the syndrome of cortisol excess are the 1-mg overnight dexamethasone suppression test and the 24-hour urine-free cortisol. The tests used to establish a precise etiology of the cortisol excess are the ACTH level, high-dose dexamethasone suppression test, CT and MRI scanning, and occasionally sampling of the petrosal venous sinus, which drains out of the pituitary.

The 1-mg overnight dexamethasone suppression test is used to establish a diagnosis of Cushing syndrome or glucocorticoid excess. If you give a milligram of dexamethasone at 11 P.M., the cortisol level at 8 A.M. should come to normal if there is the normal ability to suppress ACTH production over several hours. The problem with this test is that there can be falsely abnormal or positive tests. Any drug that increases the metabolic breakdown of dexamethasone will prevent its ability to suppress cortisol levels. Examples of drugs increasing the metabolism of dexamethasone are phenytoin, carbamazepine, and rifampin.

Stress increases glucocorticoid levels. The 1-mg overnight dexamethasone suppression test can be falsely positive in stressful conditions such as starvation, anorexia, bulimia, alcohol withdrawal, or depression. An abnormality on the 1-mg overnight test should be confirmed with a 24-hour urine-free cortisol. The 24-hour urine-free cortisol is more accurate.

A third screening test for Cushing is the midnight salivary cortisol. In normal patients, cortisol is at its lowest at midnight. In Cushing patients, cortisol is abnormally elevated at midnight.

The precise etiology of the Cushing syndrome is first established by using ACTH levels, sometimes in combination with high-dose dexamethasone suppression testing. ACTH levels are elevated with either a pituitary source of ACTH such as an adenoma or with an ectopic source. High-dose dexamethasone suppression testing can distinguish the difference. The output of a pituitary adenoma will suppress with high-dose dexamethasone. The output of an ectopic source will not suppress with high-dose dexamethasone.

If the ACTH level is low, then the etiology is most likely from an adrenal tumor such as an adenoma, cancer, or from adrenal hyperplasia. When the adrenal gland is the source of increased cortisol production, there is feedback inhibition on the pituitary and the ACTH level is suppressed.

When there is a low ACTH level, the precise etiology is confirmed with a CT scan of the adrenals.

When there is a high ACTH level, the precise etiology is confirmed with an MRI of the pituitary looking for an adenoma or a CT scan of the chest looking for an ectopic focus. If neither of these show a lesion or the MRI of the brain is equivocal, then inferior petrosal sinus sampling should be done to see if there is increased ACTH coming out of the brain.

Single random cortisol levels are not reliable.

- High plasma ACTH levels = pituitary or ectopic source
- Low plasma ACTH levels = adrenal tumors or hyperplasia

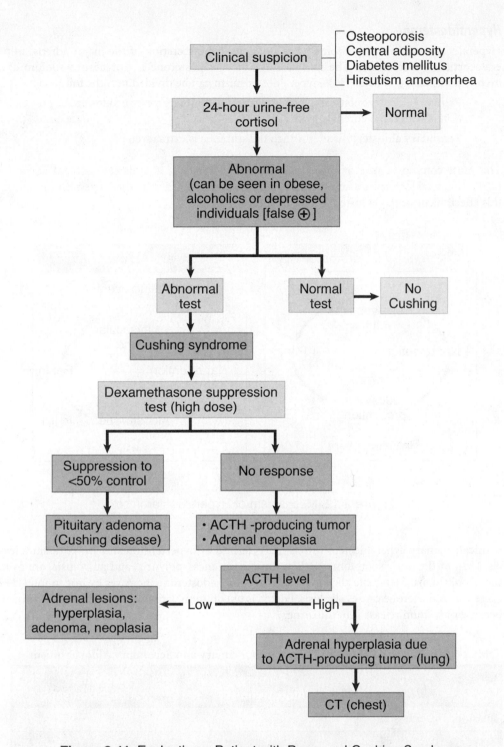

Figure 2-11. Evaluating a Patient with Presumed Cushing Syndrome

Management. Depends on the etiology, and can be surgical or medical. Unresectable adrenal tumors are treated with ketoconazole or metyrapone.

Hyperaldosteronism

Hyperaldosteronism is a syndrome associated with hypersecretion of the major adrenal mineralocorticoid, aldosterone. The normal function of aldosterone is to reabsorb sodium and excrete potassium and acid (H^+). Hyperaldosteronism can be divided into the following:

- **Primary aldosteronism**, in which the stimulus for the excessive aldosterone production is within the adrenal gland
- **Secondary aldosteronism**, in which the stimulus is extraadrenal

The most common cause of primary hyperaldosteronism is a unilateral adrenal adenoma (70%). Bilateral hyperplasia accounts for 25–30%. Excessive black licorice ingestion can mimic this effect. Licorice has aldosterone-like qualities.

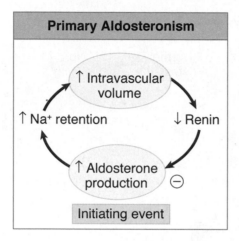
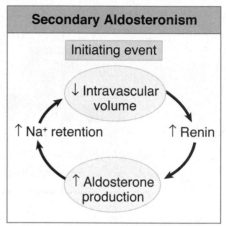

Figure 2-12. Mechanism of Hyperaldosteronism

Clinical. Primary hyperaldosteronism is characterized by hypertension and low potassium levels. Most of the other symptoms, such as muscle weakness, polyuria, and polydipsia, are from the hypokalemia. Metabolic alkalosis occurs because aldosterone increases hydrogen ion (H+) excretion. Aldosterone causes alkalosis. Edema is uncommon with primary hyperaldosteronism because of sodium release into the urine.

Table 2-7. Clinical and Laboratory Findings in Primary and Secondary Aldosteronism

	Primary Aldosteronism	Secondary Aldosteronism
Diastolic hypertension	+	–
Muscle weakness	+	+/–
Polyuria, polydipsia	+	+/–
Edema	–	+/–
Hypokalemia	+	+
Hypernatremia	+	–
Metabolic alkalosis	+	+

Diagnosis. The preliminary screen for hyperaldosteronism is a plasma aldosterone concentration (PAC) and plasma renin activity (PRA). A positive screen is a PAC/PRA ratio >20:1 and a PAC >15. To confirm hyperaldosteronism, an NaCl challenge is required. This can be via normal saline, NaCl tabs, or fludrocortisone. After an NaCl challenge, PAC should be suppressed as in a normal individual. If PAC is still elevated, this confirms the diagnosis.

Management. Adrenal adenomas are removed surgically. Bilateral hyperplasia is treated with spironolactone, which blocks aldosterone.

Bartter Syndrome. The exception of secondary hyperaldosteronism without edema or hypertension is Bartter syndrome. Bartter syndrome is caused by a defect in the loop of Henle in which it loses NaCl. This is due to a defect in the Na-K-2Cl cotransporter. This is like having a furosemide-secreting tumor.

In Bartter syndrome there is juxtaglomerular hyperplasia, normal to low blood pressure, no edema, severe hypokalemic alkalosis, defect in renal conservation of sodium or chloride, and renal loss of sodium, which stimulates renin secretion and aldosterone production.

Syndromes of adrenal androgen excess

Syndromes of adrenal androgen excess result from excess production of dehydroepiandrosterone (DHEA), and androstenedione, which are converted to testosterone in extraglandular tissues. The elevated testosterone accounts for most androgenic effects.

Clinical Signs and Symptoms. Hirsutism, oligomenorrhea, acne, and virilization. Etiology includes congenital adrenal hyperplasia, adrenal adenomas (rare), and adrenal carcinomas.

Congenital adrenal hyperplasia (CAH)

Definition. Congenital adrenal hyperplasia is a syndrome associated with increased adrenal androgen production because of enzymatic defects.

Etiology. CAH is the most common adrenal disorder of infancy and childhood. CAH arises from autosomal recessive mutations, which produce deficiencies of enzymes necessary for the synthesis of cortisol.

Common Enzymatic Defects Associated with CAH. Enzymatic defects include C-21 hydroxylase deficiency in 95% of all cases. C-21 hydroxylase deficiency is associated with reduction in aldosterone secretion in one-third of patients. Adrenal virilization occurs with or without an associated salt-losing tendency, owing to aldosterone deficiency, which leads to hyponatremia, hyperkalemia, dehydration, and hypotension.

Patients are female at birth with ambiguous external genitalia (female pseudohermaphrodism), enlarged clitoris, and partial or complete fusion of the labia. Postnatally CAH is associated with virilization. Patients may be male at birth with macrogenitosomia; postnatally this is associated with precocious puberty.

C-11 hydroxylase deficiency can also occur. The mineralocorticoid manifestations in C-11 deficiency can be 'biphasic.' In early infancy, despite having excessive mineralocorticoid hormones, patients sometimes present with relative 'salt wasting' (aldosterone deficiency). This is because some infants have inefficient salt conservation as well as immature aldosterone production. During this phase, infants can present with hypotension and hyperkalemia (very similar to 21 hydroxylase deficiency). Later in life (childhood and adulthood), there is better ability to hold onto salt, so the patient develops the typical C-11 deficiency syndrome: hypertension and hypokalemia.

Note

The 'biphasic' presentation is rare. Overall, when you think about 11 deficiency, think mineralocorticoid excess (hypertension and hypokalemia) with low cortisol production (remember you need C-11 for the final step in converting to cotrisol).

C-17 hydroxylase deficiency can occur as well, and is characterized by hypogonadism, hypokalemia, and hypertension resulting from increased production of 11-deoxycorticosterone.

Diagnosis. CAH should be considered in all infants exhibiting failure to thrive, especially those with episodes of acute adrenal insufficiency, salt wasting, or hypertension. The most useful measurements are of serum testosterone, androstenedione, dehydroepiandrosterone, 17-hydroxyprogesterone, urinary 17-ketosteroid, and pregnanetriol.

Management. Treatment is glucocorticoid (hydrocortisone) replacement.

Hypofunctioning of the Gland

Adrenal insufficiency

Definition. Adrenal insufficiency can be divided into **primary adrenocorticoid insufficiency** (**Addison disease**) and **secondary failure in the elaboration of ACTH**. Primary adrenocortical insufficiency is a slow, usually progressive disease due to adrenocorticoid hypofunction.

Etiology. The etiology of Addison disease can be secondary to anatomic destruction of the gland (chronic and acute). Idiopathic atrophy is the most common cause of anatomic destruction, and autoimmune mechanisms are probably responsible. Autoimmune destruction accounts for 80% of cases. Anatomic destruction can also be secondary to surgical removal, infection (TB, fungal, cytomegalovirus), hemorrhagic, trauma, and metastatic invasion. Metabolic failure in hormone production can also lead to Addison disease and can be secondary to CAH, enzyme inhibitors, and cytotoxic agents (mitotane).

Clinical Findings. The clinical findings in Addison disease include weakness, paresthesias, cramping, intolerance to stress, and personality changes such as irritability and restlessness. Chronic disease is characterized by a small heart, weight loss, and sparse axillary hair. Hyperpigmentation of the skin can occur and appears as diffuse brown, tan, or bronze darkening of both exposed and unexposed body parts. Arterial hypotension is seen and is often orthostatic owing to lack of effect of cortisol on vascular tone. Abnormalities of GI function are found, and symptoms vary from mild anorexia with weight loss to nausea, vomiting, diarrhea, and abdominal pain. Acute Addisonian crisis is characterized by fever and hypotension. A low sodium with a high potassium level and mild acidosis are also present.

Diagnosis. The diagnosis of Addison disease is made through rapid ACTH administration and measurement of cortisol. Laboratory findings include white blood cell count with moderate neutropenia, lymphocytosis, and eosinophilia; elevated serum potassium and urea nitrogen; low sodium; low blood glucose; and morning low plasma cortisol.

The definitive diagnosis is the cosyntropin or ACTH stimulation test. A cortisol level is obtained before and after administering ACTH. A normal person should show a brisk rise in cortisol level after ACTH administration.

Differences between primary and secondary adrenal insufficiency:
- Hyperpigmentation (occurs only with primary insufficiency)
- Electrolyte abnormalities
- Hypotension

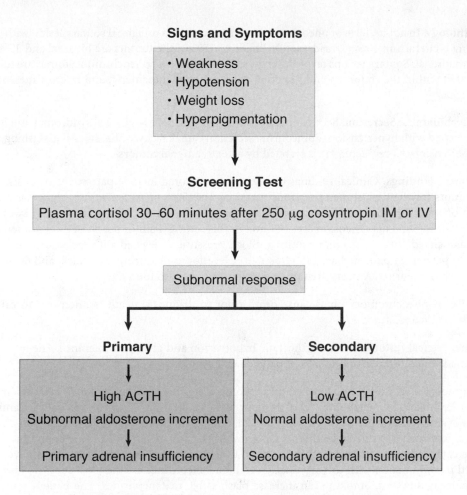

Signs and Symptoms

- Weakness
- Hypotension
- Weight loss
- Hyperpigmentation

Screening Test

Plasma cortisol 30–60 minutes after 250 μg cosyntropin IM or IV

Subnormal response

Primary

High ACTH

Subnormal aldosterone increment

Primary adrenal insufficiency

Secondary

Low ACTH

Normal aldosterone increment

Secondary adrenal insufficiency

Figure 2-13. Diagnosis of Adrenal Insufficiency

Management. The management of Addison disease involves glucocorticoid, mineralocorticoid, and sodium chloride replacement, in addition to patient education.

Adrenal Crisis. In an adrenal crisis, fever, vomiting, abdominal pain, altered mental status, and vascular collapse may occur. Get a cortisol level, then rapidly administer fluids and hydrocortisone. This may occur in:

- Previously undiagnosed patient with adrenal insufficiency who has undergone surgery, serious infection, and/or major stress
- Bilateral adrenal infarction or hemorrhage
- Patient who is abruptly withdrawn from chronic glucocorticoid therapy

Pheochromocytoma

Definition. A rare, usually benign, tumor that arises from the chromaffin cells of the sympathetic nervous system. The **rule of 10%** applies in pheochromocytoma with 10% being extraadrenal, 10% malignant, 10% in children, and 10% bilateral or multiple (>right side). Also, 10% are not associated with hypertension.

Epidemiology. Pheochromocytoma occurs in approximately 0.1% of the hypertensive population. Familial pheochromocytoma occurs in 5% of cases, and is transmitted as an autosomal dominant trait alone or in combination with MEN type II or III, von Recklinghausen neurofibromatosis, or von Hippel-Lindau retinal cerebellar hemangioblastomatosis.

Pathology. In adults, 80% of pheochromocytomas occur as a unilateral solitary lesion with 10% being bilateral and 10% extraadrenal. In children, 25% of the tumors are bilateral and 25% are extraadrenal. Solitary lesions favor the right side. Extraadrenal pheochromocytomas are mostly located within the abdomen and near the celiac, superior mesenteric, and inferior mesenteric ganglia.

Catecholamine Secretion. Secretion of dopamine occurs more in familial syndromes and is not associated with hypertension. Epinephrine secretion causes tachycardia, sweating, flushing, and hypertension. Norepinephrine is secreted by all extraadrenal tumors.

Clinical Findings. Clinical findings of pheochromocytoma include paroxysms or crisis. This accounts for the typical manifestations occurring in >50% of patients. The attack has a sudden onset, lasting from a few minutes to several hours or longer. Headache, profuse sweating, palpitations, and apprehension are common in this setting. Pain in the chest or abdomen may be associated with nausea and vomiting. Blood pressure is elevated with tachycardia in crisis. Forty percent of patients have blood pressure elevation only during the attack, and 60% have stable hypertension. Anxiety, tremor, and weight loss are also found.

>33% of pheochromocytomas cause death prior to diagnosis; death is often due to cardiac arrhythmia and stroke.

Other clinical features include orthostatic hypotension and glucose intolerance. The hyperglycemia is only found in about 33% of patients and is mild.

Diagnosis. Diagnosis is established by demonstrating increased amounts of catecholamines or catecholamine metabolites in a 24-hour urine collection. Urinary-free catecholamines, urinary metanephrines, vanillylmandelic acid, and plasma catecholamines are tests of choice. Metanephrines are catecholamine metabolites. A 24-hour urinary VMA, metanephrines, and free catecholamines are the best initial tests. Recently, plasma metanephrine levels have been used in conjunction with urinary tests. Overall, metanephrines are the most sensitive and specific individual test. Smoking can increase plasma-free metanephrines. The patient must not smoke at least 4 hours before the test.

Clonidine should suppress epinephrine levels. Failure of epinephrine levels to fall after clonidine administration is highly suggestive of pheochromocytoma. A clonidine-suppression test is used when the above screening tests are equivocal.

When the catecholamine or metanephrine levels are abnormal, the tumor is confirmed with CT or MRI scan. MIBG (metaiodobenzylguanidine) scanning is used to locate a pheochromocytoma not found on a CT scan. If the biochemical tests (catecholamines, metanephrines) are positive and the CT scan does not show the location of the pheochromocytoma, then do an MIBG scan.

Differential Diagnosis. The differential diagnosis of pheochromocytoma includes essential hypertension, anxiety attacks, factitious crisis, intracranial lesions, and autonomic epilepsy.

Management. The most important step in management of pheochromocytomas involves controlling the blood pressure by using alpha-adrenergic blocking agents (phentolamine, phenoxybenzamine). **No other antihypertensive drugs should be used before adequate control of blood pressure is accomplished with alpha blockade.**

Curative surgical removal of the pheochromocytoma is performed only after stabilization of blood pressure.

DISEASES OF THE TESTES, HYPOGONADISM

Definition. In hypogonadism there is decreased function of the testes or ovaries, resulting in the absence or impairment of secondary sexual characteristics and infertility.

Etiology

- **Primary hypogonadism** (hypergonadotropic: increased LH, FSH) can result from Klinefelter syndrome (small testes, eunuchoid, 47XXY), anorchia, surgical or accidental castration or radiotherapy, infections (mumps, TB, leprosy), or chemotherapeutic agents.

- **Secondary hypogonadism** (hypogonadotropic: low LH, FSH) can result from hypopituitarism secondary to idiopathic causes or tumors, hypothalamic lesions, and Kallmann syndrome (hypogonadic hypogonadism, associated with decreased sense of smell).

Clinical Findings. Clinical findings include prepubertal hypogonadism, which is most often caused by a specific gonadotropic deficiency of the pituitary. External genitalia are underdeveloped, voice is high-pitched, beard does not grow, and the patient lacks libido and potency. As an adult, the patient has a youthful appearance, with obesity, disproportionately long extremities, lack of temporal recession of the hairline, and a small Adam's apple. Gynecomastia is sometimes seen. The skin is fine-grained, wrinkled, and free of acne. The testes may be absent from the scrotum. Bone age is retarded. Urinary 17-ketosteroid is low to normal, and serum testosterone is below normal. Serum FSH and LH are low in hypothalamic or pituitary origin and elevated in primary testicular failure. Treatment is with testosterone.

Postpubertal hypogonadism can be caused by any pituitary lesion or testes that may be damaged by trauma, radiation, infection, or drugs. Libido and potency are lost. Hair growth is retarded. Vasomotor symptoms including flushing, dizziness, and chills can occur. Lack of aggressiveness and interest, sterility, muscle aches, and back pain are also seen. The skin on the face is thin and finely wrinkled. Urinary and plasma testosterone levels are low. Urinary and serum FSH and LH are low with pituitary lesions and high with pituitary testicular failure. Serum prolactin is often elevated in hypothalamic or pituitary lesions. Treatment is with testosterone.

Klinefelter syndrome is the most common primary developmental abnormality causing hypogonadism (testicular damage). This syndrome affects 1 of every 400–500 males. It is caused by one or more supernumerary X chromosomes. Eighty percent of patients have a 47,XXY karyotype. Gynecomastia is found with elevated levels of LH and FSH. Sterility and lack of libido are present. The testes are small and thin. Mental retardation may be present. Urinary 17-ketosteroids are low normal or normal, serum testosterone is low to normal, LH and FSH are elevated, and serum estradiol is elevated. Treatment is testosterone replacement.

Note

Males affected by Klinefelter syndrome have a 20× increased risk of breast cancer.

Rheumatology 3

EVALUATING A PATIENT WITH ARTHRITIS

When a patient presents with joint swelling, a differential diagnosis is generated based on the answers to the following questions:

1. What is the distribution of joint involvement and how many joints are involved?

Polyarticular symmetric involvement is characteristically seen with rheumatoid arthritis (RA), systemic lupus erythematosus (SLE), parvovirus B19, and hepatitis B. On the other hand, monoarticular arthritis is consistent with osteoarthritis, crystal-induced arthritis (gout, pseudogout), septic arthritis (gonococcus), trauma, and hemarthrosis.

Migratory arthropathy (inflammation and pain migrates from joint to joint, while the previous involved joints improve) is caused by rheumatic fever, disseminated gonococcal infection, and Lyme disease. Oligoarticular asymmetric arthritis is common with the spondyloarthropathies (ankylosing spondylitis) and osteoarthritis involving the small joint of the upper extremities and rarely as a presentation of polyarticular gout.

2. Are the symptoms acute or chronic?

Osteoarthritis is a chronic disease; the patients have symptoms for months to years. Patients with septic arthritis or crystal-induced arthropathies have short-lived symptoms, commonly only a few days.

3. Does the patient have systemic symptoms (beyond the arthritis)?

SLE presents with lung (pleural effusions), kidney (proteinuria and renal failure), CNS (vasculitis, strokes, and change in personality), skin (malar and photosensitivity rash), and hematologic (immune-mediated anemia, thrombocytopenia) manifestations.

Sjögren syndrome has keratoconjunctivitis sicca (dry eyes/mouth) and parotid enlargement.

Systemic sclerosis has skin involvement and Raynaud phenomenon.

Wegener granulomatosis presents with upper respiratory (sinusitis and rhinitis), lower respiratory (lung nodules and hemoptysis), and renal (necrotizing glomerulonephritis) involvement.

OA, on the other hand, presents with absence of systemic symptoms.

4. Is there evidence of joint inflammation?

Evidence of joint inflammation includes: joint stiffness in the morning >1 hour, joint erythema and warmth, and elevated erythrocyte sedimentation rate (ESR) and C-reactive protein. An example of inflammatory arthritis is rheumatoid arthritis, while OA is typically noninflammatory.

Do not go further into a history unless you have answered the above 4 questions.

Examples
- A 62-year-old man presents with right knee pain.
- A 24-year-old woman presents with bilateral wrist, MCP, PIP joint swelling, and pain.
- A 32-year-old man presents with knee swelling after you had seen him one week ago for left wrist pain and swelling, which has now resolved.
- A 29-year-old man has right knee pain and swelling and left hip pain.

TESTS IN RHEUMATOLOGIC DISEASES

Joint Aspiration

If there is fluid in the joint, it needs analysis immediately.

The basic tests to run on the synovial fluid are the 3 Cs (cell count, crystals, and cultures) and the Gram stain.

Synovial fluid may be stratified according to the number of cells:
- OA and traumatic arthritis have 200–2,000 WBCs/mm^3 in the synovial fluid
- Inflammatory diseases (RA, gout) have 5,000–50,000 WBC/mm^3
- Septic arthritis has >50,000 WBC/mm^3

Table 3-1. Synovial Fluid Analysis in Different Rheumatologic Diseases

Disease	WBCs	Crystals/Polarization
DJD	<2,000	Negative traumatic
Inflammatory	5,000–50,000	Gout: needle-shaped, negative birefringent Pseudogout (CPPD): Rhomboid-shaped, positive birefringent
Septic	>50,000	Negative (Gram stain and culture usually negative for GC but positive in *Staph*, strep, and gram-negatives)

There are a few exceptions to the above:
- Septic arthritis may sometimes present with <50,000 WBC/mm^3 in the joint aspirate if antibiotics are given before the joint aspiration. Septic arthritis should be considered a possibility in a patient with >5,000 WBC/mm^3 in the synovial fluid, monoarticular arthritis, but absence of crystals.
- Gout and pseudogout uncommonly present with >50,000 WBC/mm^3 in the absence of infection. Consider this possibility if there is evidence of crystals in the aspirate.
- Culture of joint fluid is positive in only 50% or less of gonococcal arthritis.

Antinuclear Antibodies

Antinuclear antibodies (ANA) are antibodies that have the capability of binding to certain structures within the nucleus of the cells. ANAs are found in patients whose immune system may be predisposed to generate antibodies against their own body tissues. This is referred to as autoimmunity.

Although ANAs are found in patients with SLE, Sjögren syndrome, and systemic sclerosis, they may also be found in approximately 5% of normal people. When ANAs are present in normal people, they are usually in low titers (<1:80).

The ANA test is performed by exposing the antibodies in the serum of the blood to the laboratory test cells. It is then determined whether or not antibodies are present that react with various parts of the nucleus. Fluorescent techniques are now more frequently used, thus the test may be referred to as a fluorescent antinuclear antibody test (FANA).

ANAs present in different patterns depending on the staining of the cell nucleus: homogeneous, speckled, nucleolar, and peripheral (or rim). While these patterns are not specific for any one disease, certain diseases can more frequently be associated with one pattern or another. For example, the peripheral (rim) pattern may be seen with SLE, while the nucleolar pattern is more commonly seen in systemic sclerosis. The speckled pattern is more commonly seen in normal people.

Also, subsets of ANAs are associated with specific autoimmune diseases and are thus used to further diagnose these diseases. For example, anti ds-DNA and anti-SM antibodies are found in patients with SLE; anti-histone antibodies are found in patients with drug-induced lupus. (*See* Tables 3-2 and 3-3.)

Table 3-2. ANA Patterns

Peripheral (Rim)	SLE
Diffuse	Nonspecific
Speckled	Nonspecific
Centromere	CREST
Nucleolar	Systemic sclerosis

Table 3-3. Specific ANAs

Anti-ds-DNA (native DNA)	SLE only (60%); an indicator of disease activity and lupus nephritis
Anti-SM	SLE only (25–30%)
Anti-histone	Drug-induced lupus (95%)
Anti-Ro (SSA)	Neonatal lupus, Sjögren and in the 3% of ANA-negative lupus
Anti-LA (SSB)	Sjögren
Anti-centromere	CREST
Anti-RNP	100% mixed connective tissue disease (MCTD)

Clinical Correlate

Overall, >95% of SLE patients have positive ANA test results, which makes a negative ANA result a good rule-out test for SLE.

Interpret a positive ANA test in the context of the clinical symptoms, i.e., a positive ANA in an asymptomatic patient with no other abnormal tests is likely to be a false–positive (5% of the population); a positive ANA in a patient with arthritis, proteinuria, and pleural effusion is likely to be associated with SLE.

Rheumatoid Factor

Rheumatoid factor (RF) is an autoantibody against the Fc portion of IgG. Rheumatoid factors are found in approximately 70% of patients with RA. However, these antibodies are not specific for RA and are found in 5% of healthy adults (the prevalence increases with age, sometimes seen in up to 20% of people >65 years of age).

Therefore, RF is neither sensitive nor specific for the diagnosis of RA.

The presence of RF can be of prognostic significance, since patients with high titers tend to have more aggressive disease with extraarticular manifestations.

Antineutrophil Cytoplasmic Antibodies

Antineutrophil cytoplasmic antibodies (ANCAs) are antibodies directed against certain proteins in the cytoplasm of neutrophils. The cytoplasmic (c) ANCA refers to the diffuse staining pattern observed when serum antibodies bind to indicator neutrophils; it is seen in >90% of patients with Wegener granulomatosis. Perinuclear (p) ANCA refers to a localized staining pattern observed on the indicator neutrophils, the major target of these antibodies being the enzyme myeloperoxidase; it is found in PAN and Churg-Strauss but is a nonspecific test.

Antiphospholipid Antibody Syndrome

Antiphospholipid antibody syndrome (lupus anticoagulant or anticardiolipin antibodies) is a hypercoagulable state associated with a group of antibodies that are directed against phospholipids or cardiolipins. It is unclear whether the antibodies are directly involved in the etiology of the clotting disorder associated with this syndrome. The nature of these antibodies causes the common laboratory abnormalities associated with the syndrome, i.e., elevated partial thromboplastin time (PTT) and false-positive RPR or VDRL. Clinically, it presents with spontaneous abortions in otherwise healthy women or thromboembolism (pulmonary embolism, DVT) in other patients. Two first-trimester spontaneous abortions suggest antiphosolipid antibodies.

RHEUMATOID ARTHRITIS

A 26-year-old woman with no prior medical history presents with a 3-week history of joint swelling and stiffness. She informs you that she has had stiffness for about 2 h every morning since these symptoms started and that the symptoms improve as the day progresses. She denies back stiffness or back pain. She has fatigue and low-grade fever. On the examination the wrist, MCPs, and PIPs are red and swollen on both hands. The DIPs are not involved. There is fluid in the wrist joints. Otherwise the examination is normal.

Definition. RA is a chronic inflammatory multisystemic disease with the main target being the synovium. The hallmark of RA is inflammatory synovitis that presents in a symmetric distribution. The intense joint inflammation that occurs has the potential to destroy cartilage and cause bone erosions and eventually deform the joint.

Anti-CCP (cyclic citrullinated peptide) is also positive in RA and carries a very high specificity.

Etiology/Epidemiology. The cause of RA is unknown. RA may be triggered as a reaction to an infectious agent (mycoplasma, parvovirus) in a susceptible host.

Of the environmental factors, only cigarette smoking seems to be associated with RA. Women are affected 3× more than men, and in 80% of cases the age of onset is between 35 and 50 years.

Pathogenesis. An initiation phase of nonspecific inflammation occurs, followed by an amplification phase resulting from T-cell activation, and finally the stage of chronic inflammation and tissue injury.

The predominant infiltrating cell is the *T lymphocyte*. Diseases like human immunodeficiency virus (HIV), in which T cells are decreased, will characteristically improve preexisting RA; this is also the reason why *RA is very rare in patients with HIV*.

Recent studies have shown that excessive amounts of the pro-inflammatory cytokines—tumor necrosis factor alpha (TNF-a), interleukin-1, and interleukin-6 (IL-6)—mediate most of the pathogenic features of rheumatoid arthritis. This underscores the focus of new treatment modalities on inhibiting these cytokines (see TNF inhibitors on following pages).

Presentation. Diagnostic criteria—need 4 of the following diagnostic criteria.

- Morning stiffness (>1 h) for 6 weeks
- Swelling of wrists, MCPs, PIPs for 6 weeks
- Swelling of 3 joints for 6 weeks
- Symmetric joint swelling for 6 weeks
- RF positive or anti-cyclic citrullinated peptide
- CRP or ESR

X-ray abnormalities and nodules are not necessary for the diagnosis of RA.

Criteria. RA is a chronic inflammatory symmetric arthropathy. There needs to be involvement of multiple joints, but some joints are *never* involved in RA:

- DIPs
- Joints of the lower back

Because RA is a systemic disease, ~70% of patients present with constitutional symptoms—fatigue, anorexia, weight loss, generalized weakness—before the onset of the arthritis.

Extraarticular Manifestations

- Damage to the ligaments and tendons
  - Radial deviation of the wrist with ulnar deviation of the digits
  - Boutonnière deformity
  - Swan-neck deformity
- Rheumatoid nodules
  - Initial event caused by focal vasculitis
  - 20–30% of patients with RA; usually occur in areas of mechanical stress (olecranon, occiput, Achilles tendon)
  - Methotrexate may flare this process

Note

In 2010, a new set of criteria was proposed by the American College of Rheumatology and the European League against Rheumatism which focuses more on serologies, acute phase reactants, number of joints involved, and duration of joint involvement over 6 weeks. This leads to a point system.

For the moment, the 1987 criteria are not obsolete.

- Felty syndrome (RA + splenomegaly + neutropenia)
- Caplan syndrome (RA + pneumoconiosis)

Laboratory Findings
- RF or anti-CCP
- Anemia
- ESR or C-reactive protein (CRP)
- X-rays
- Synovial fluid analysis

Diagnosis. The diagnosis is based on the use of clinical criteria; there is no single test or finding that will diagnose RA. Anti-CCP is more specific than RF.

Treatment. None of the nonsteroidal antiinflammatory drugs (NSAIDs) have been shown to be better than aspirin in RA, but they have fewer GI side effects.

There is no single NSAID superior to other agents, and the newer agents have not been shown to have a decreased incidence in toxicity (GI, renal, etc.).

Cyclooxygenase 2 (COX-2) inhibitors are a type of NSAID which selectively blocks the COX-2 enzyme at the site of inflammation. The benefit of COX-2 inhibitors is that they do not inhibit COX-1, an enzyme that helps with the production of the protective stomach lining. The non-selective (traditional) types of NSAIDs block both COX-2 and COX-1, which can lead to increased risk for GI side effects (bleeding, etc.).

Because of the increased risk of MI, both rofecoxib and valdecoxib have been recalled; currently only celecoxib is available.

Other drugs in RA:
- Glucocorticoids (usually for short courses only)
- Disease-modifying agents: antimalarials, gold, sulfasalazine, methotrexate (MTX), and tumor necrosis factor (TNF) receptor inhibitors

Disease-modifying Anti-rheumatic Drugs

The best initial DMARD is methotrexate (MTX). If MTX does not control disease, an anti-TNF medication is added to treatment.

Table 3-4. Adverse Effects of DMARD

Drug	Profile/Side Effects	Screening Tests for Toxicity
Hydroxychloroquine	Retinopathy	Regular eye examination
MTX (methotrexate; most utilized agent and mainstay of treatment)	Rapid onset of action; hepatitis and hepatic fibrosis; pneumonitis; may flare rheumatoid nodules	CBC and liver enzymes every 4–8 weeks

Hydroxychloroquine and sulfasalazine are used in early, mild disease. Steroids are used briefly to control disease while waiting for methotrexate to work.

Biologic Agents. Tumor necrosis factor (TNF) inhibitors. Tumor necrosis factor alpha (TNF-α) is a pro-inflammatory cytokine produced by macrophages and lymphocytes. It is found in large quantities in the rheumatoid joint and is produced locally in the joint by synovial macrophages and lymphocytes infiltrating the joint synovium. TNF inhibitors relieve the signs and symptoms of RA, and slow or halt radiographic damage. These drugs have been shown to be effective in patients who were thought to be resistant to all methotrexate.

Latent assessment and treatment for TB is required before use of any of these agents.

There are 3 TNF inhibitors approved for the treatment of RA:

- Infliximab (Remicade) is a monoclonal antibody to TNF-α that binds to TNF-α in the joint and in the circulation. The combination of infliximab and methotrexate is very effective in reducing clinical manifestations of disease. Infliximab is given as an IV infusion. Cases of sepsis, disseminated tuberculosis, and other opportunistic infections have been reported for patients treated with infliximab or other anti-TNF therapy.

- Adalimumab (Humira) is an anti-TNF mAb that differs from infliximab in that its sequences are entirely human.

- Etanercept (Enbrel) is a human fusion protein that is entirely human, and anti-etanercept antibodies are relatively uncommon.

Complications/Follow-Up. Aggressive disease is likely to occur with the following features: high titers of RF, diffuse rheumatoid nodules, early joint erosions, late age of onset, and certain subtypes of the HLA-DR4.

Atlantoaxial subluxation may occur in patients with RA when there is excessive movement at the junction between the atlas (C1) and axis (C2), due to either a bony or ligamentous abnormality. In RA, the incidence of cervical involvement has been reported to be 25–80% and results from pannus formation at the synovial joints between C1 and C2. Neurologic symptoms occur when the spinal cord is involved (paraplegia, quadriplegia). Commonly, patients have subtle symptoms, which include neck pain (occipital), C2 radicular pain (paresthesias of the hands and feet), and myelopathy.

Consider this diagnosis in patients who have RA and neck pain, paresthesias, etc. The first test to do when considering the diagnosis is an x-ray of the cervical spine (order multiple views of the cervical spine, including an open-mouth view). You may further investigate with a CT scan or an MRI. Refer always to a spine surgeon (orthopedic specialist or neurosurgeon) if the radiologic testing is positive. All patients with RA should be screened with a plain x-ray for C1–C2 subluxation before intubation or anesthesia is performed.

If a patient with RA presents with a swollen painful calf, consider a ruptured Baker cyst. Baker cyst is the extension of inflamed synovium into the popliteal space.

Note

Screen for TB before using TNF inhibitors.

Clinical Pearl

- Consider atlantoaxial subluxation in patients with RA who complain of occipital headaches and upper extremity tingling and numbness.

- Always rule out subclinical subluxation in patients with RA who are undergoing surgery and intubation electively.

SYSTEMIC LUPUS ERYTHEMATOSUS

A 35-year-old woman is brought for the evaluation of confusion lasting 1 day. Her friends and family inform you that "she did not know how to come home from work" and that lately "she has not been herself." You find that the patient has elevated blood pressure, decreased air entry on the right lung base with dullness to percussion, and symmetrical joint swelling of the wrists and MCPs. A chemistry profile shows an elevated creatinine of 2.4 mg/dL, and there is protein in the urine on the urinalysis.

Definition. SLE is a systemic disease in which tissues and multiple organs are damaged by pathogenic autoantibodies and immune complexes.

Etiology/Pathogenesis. SLE is of unknown etiology.

- Ninety percent of cases are women.
- The abnormal immune response probably depends on interactions between a susceptible host and environmental factors.

Ultraviolet (UV)-B light is the only environmental factor known to cause flares.

Presentation. Diagnostic criteria—need 4 to diagnose.

- Malar rash
- Discoid rash
- Photosensitivity
- Oral ulcers
- Arthritis
- Serositis (pleuritis or pericarditis)
- Renal involvement
- Neurologic disorder (seizures or psychosis)
- Hematologic disorder (hemolytic anemia, leukopenia, thrombocytopenia)
- Immunologic disorder (anti-ds DNA, anti-SM, and other ANAs)

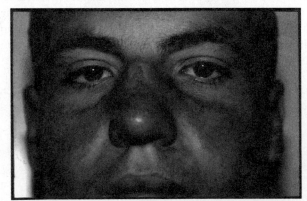

Copyright 2007 Gold Standard Multimedia Inc.

Figure 3-1. Malar Rash Associated with SLE

Summary of Criteria

- Arthritis is identical to that of RA except that it is non-erosive.

- Both the malar rash and photosensitivity rash (diffuse, maculopapular) flare with exposure to UV-B light (thus are considered photosensitive) and resolve with no scarring of the skin. The discoid lupus (DLE) is a circular rash with a raised rim that occurs over the scalp and face; it can be disfiguring because of central atrophy and scarring. Only 5% of patients with DLE will go on to develop SLE.

- All patients with renal involvement must undergo renal biopsy before treatment is initiated.

- Change of personality and psychosis may be manifestations of CNS lupus. Seizures, paralysis, and aphasia may follow.

- Libman-Sacks endocarditis is a noninfectious endocarditis that is occasionally seen in lupus patients.

Diagnosis

- A positive ANA supports the diagnosis but is not specific for SLE.
- Complement levels (C3, C4) are _____ in patients with active lupus.
- Elevated levels of ds-DNA antibodies are seen with active lupus.

Treatment. Since there is no cure for SLE, treatment is aimed at controlling symptoms. NSAIDs are used to treat arthritis and pleurisy. Corticosteroid creams are used to treat skin rashes. Antimalaria drugs (hydroxychloroquine) and oral corticosteroids may also be used for skin and arthritic symptoms. Cytotoxic drugs (azathioprine, cyclophosphamide) are used with severe symptoms (lupus nephritis, heart and lung involvement, hemolytic anemia, central nervous system involvement, etc.), along with corticosteroids. Mycophenolate is often used to treat lupus nephritis.

All patients should be advised to wear protective clothing, sunglasses, and sunscreen when in the sun. Belimumab is an inhibitor of B-cell activation. Belimumab is an IgG monoclonal antibody given intravenously to prevent B-cell activation.

Prognosis. The prognosis of patients with SLE has improved significantly in recent years with a 10-year survival rate >85%. People with severe involvement of the CNS, kidney, heart, and lungs have a worse prognosis in terms of overall survival and disability. Lupus nephritis is probably the most common cause overall of disability in patients with SLE.

Pregnancy and SLE

- Fertility rates are normal in patients with SLE, but spontaneous abortions and still-births are more common when compared with normal patients.

- One reason for the spontaneous abortions in these patients may be anti-phospholipid antibodies, which cause placental infarcts. This is treated with low-molecular weight heparin (LMWH) during pregnancy.

- It is unclear whether lupus worsens with pregnancy. In the case of a lupus flare during pregnancy, steroids may be used safely to suppress the disease.

- All pregnant patients with lupus need to be screened for SSA/anti-Ro antibodies. These antibodies cross the placenta and are passively transferred to the fetus, causing neonatal lupus and heart block.

DRUG-INDUCED LUPUS

Drug-induced lupus erythematosus is a side effect of use of certain medications. There are over 40 drugs that are implicated to cause drug-induced lupus, but the drugs most commonly associated are: hydralazine, isoniazid, procainamide, and quinidine. The most common symptoms are: arthritis, fatigue, fever, and rarely pleurisy. Acute onset SLE is usually not confused with drug-induced lupus, due to the lack of skin disease, kidney disease, and the milder symptoms seen in the latter. Also, photosensitivity, hair loss, and central nervous system disease are uncommon in drug-induced lupus.

Answer to question on previous page

decreased

Patients with drug-induced lupus develop ANAs, although those with drug-induced lupus related to quinidine often are ANA-negative. The ANAs in drug-induced lupus are autoantibodies that react with a histone-DNA complex, which is the major component of the nucleus (anti-histone antibodies).

Anti-histone antibody testing is a sensitive marker for the diagnosis of drug-induced lupus. Hydralazine is the exception, as only about one-third of patients will have positive anti-histone antibodies.

Once the suspected medication is stopped, symptoms resolve within one to two weeks. This confirms the diagnosis of drug-induced lupus with certainty.

SCLERODERMA

> A 36-year-old woman comes to you because of skin tightness and painful fingertips with exposure to cold for >1 year. The physical examination discloses a BP of 165/100 and diffuse shiny, thickened skin. The examination is otherwise normal. The laboratory tests reveal an elevated serum creatinine.

Definition. Systemic sclerosis (SSc) is a chronic multisystem disease characterized clinically by thickening of the skin caused by accumulation of connective tissue and by involvement of visceral organs (GI, lungs, kidneys).

Presentation. All patients have Raynaud phenomenon and skin thickening. The Raynaud phenomenon occurs because of vascular damage and diminished blood flow to the extremities.

GI features include esophageal dysmotility, hypomotility of the small intestine with bacterial overgrowth and malabsorption, and dilatation of the large intestine with formation of large diverticula.

Pulmonary features include pulmonary fibrosis with restrictive lung disease and cor pulmonale. Pulmonary involvement is now the leading cause of death in SSc.

Renal features include the scleroderma renal crisis in which malignant hypertension develops and causes acute renal failure. This was the most common cause of death but now is easily treated with angiotensin-converting enzyme (ACE) inhibitors.

The term "scleroderma renal crisis" has been used to characterize the renal involvement in scleroderma, in which malignant hypertension occurs over days to weeks and is associated with acute renal failure (rapid rise in creatinine and proteinuria). The ACE inhibitors (enalapril, lisinopril, etc.) have been effective in reducing the devastating consequences of renal crisis in patients where treatment is initiated before the onset of renal failure.

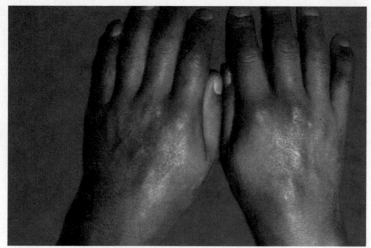

Copyright 2007 CMSP—Custom Medical Stock Photo.

Figure 3-2. Shiny Skin of Scleroderma

CREST syndrome, a variant of scleroderma, is now called limited scleroderma or limited cutaneous systemic sclerosis. The acronym CREST represents the hallmarks of the disease: **C**alcinosis, **R**aynaud, **E**sophageal dysfunction, **S**clerodactyly, and **T**elangiectasias. Calcinosis is a condition in which calcium deposits occur in soft tissues usually in the fingers (especially proximal inter-phalangeal joints), knees, and elbows. These deposits occur near the skin surface and may ulcerate and become infected. Sclerodactyly refers to skin thickening, primarily affecting the fingers and toes.

Patients with limited scleroderma generally have skin involvement that does not extend above the elbow or above the knee. Rarely in some patients, the face may be affected. Limited disease generally progresses slowly compared to the diffuse cutaneous form of scleroderma, which is more likely to affect internal organs, although pulmonary arterial hypertension may occur in 25–50% of persons with limited scleroderma. Interstitial lung disease may occur in 10% of this population.

In patients with limited scleroderma, the ANA test is positive, showing a pattern of anticentromere antibodies in up to 90% of patients. Antibodies to Scl-70 are usually negative in limited scleroderma and positive in diffuse scleroderma.

Raynaud phenomenon is defined as episodes of pallor or cyanosis in response to cold or emotional stimuli. The pallor is caused by vasoconstriction of blood vessels (arteries and arterioles) that results in reduced blood flow, while cyanosis is created by deoxygenation of slow-flowing blood. After rewarming the hands, the blood flow will rebound (hyperemia) and the skin will appear reddened or blushed.

It is common for patients with Raynaud phenomenon to complain of cold sensitivity and to have other areas of the skin involved, including the ears, nose, and lower extremities. Episodes come as sudden attacks and are most often triggered by rapid changes in ambient temperature. Attacks may begin in one or two fingers but typically involve all fingers and/or toes symmetrically and bilaterally.

Primary Raynaud phenomenon (Raynaud disease) denotes a patient without an associated underlying disease. Secondary Raynaud phenomenon is used to describe patients with a defined secondary or associated disease (e.g., scleroderma). One test that allows the differentiation between primary and secondary Raynaud is the nailfold capillaroscopy test (done by placing a

Note

Remember, CREST is now called limited scleroderma.

drop of oil on the patient's nailfold at the base of the fingernail). Examination of this area under a microscope is then conducted to look for any capillary changes. Enlarged, dilated, or absent nailfold capillaries are noted among patients with scleroderma and other autoimmune diseases.

About 5% of the general population has symptoms and signs consistent with Raynaud phenomenon. It is more common among young women, about 30% have a first-degree relative with Raynaud, and most have primary Raynaud phenomenon without any defined cause or associated systemic disease.

Treatment. There is no cure for SSc. For the skin manifestations, D-penicillamine may be used. For severe Raynaud phenomenon, use calcium-channel blockers, specifically nifedipine; for hypertension, angiotensin-converting enzyme inhibitors are the drugs of choice.

SJÖGREN SYNDROME

> A 42-year-old woman presents to your office with some peculiar symptoms lasting 1 year. She feels there is constantly something in her eyes—like dust or sand—and that dry and solid foods are painful to swallow. You are perplexed by her complaints but decide to examine her and find that she has bilateral parotid enlargement The exam is otherwise unremarkable. An ANA test is positive. What specific ANAs would you expect to be positive in this patient?

Definition. Sjögren syndrome is a chronic autoimmune disease characterized by lymphocytic infiltration of the exocrine glands, resulting in xerostomia and dry eyes. Sjögren may be seen alone (primary) or with other autoimmune diseases (secondary) such as RA, primary biliary cirrhosis, or SLE.

As Sjögren syndrome progresses, it becomes a systemic disease involving major organs (lungs, kidneys, etc.) and may eventually evolve into a lymphoproliferative disease—malignant lymphoma.

Presentation. Patients complain of itchy eyes, sandy feeling under their eyes (because of decreased lacrimal production and destruction of the corneal epithelium—keratoconjunctivitis sicca), and difficulty swallowing food.

Also look for increase in dental caries and parotid enlargement.

Diagnostic Tests. Schirmer's test will show decreased tear production, and the rose Bengal stain will document corneal ulcerations. ANAs will be positive and specifically anti-Ro (SSA) and anti-La (SSB).

Lymphocytic infiltration of the salivary glands will be noted on the biopsy.

Treatment. There is no cure for this disease. Symptomatic treatment includes artificial tears.

Pilocarpine and cevimeline increase acetylcholine and increase tear and saliva production.

All of the diseases we just reviewed have an arthritis that is symmetric and polyarticular. RA is a disease that involves mostly the joints; the others—SLE, SSc, and Sjögren syndrome—usually have arthritis plus multiple organ involvement.

For the rheum wizards: There are a few other diseases that may cause symmetrical polyarthropathy—know Parvovirus B19 and hepatitis B.

SERONEGATIVE ARTHROPATHIES, SPONDYLOARTHROPATHIES

A 27-year-old man presents with complaints of severe lower back stiffness and pain that have been bothering him for the past 5 years. The stiffness is most apparent in the morning when he wakes up, lasting sometimes >2 h. The only thing improving these problems is exercise. On examination he has a 2/6 murmur over the second right intercostal space and decreased range-of-motion of the lumbar spine.

Definition. The spondyloarthropathies are a group of disorders that share certain clinical features and an association with the B-27 allele. The similarities among these diseases suggest that these disorders share pathogenic mechanisms.

There are 4 diseases that have 4 similar clinical and laboratory characteristics:

Table 3-5. Seronegative Arthropathies

Diseases	Characteristics
Ankylosing spondylitis	• Seronegative (ANA negative, RF negative)
Reactive arthritis	• Involve lower back and sacroiliac joints
Psoriatic arthritis	• HLA-B27
Enteropathic arthropathy	• Extraarticular manifestations

All of the above diseases have most of the 4 characteristics plus a few others that are disease-specific.

Ankylosing Spondylitis

Definition. Ankylosing spondylitis (AS) is an inflammatory disorder of unknown etiology that affects primarily the axial skeleton and peripheral joints. AS usually starts by the second to third decade (very rare age >40).

Prevalence in men is 3–4 times that of women—this is one of the few collagen vascular diseases that affects men more than women. 90% of patients are positive for HLA B-27.

Presentation. AS will usually present with **chronic lower back pain** in a young man (in his late twenties to early thirties). The giveaway is the **morning stiffness** lasting at least **1 h** that **improves with exercise.**

The cervical spine is rarely if ever affected and only late in the disease.

Extraarticular manifestations are common in AS: anterior uveitis, aortic insufficiency sometimes leading to CHF and third-degree heart block.

On examination there will be evidence of decreased spine mobility: positive Schober test (measures spine flexion) and sometimes obliteration of the lumbar lordosis. Because of this, spine fractures are sometimes seen in patients with AS after minimal trauma (know that spine fractures occur with insignificant stress in older people with osteoporosis and young people with long-standing inflammatory disease of the spine, e.g., AS).

X-rays show evidence of sacroiliitis (this is the earliest finding) and eventual fusing of the sacroiliac joint. Chronic spine inflammation will eventually cause the bamboo spine and squaring of the vertebral bodies.

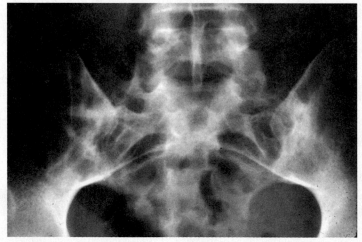

SIU BIOMED COMM 2007—Custom Medical Stock Photo.

Figure 3-3. X-ray of Pelvis in AS Demonstrating Sacroilitis

Diagnosis. The diagnosis of AS is based on clinical and x-ray findings. The HLA-B27 is not commonly used as a diagnostic test.

Treatment. NSAIDs, physical therapy, and exercise. The most promising medications used in the treatment of AS and other spondyloarthropathies are the TNF blockers (infliximab, adalimumab, etanercept). These biologic agents are recommended for axial disease.

Unlike RA, anti-TNF medications are used first and methotrexate used later. Anti-TNF drugs work better for axial disease.

Reactive Arthritis

Reactive arthritis (ReA) is a seronegative arthropathy that occurs as a complication from an infection somewhere in the body. There are 2 types of infection causing 2 different syndromes.

- One (Reiter syndrome) occurs after a nongonococcal urethritis (chlamydia, ureaplasma). These patients have distinct mucocutaneous manifestations: keratoderma blennorrhagica, circinate balanitis, oral or genital ulcers, conjunctivitis, and arthritis.

- The other ReA occurs after an infectious diarrhea caused by Campylobacter, Shigella, or Salmonella organisms (think of the organisms that cause enteroinvasive diarrheas; these are the same ones that cause ReA). The most common is Campylobacter.

Diagnosis is based on clinical criteria. X-ray findings will be consistent with a seronegative spondyloarthropathy.

Treatment. Treatment is the same as for AS. There are studies that support an accelerated recovery of Reiter syndrome caused by a chlamydial infection from prolonged tetracycline use (~3 weeks' duration). There are also studies to support the notion that prompt antibiotic use in urethritis will decrease the chance of Reiter syndrome (this is the only exception to the rule that the seronegative arthropathies are untreatable diseases).

A severe form of Reiter syndrome and reactive arthritis has been described in HIV patients. The skin manifestations are particularly aggressive in these patients and improve with antiretroviral medications.

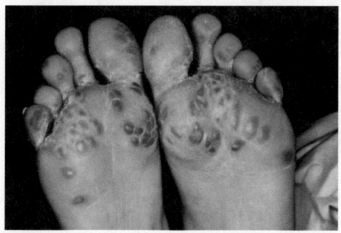

phil.cdc.gov.

Figure 3-4. Keratoderma Blenorrhagica Sometimes
Seen with Reiter Syndrome

Psoriatic Arthritis

Commonly involves the DIP joints when associated with psoriatic nail disease (pitting of the nails); this involvement may sometimes cause the characteristic sausage-shaped digit. Here, the peripheral arthritis is deforming.

Enteropathic Arthropathy

Occurs with ulcerative colitis and Crohn's disease; sometimes the arthritis occurs with flares of the inflammatory bowel disease. Patients sometimes develop characteristic skin lesions: pyoderma gangrenosum and erythema nodosum.

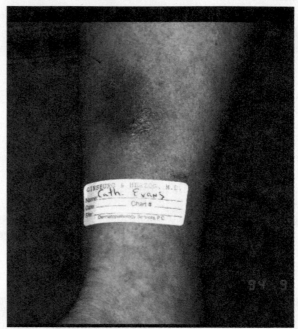

Gold Standard Multimedia Inc. 2007

Figure 3-5. Erythema Nodosum, Characteristic of Some Rheumatic Disorders

OSTEOARTHRITIS

A 64-year-old man comes to you for the evaluation of knee pain. He tells you that he has had right knee pain for many years but recently it has gotten worse. He denies constitutional symptoms and other joint pain except for his left second and third DIPs. He has not noticed stiffness in the morning. On examination you hear crepitations as you move his right knee, but otherwise there is no evidence of swelling, warmth, or erythema of the knee. Laboratory testing is unremarkable.

Definition. Osteoarthritis (OA) is the most common joint disease in humans. The target tissue in OA is articular cartilage. There is destruction of cartilage along with secondary remodeling and hypertrophy of the bone. OA, unlike RA, is not an inflammatory disease.

Knee OA is the leading cause of chronic disability in the elderly.

Major risk factors for OA include age, female sex, genetic factors, major joint trauma, repetitive stress, and obesity (the last 3 factors are potentially modifiable).

The classification involves stratification of OA into idiopathic—the most common form and where no predisposing factor is evident—and secondary, which is attributable to an underlying cause, e.g., other arthropathies (gout), endocrine diseases (diabetes mellitus, acromegaly), deposition diseases (hemochromatosis), and mechanical factors (valgus or varus deformity, unequal lower extremity length). (Remember that any disease that will cause stress or trauma to a joint may eventually cause secondary OA.) Secondary OA is pathologically indistinguishable from idiopathic OA.

The most common joint to be affected is the knee; the second most common joint affected is the base of the thumb.

Presentation. The major joints involved in OA are the weight-bearing joints (hip and knee) and the small joints of the fingers (PIPs and DIPs). These joints are affected in an oligoarticular-asymmetric or monoarticular pattern. The joint involvement is very slow, progressive, and irreversible. Because the cartilage fails and there is increased pressure on articular bone, joint pain increases with exercise and is relieved by rest. Morning stiffness is always <20–30 min. Crepitations may be noted with movement of the joint. There are no systemic manifestations in OA.

Laboratory Tests. These are always normal, especially indices of inflammation. Thus, ESR and C-reactive protein are always normal in OA. (Remember, if ESR is elevated, some other process is complicating OA, e.g., septic joint, or it's not OA.) X-ray findings include osteophytes and unequal joint space. Osteophytes (spurs) are the reparative efforts by the bone; when these occur in the PIPs they are called Bouchard's nodes, whereas similar changes occurring in the DIPs are called Heberden's nodes.

Diagnosis. Made on clinical and x-ray findings.

Treatment. Aimed at reducing pain and maintaining mobility, since there is no cure for OA.

Nonpharmacologic Measures. Reduction of joint loading can be achieved by correction of poor posture and weight loss. Physical therapy and exercise programs should be designed to maintain range of motion, strengthen periarticular muscles, and improve physical fitness.

Drug Therapy. Therapy is palliative because no agent has been shown to change the natural course of the disease. Although limited studies have claimed a chondroprotective effect of certain NSAIDs, well-done studies have not documented such an effect. NSAIDs should only be used to alleviate pain.

In double-blinded placebo trials, there was no difference in relief of joint pain among acetaminophen (4,000 mg/d), analgesic doses of ibuprofen (1,200 mg/d), and antiinflammatory doses of ibuprofen (2,400 mg/d). Although the first drug to use for pain in OA is acetaminophen, it is reasonable to add on analgesic doses of NSAIDs if there is no relief. Cautious dosing should be prescribed in elderly patients because they are at highest risk for the side effects associated with NSAIDs, especially GI (ulcers, hemorrhage, etc.). COX-2 inhibitors may be used in patients who are at high risk for GI complications (only available agent is celecoxib).

Another modality that has been shown to benefit patients with OA is the use of capsaicin cream, which depletes local sensory nerve endings of substance P. Some patients do feel local burning.

Orthopedic surgery and joint arthroplasty is reserved for cases in which aggressive medical treatment has been unsatisfactory, especially if the patient's quality of life has been decreased.

Note

There are rare cases of erosive OA, polyarticular OA, and OA with inflammatory features. These are exceptions, and you do *not* need to know them.

Intraarticular injection of hyaluronic acid has been approved for treatment of knee OA that hasn't responded to pharmacologic treatment. Despite this, the efficacy of hyaluronic acid has been questioned since a large clinical trial failed to demonstrate superiority over intraarticular injections of saline. Similarly glucosamine and chondroitin sulfate are not routinely used in the treatment of OA since in 4 recent randomized, double blind trials both of these agents were no more effective than placebo.

Also, clinical trial results based on analysis of x-rays suggested the possibility of glucosamine being chondroprotective. Since the radiologic methods employed in the trial were limited, there was concern about the interpretation of such data. A current multicenter trial sponsored by the National Institutes of Health is under way in order to address this question.

CRYSTAL-INDUCED ARTHROPATHIES

Definition. The crystal-induced arthropathies, monosodium urate (MSU), calcium pyrophosphate (CPPD), calcium oxalate (CaOx), and calcium hydroxyapatite (HA), are caused by microcrystal deposition in joints. In spite of differences in crystal morphology, they have identical clinical presentations and can only be distinguished by synovial fluid analysis.

Gout

Gout is a disease that affects middle-aged men and presents most commonly with acute monoarthritis (women represent only about 5–15% of all patients with gout; premenopausal women make up 17% of all women with gout). As gout becomes chronic, multiple joints may be involved, and deposition of urate crystals in connective tissue (tophi) and kidneys may occur.

The metatarsophalangeal joint of the first toe is commonly affected (podagra), but other joints like the knee, ankle, PIPs, or DIPs may be initially involved. The first episode commonly occurs at night with severe joint pain waking the patient from sleep. The joint rapidly becomes warm, red, and tender (it looks exactly like cellulitis). Without treatment the joint pain goes away spontaneously within 3–14 days.

Certain events that precipitate gout sometimes precede the attack: excessive alcohol ingestion, red meat intake, trauma, surgery, infection, steroid withdrawal, drugs (diuretics, such as HCTZ [hydrochlorothiazide] and furosemide; anti-TB medicines, such as pyrazinamide and ethambutol), and serious medical illnesses.

MSU deposition causes an intense inflammatory process—red, warm joint. Thus, on an x-ray of a joint that has been involved in multiple gouty attacks you would expect to find _____.

Diagnosis. The serum uric acid during the acute attack may be normal or low. On the other hand, many people have elevated serum uric acid levels and never develop gout. Thus, the serum uric acid level is of no value in the diagnosis of acute urate arthropathy. This is why the diagnosis is made by the analysis of synovial fluid.

On synovial fluid analysis, the MSU crystals are _____ birefringent and _____ shaped. The number of WBCs should be between _____.

Treatment

Acute gouty arthritis: The goal is to decrease inflammation and thus prevent erosions and joint destruction; also in this stage it is very important to avoid any fluctuations in serum uric acid levels.

- NSAIDs
- Steroids, oral, rarely intraarticular, in elderly patients who cannot tolerate NSAIDs or colchicine or in patients with renal impairment
- Colchicine is rarely to be used in acute gout but is still available.

Chronic hypouricemic therapy: The goal here is to decrease uric acid levels. This is usually required for life and initiated in patients who have had recurrent gouty attacks that cannot be corrected by low-purine diet, limitation of alcohol, avoiding diuretics, etc. Unlike acute gout, here the uric acid level may be helpful in following the effect of hypouricemic treatment.

- Allopurinol can be used in overproducers, undersecretors, or patients with renal failure or kidney stones
- Febuxostat is used in those intolerant of allopurinol.
- Pegloticase dissolves uric acid: used in refractory disease
- Probenecid can be used in the undersecretors (>80% of adults) only. Rarely used today.

A 32-year-old man comes with a history of right ankle swelling that occurred the night before. He has noticed that his ankle has been red, warm, and very painful. He occasionally drinks alcohol. On examination you find a red swollen ankle with evidence of an effusion. The range of motion is restricted.

What is the first step in this patient? *Aspiration*

What do we do after confirming the diagnosis? *Treat with NSAIDs*

Six months after the first episode he comes back to your office with left knee swelling. A red, warm knee is noted on examination.

What is the first step now? *Aspiration again*

What do you do after confirming the diagnosis? *NSAIDs*

On a routine visit the same patient has had 4 documented episodes of gout despite limiting alcohol and diet.

What would be the appropriate next step here? *Consider allopurinol or probenecid*

You have decided to place him on allopurinol. He does very well for more than 2 years with no gouty attacks. He then experiences another episode of right ankle swelling.

Note

Allopurinol should not be initiated during an acute crisis. However, if a patient has been taking allopurinol and an acute attack occurs, it should not be discontinued.

Clinical Pearl

Use primarily allopurinol in the chronic treatment of gout.

Answers to question on previous page

- erosive calcifications
- negative; needle; 5,000 and 50,000

Pseudogout

Definition and Pathogenesis. CPPD crystal deposition is more common in the elderly population and in people who have preexisting joint damage.

A small percentage of the patients have metabolic abnormalities that are associated with CPPD deposition (secondary). Remember the 4 Hs: hyperparathyroidism, hemochromatosis, hypophosphatemia, hypomagnesemia. The presence of pseudogout in a patient <50 years of age should raise suspicions about one of these metabolic abnormalities.

Clinical Manifestations. Pseudogout may have an acute presentation like gout. It may also present in an asymptomatic and chronic form. The knee is the most commonly affected joint; other joints commonly affected are the wrist, shoulder, and ankle.

Diagnosis. Definitive diagnosis requires the typical rectangular, rhomboid, positive birefringent crystals on synovial fluid evaluation.

Radiographs may reveal linear radiodense deposits in joint menisci or articular cartilage (chondrocalcinosis). (Do not forget to look at an x-ray of chondrocalcinosis before going to the exam.)

Treatment. The treatment is the same as gout. Prevention of frequent recurrences may be treated with low doses of colchicine.

SEPTIC ARTHRITIS

A 67-year-old woman with history of RA for many years presents with right shoulder pain and swelling for 2 days. She has low-grade fever. The examination reveals decreased passive and active range of motion of the right shoulder joint, as well as erythema. She asks you if this is related to an RA flare and if she should start steroids to decrease the pain.

What is the next step? *Do an arthrocentesis*

The most common cause of infectious arthritis is gonorrhea, and gonococcal arthritis accounts for 70% of episodes in patients age <40. Women are at greater risk during menses and pregnancy and are 2–3 times more likely than men to develop disseminated arthritis.

In older patients, *Staphylococcus aureus* is a common cause of infectious arthritis and occurs in patients with preexisting joint destruction from other rheumatic diseases. Patients with RA have the highest risk because of chronic inflamed or destroyed joints, steroid therapy, and frequent skin breakdown over deformed joints.

Acute bacterial infection may cause rapid cartilage destruction, and thus a patient presenting with monoarticular arthritis needs prompt diagnosis. This is done by arthrocentesis. Further, *Staph* or Strep must be cleaned out of the joint space by arthocentesis or arthroscopy.

Remember that most infected joints with gonococcal will not have positive cultures, and the Gram stain will be negative.

Treatment. Treatment should focus on the likely etiology. For example, a 30-year-old woman with acute monoarticular arthritis who is found to have >50,000 WBCs in the synovial fluid without crystals should be treated with ceftriaxone. A 72-year-old man with RA with the same findings should be treated with nafcillin or vancomycin.

This disease is discussed further in the Infectious Diseases chapter.

VASCULITIS SYNDROMES

Definition. Vasculitis is an inflammatory process involving the blood vessels that results in decrease of the lumen diameter and eventual ischemia of the tissues supplied.

The vasculitis syndromes are stratified according to the types of vessels involved.

Wegener Granulomatosis

Wegener granulomatosis is a small vessel vasculitis that can involve any organ system but mainly affects the respiratory tract (sinuses, nose, trachea, and lungs) and kidneys.

The most common sign of Wegener granulomatosis is involvement of the upper respiratory tract, which occurs in nearly all patients. Symptoms include rhinitis, sinusitis, and, rarely, nasal ulcers. A common sign of the disease is chronic rhinitis that does not respond to usual treatment and that becomes increasingly worse.

The lungs are affected in most people despite lack of symptoms. If symptoms are present, they include cough, hemoptysis, and dyspnea. Kidney involvement occurs in >80% of people with this disorder and is a major cause of morbidity and mortality. Arthritis occurs in about 60% of the cases.

Patients with Wegener granulomatosis usually have the presence of antineutrophil cytoplasmic antibodies (C-ANCA). Although a positive ANCA test is useful to support a suspected diagnosis of Wegener granulomatosis, it is never diagnostic. Also, the C-ANCA test may be negative in some people with active Wegener. The only way to confirm the diagnosis is by performing a biopsy of an involved organ (usually the nasal septum), which demonstrates the presence of vasculitis and granulomas.

The standard treatment consists of a combination of a glucocorticoid and an immunosuppressive agent (cyclophosphamide). In a study of 158 patients who were treated with prednisone and cyclophosphamide at the National Institutes of Health (NIH), 90% markedly improved; after years of follow-up, 80% of the patients survived.

Polyarteritis Nodosa (PAN)

PAN is a multisystem disease that may present with nonspecific complaints such as fever, malaise, weight loss, anorexia, and abdominal pain. The disease can affect nearly any site in the body, except the lungs. It has a predisposition for organs such as the skin, kidney, nerves, and GI tract. Peripheral neuropathies are very common (70%). This includes tingling, numbness, and/or pain in the hands, arms, feet, and legs, and mononeuritis (e.g., foot drop). GI manifestations are also common, such as abdominal pain and GI bleeding (occasionally is mistaken for inflammatory bowel disease). A minority of patients with PAN have an active hepatitis B infection.

The diagnosis is made by biopsy of involved organs, taken more commonly from skin, symptomatic nerves, or muscles. The diagnosis is confirmed by a biopsy showing pathologic changes

Clinical Pearl

In patients with PAN, exclude co-existing chronic active viral hepatitis.

in medium-size arteries. An angiogram of the abdominal vessels may also be very helpful in diagnosing PAN since aneurysms affecting the arteries of the kidneys and/or GI tract are found.

Before the availability of effective therapy, untreated PAN was usually fatal within weeks to months. Most deaths occurred as a result of kidney failure, or heart or GI complications. Effective treatment is now available for PAN and consists of high doses of corticosteroids, along with immunosuppressive drugs (cyclophosphamide).

Churg-Strauss Syndrome

This syndrome shares many of the clinical and pathologic features of PAN and can involve any organ. The cardinal manifestations of Churg-Strauss syndrome are asthma, eosinophilia, and lung involvement (for the sake of remembering this syndrome, you may consider this Churg-Strauss as PAN in an asthmatic patient). The typical patient with Churg-Strauss is a middle-aged individual with new-onset asthma. Asthma symptoms may begin long before the onset of vasculitis. Other symptoms include: mononeuropathy (mononeuritis multiplex similar to PAN), transient pulmonary infiltrates on chest x-rays, paranasal sinus abnormalities, nasal polyps, and allergic rhinitis.

Diagnosis is made by biopsy and treatment is similar to PAN (combination of prednisone and cytotoxic agent).

PAN and Churg-Strauss syndrome both involve the small- and medium-sized arteries.

Temporal Arteritis (TA)

TA, also known as giant cell arteritis, is a vasculitis affecting the large arteries that supply the head, eyes, and optic nerves. New-onset headache in any patient age >50 prompts consideration of this diagnosis, which if left untreated may result in permanent vision loss.

The most common symptoms of giant cell arteritis are headache and pain that usually occurs in one or both temples. Other common symptoms include scalp tenderness (pain when combing hair), jaw claudication (jaw pain when chewing), decreased vision or blurry vision, tongue numbness, or, rarely, sudden loss of vision. Sometimes the patient may have proximal stiffness (neck, arms, hips) due to polymyalgia rheumatica, a coexisting condition with TA. Over 25% of patients with TA also have polymyalgia rheumatica.

The erythrocyte sedimentation test (ESR) is the first test to do in patients suspected to have TA. Since the ESR is always increased in TA, all patients will have an elevated ESR (100% sensitive). The diagnosis is always confirmed by biopsy of the temporal arteries in which the characteristic giant cells are demonstrated. In the patient whom you suspect to have TA, if the ESR is elevated, corticosteroids should be started immediately, before the temporal artery biopsy is performed. Do not withhold treatment waiting for the biopsy to be done.

Clinical Pearl

Always consider TA in patients with new-onset headache who are age >50–60.

> A 72-year-old woman comes to you because she has been bothered by a right-sided headache for the past 4 weeks. She has never had migraine headaches and denies blurry vision, nausea, or vomiting. The headache does not get worse any specific time of the day. She has noticed a feverish feeling and hip stiffness along with the headache.

What is the first step? *Do an ESR; if elevated, start prednisone*

INFLAMMATORY MYOPATHIES

A 42-year-old woman is admitted to your service with severe proximal weakness for 2 months. Her examination shows a diffuse lilac rash over the sun-exposed areas. The motor strength is 3/5 in the upper and lower proximal muscle groups.

Definition. The inflammatory myopathies are inflammatory muscle diseases that present with progressive muscle weakness. They include polymyositis, dermatomyositis, and inclusion body myositis.

Clinical Findings. Patients report difficulty with tasks that involve the proximal muscles: lifting objects, combing hair, getting up from the chair, etc. Fine-motor tasks that involve the distal muscles, e.g., writing, are only affected late in the disease. Ocular muscles are never involved; this feature differentiates the inflammatory myopathies from myasthenia gravis and Eaton-Lambert syndrome.

Dermatomyositis will also have skin involvement; the heliotrope rash is a purple-lilac discoloration of the face, eyelids, and sun-exposed areas of the body. Gottron's papules are the scaly lesions seen sometimes over the knuckles.

Laboratory Findings. The inflammatory destruction of muscles causes an elevation of the muscle enzymes (sometimes up to 50-fold), creatine phosphokinase (CPK), and aldolase. These are the most sensitive tests to perform in patients suspected of inflammatory myopathies.

Autoantibodies (anti-Jo-1) occur in patients with inflammatory myopathies, which supports the possible autoimmune origin of these diseases.

Diagnosis. Electromyography shows evidence of myopathic potentials characterized by short-duration, low-amplitude units. Diagnosis is confirmed by muscle biopsy.

Treatment. Steroids are useful in polymyositis and dermatomyositis. Inclusion body myositis is resistant to immunosuppressive therapy.

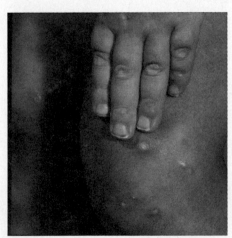

Courtesy of Dr. Muhammad Al-Lozi,
Washington University Dept. of Neurology.

Figure 3-6. Gottron's Papules, a Feature of Dermatomyositis

Gastroenterology 4

DISEASES OF THE ESOPHAGUS

The majority of diseases of the esophagus result in dysphagia. Dysphagia refers specifically to difficulty swallowing. Only a few of the diseases of the esophagus result in pain on swallowing, called odynophagia. Both dysphagia and odynophagia will result in weight loss if the symptoms persist for more than a few days. The mere presence of dysphagia or odynophagia is not sufficient to help one establish a diagnosis. The basic questions are, What additional information has to be added to this presentation to sufficiently answer the question, and, Which of the following is the most likely diagnosis?

In general, a barium swallow or barium esophagram is a good answer to questions asking for the best initial test. This is not an absolute answer, however, and if there are clear signs of obstruction, then the answer could also be upper endoscopy as the best initial test.

Achalasia

A 32-year-old woman with no past medical history comes to your office for the evaluation of "difficulty swallowing" foods. She has had this problem for almost a year, and it is most difficult for her to eat solids. Her symptoms have not worsened at all over this time period, and her weight has been stable. Physical examination is unremarkable. What is the next step in evaluation?

Pathogenesis. Achalasia is the idiopathic loss of the normal neural structure of the lower esophageal sphincter (LES). The LES is usually contracted to prevent the acidic gastric contents from refluxing backward into the esophagus. For swallowing to occur, there is normally a relaxation process of the LES in order to allow food to pass into the stomach. Inhibitory neurons are stimulated, blocking the impulses that cause constriction. In achalasia, these inhibitory neurons have been lost, as well as the ability to relax the LES. The vast majority of cases are of unknown etiology. A very small number can be from Chagas disease, gastric carcinoma, or diseases that can infiltrate into the area, such as lymphoma.

Clinical Presentation. Achalasia presents with progressive dysphagia to both solids and liquids simultaneously and can have regurgitation several hours after eating. There can also be weight loss. Achalasia has no relationship with alcohol or tobacco use. This is different from esophageal cancer, which not only usually presents with dysphagia to solid foods that progresses to difficulty swallowing liquids, but also is more common in older patients with a long history of alcohol and tobacco use.

Diagnosis. Esophagogastroduodenoscopy (EGD) is done for alarm symptoms: onset after age 60, anemia, heme-positive stools, >6-month duration of symptoms, and weight loss. Although a chest x-ray may show an air-fluid level in the dilated esophagus, plain radiography is insufficiently accurate to be very useful. Barium esophagography is very accurate and shows dilation of the esophagus, which narrows into a "bird's beak" at the distal end. The most accurate test overall (gold standard) is esophageal manometry. Manometry shows increased lower esophageal (LES) resting pressure.

Treatment. The best initial therapy is with pneumatic dilation or surgery. Pneumatic dilation should be effective in 80 to 85% of patients. The procedure gives a 3–5% risk of perforation. Botulinum toxin injections into the LES are used in those patients not willing to undergo pneumatic dilation, or in whom it has failed. Although the *botulinum* toxin is relatively benign, the main limiting factor in its use is a need for additional injections in a few months. Fifty percent will relapse in 6 to 9 months, and all patients will need reinjection after 2 years. Botulinum toxin is also used in patients who are poor surgical candidates, e.g., the elderly with multiple comorbid conditions who would not tolerate surgery. If both pneumatic dilation and *botulinum* toxin injections fail, then surgical myotomy is performed. Myotomy is performed laparoscopically and results in reflux in 20% of patients as a complication of therapy.

Esophageal Cancer

A 62-year-old man comes for evaluation of progressive "difficulty swallowing solids and, recently, semisolids" for 4 months. He has noticed a 20-lb weight loss. His past medical history is significant for reflux esophagitis for 15 years and a 40-pack-year smoking history. On the physical examination, a 1.5-cm, left supraclavicular lymph node is found. The remainder of the physical examination is unremarkable.

Pathogenesis. Esophageal cancer is linked to the synergistic, carcinogenic effect of alcohol and tobacco use for cases of squamous cell cancer in the proximal two-thirds of the esophagus. Adenocarcinoma is found in the distal third of the esophagus and is associated with long-standing gastroesophageal reflux disease and Barrett esophagus. The rate of development of cancer from Barrett esophagus is between 0.4 and 0.8% per year. Squamous and adenocarcinoma are now of equal frequency.

Clinical Presentation. Esophageal cancer presents with progressive dysphagia first for solid food, then for liquids. Weight loss is prominent. Rarely, halitosis, regurgitation, and hoarseness occur. Hypercalcemia may arise, as it can with most cancers.

Diagnosis. Although a barium swallow can be done first, endoscopy is mandatory because this is a diagnosis that requires a tissue biopsy. CT scanning detects the degree of local spread, and bronchoscopy detects asymptomatic spread into the bronchi. Endoscopic U/S is performed for staging.

Treatment. The only truly effective therapy for esophageal carcinoma is surgical resection if the disease is sufficiently localized to the esophagus. Only 25% of patients are found to be operable. Five-year survival is 5–20%. Chemotherapy with a 5-fluorouracil-based chemotherapy is combined with radiation to control locally metastatic disease.

Scleroderma (Progressive Systemic Sclerosis)

Pathogenesis. As many as 80 to 90% of patients with scleroderma will develop diminished esophageal peristalsis from the atrophy and fibrosis of the esophageal smooth muscle.

Clinical Presentation. Although there is dysphagia, the main clue to the diagnosis is simply the presence of gastroesophageal reflux symptoms in a person with a history of scleroderma. The LES will neither contract nor relax and basically assumes the role of an immobile open tube.

Diagnosis. Barium studies are generally unnecessary. The most accurate diagnostic test is motility studies.

Treatment. Therapy is with proton-pump inhibitors, such as omeprazole. Metoclopramide is a promotility agent that has some modest efficacy.

Diffuse Esophageal Spasm and Nutcracker Esophagus

A 34-year-old man complains of "crushing" chest discomfort for 1 hour. He has no significant medical history. The ECG is normal. He is given sublingual nitroglycerin in the emergency room that improves his chest pain almost immediately.

Pathogenesis. Esophageal spastic disorders are idiopathic abnormalities of the neural processes of the esophagus. Fundamentally, diffuse esophageal spasm and nutcracker esophagus are the same disease. The only difference may be in the manometric pattern.

Clinical Presentation. These patients present with intermittent chest pain and dysphagia. The pain can simulate that of a myocardial infarction, but it bears no relationship with exertion. There is no relationship with eating, ruling out odynophagia. The pain can be precipitated by drinking cold liquids.

Diagnosis. Barium studies may show a "corkscrew"' pattern at the time of the spasm. The most accurate test is manometric studies, which will show high-intensity, disorganized contractions. Because the contractions are disorganized, they do not lead to the forward flow of food and peristalsis.

Treatment is with calcium-channel blockers, such as nifedipine, and nitrates.

Rings and Webs

Pathogenesis. Schatzki's ring and Plummer-Vinson syndrome reveal thin, epithelial membranes made out of squamous epithelial cells. Neither of them is progressive in nature, distinguishing both of these conditions from achalasia.

Schatzki's ring is more common and leads to intermittent dysphagia and is not associated with pain. It is also more distal and located at the squamocolumnar junction proximal to the lower esophageal sphincter.

Plummer-Vinson syndrome (PVS) is more proximal and is located in the hypopharynx. The dysphagia is sometimes with liquids as well. Plummer-Vinson syndrome is associated with iron-deficiency anemia and squamous cell cancer; it most often occurs in middle-aged women.

Diagnosis. Both disorders are best diagnosed with a barium swallow or barium esophagram.

Treatment. Plummer-Vinson syndrome may respond to treatment of the iron deficiency. Both are treated with dilation procedures.

Esophagitis

Pathogenesis. Esophagitis refers to either infection or inflammation of the esophagus. The most common infection is from *Candida albicans*. When *Candida* esophagitis occurs, it is almost exclusively in patients who are HIV positive with a CD4 count <200/mm^3, usually even <100/mm^3. Diabetes mellitus is the second most common risk for developing *Candida* esophagitis. Much rarer infectious etiologies of esophagitis are herpes simplex, cytomegalovirus, and aphthous ulcers. Medications and the ingestion of caustic substances are associated with the development of esophagitis. Alendronate and other bisphosphonates are most common.

Clinical Presentation. *Candida* esophagitis presents with progressive odynophagia. Although the swallowing is painful, food is still able to pass until the disease is extremely advanced. The major difference between the pain of esophagitis and the pain of spastic disorders is that in esophagitis, the pain is only on swallowing, whereas with spastic disorders the pain occurs intermittently without even needing to swallow. Esophagitis pain is simply from the mechanical rubbing of food against an inflamed esophagus as it passes by.

Diagnosis and Treatment. If the patient is HIV positive, the diagnosis is confirmed simply by seeing a response to empiric treatment with fluconazole. If the fluconazole doesn't work, then endoscopy should be performed.

Because esophagitis can also result from ingestion of medications and caustic substances, the direct effect of contact between the mucosa and the pill causes inflammation rather than infection. As with most other toxin-mediated damage to an organ, the diagnosis is based on the presentation and finding the toxin in the history. The most common pills that cause esophagitis are alendronate, quinine, risedronate, vitamin C, potassium chloride, doxycycline, NSAIDs, and iron sulfate. Pill esophagitis is managed by simply swallowing pills in the upright position and drinking enough water to flush them into the stomach. Consider pill esophagitis in a young patient who is taking medications for acne with the acute onset of odynophagia.

Zenker Diverticulum

> A 25-year-old medical student comes to seek your help because he thinks he "has bad breath." This past weekend, a most disturbing event occurred while he was watching a football game: He coughed up the chicken teriyaki he ate 2 days earlier. He claims to brush his teeth every night. The physical examination is normal. What is the next step in the evaluation of this patient?

Pathogenesis. Zenker diverticulum is the outpocketing of the posterior pharyngeal constrictor muscles at the back of the pharynx.

Clinical Presentation. This is generally a very slowly developing problem that occurs in older patients. These patients have bad breath and difficulty initiating swallowing because it is such a proximal lesion. Patients also complain of having to repeatedly clear their throats and waking up with undigested, regurgitated food on their pillow. This is particularly unpleasant because the food was usually eaten several days ago.

Diagnosis. The diagnosis is made on barium studies.

Treatment. Endoscopy and the placement of nasogastric tubes are contraindicated because of the risk of developing perforation of the pharynx. Patients with Zenker diverticulum are treated with surgical resection.

Mallory-Weiss Syndrome

Pathogenesis. Mallory-Weiss syndrome is a nontransmural tear of the lower esophagus that is related to repeated episodes of retching and vomiting.

Clinical Presentation. Although Mallory-Weiss syndrome is an esophageal disorder, the presentation is markedly different from the other problems described above. Mallory-Weiss does not present with dysphagia or odynophagia. It presents with painless upper GI bleeding. Patients develop black stool from melena if the volume of bleeding is >100 mL or with hematemesis if there is continued vomiting.

Diagnosis. These patients are diagnosed by direct visualization on upper endoscopy.

Treatment. Most of the time, Mallory-Weiss tears require no direct therapy and will resolve spontaneously. Sometimes, injection of the tear with epinephrine or performing cauterization is necessary.

EPIGASTRIC PAIN

Pathogenesis. There is no definite way to determine the etiology of epigastric discomfort or pain simply by examining the history in the majority of cases. Epigastric pain can be from ulcer disease, pancreatitis, gastroesophageal reflux disease (GERD), gastritis, and, occasionally, gastric cancer. *Helicobacter pylori* is most strongly associated with the development of duodenal ulcers, gastric ulcers, and gastritis.

Pancreatitis is the most common reason for epigastric *tenderness* and pain. Ulcer disease is associated with epigastric tenderness in <20% of patients.

Despite these diagnostic possibilities, the most common etiology of epigastric pain is, in fact, never truly determined. This is referred to as nonulcer dyspepsia, a functional disorder in which there is persistent pain in the epigastric area and all the tests are found to be normal.

Diagnosis. The hardest question is when to perform endoscopy, which is often required for a definitive diagnosis. Barium studies of the stomach, such as the upper GI series, are always less accurate than is endoscopy for problems in the stomach.

Endoscopy is indispensable in the diagnosis of cancer. Essentially, one performs endoscopy to exclude gastric cancer, as well as to determine whether a person is developing dysplasia in their lower esophagus as a result of long-standing reflux or Barrett esophagus.

H. pylori can be diagnosed with noninvasive means, such as serology, urea breath testing, and stool antigen detection. Endoscopy is not needed to determine who has *Helicobacter*, although biopsy and histology are the single most accurate tests. Make sure the patient is off proton-pump inhibitors (PPI)/Abx for 1–2 weeks prior to the test (can give false negative). *H. pylori* ELISA is not affected by PPIs. When testing for eradication, do not use ELISA. Use breath test or stool antigen.

All patients with epigastric pain and alarm symptoms, such as weight loss, dysphagia, odynophagia, or heme-positive stool, should undergo endoscopy. In addition, endoscopy is recommended for those age >45–55, essentially to exclude gastric cancer. Endoscopy is also indicated in those whose symptoms have not resolved with the use of antisecretory therapy, such as PPIs, or histamine 2 (H_2)–receptor blockers, such as ranitidine or cimetidine. H_2 blockers are only effective in two-thirds of patients.

Note

All patients with epigastric pain should generally undergo endoscopy, except for those age <45–55 with no alarm symptoms, such as bleeding, weight loss, or difficulty swallowing.

Note

There is no point in treating *Helicobacter pylori* without evidence of disease, such as gastritis or ulcer disease.

Treatment. Although endoscopy is the most accurate means of diagnosing an ulcer, one can empirically treat ulcers, reflux disease, and gastritis. Patients who do not have duodenal or gastric ulcers or gastritis should not be treated for *H. pylori*. Young, generally healthy patients can be treated empirically with H_2 blockers, liquid antacids, or PPIs, and then undergo endoscopy in the future if there is no improvement.

Gastroesophageal Reflux Disease

A 32-year-old man comes to the emergency department for substernal chest pain of 2 hours' duration. He says that he sometimes gets this pain while lying in bed at night. He is otherwise free of symptoms, except for a nonproductive cough that he has had for the past month or so. His physical examination is unremarkable. His ECG is normal. He is given sublingual nitroglycerin and notes that his chest discomfort is worsened.

Pathogenesis. Gastroesophageal reflux disease, or GERD, is caused by the abnormal flow of the acid gastric contents backward from the stomach up into the esophagus. The lower esophageal sphincter (LES) is not a true anatomic sphincter; you can't find it in a cadaver. The LES is created by the different response of the smooth muscle cells in the distal esophagus.

A number of factors can cause decreased tone or loosening of this sphincter, such as nicotine, alcohol, caffeine, peppermint, chocolate, and anticholinergics. We also know that calcium-channel blocking agents and nitrates also lower the sphincter pressure. When the tone of the LES decreases, acid is more likely to reflux backward into the esophagus, particularly when the patient is lying flat. GERD can still occur in the absence of these precipitating factors and can often simply be idiopathic in origin.

Clinical Presentation. Dyspepsia or epigastric pain can be caused by GERD, ulcer disease, pancreatitis, gastritis, and nonulcer dyspepsia. GERD can be differentiated from the others by the presence of a sore throat; a bad, metal-like taste in the mouth; hoarseness; and cough and wheezing. In addition, GERD is the one most likely to be associated with pain in the substernal area.

Diagnosis. Specific diagnostic testing is not necessary when the patient's symptoms are those described in the clinical presentation. In clear cases of epigastric pain going under the sternum and associated with a respiratory complaint or a bad taste in the mouth, therapy should be initiated immediately with antisecretory medications, such as proton-pump inhibitors (PPIs). The most accurate diagnostic test is a 24-hour pH monitor, but this is only necessary when the patient's presentation is equivocal in nature and the diagnosis is not clear. An electrode is placed several centimeters above the gastroesophageal junction, and a determination is made of what the average pH is in that area. Normal endoscopy does not exclude reflux disease.

Treatment. Therapy for GERD is primarily with PPIs, all of which are essentially equal in efficacy. Omeprazole, esomeprazole, lansoprazole, pantoprazole, and rabeprazole will all reliably increase the pH of the gastric contents to a level above 4.0. Do motility studies prior to surgery to avoid iatrogenic dysphagia.

A small number of persons, usually <5%, will not respond to PPIs and will need to undergo surgery to tighten the sphincter. Traditionally, this has been a Nissen fundoplication, which is done laparoscopically. Another method is simply placing a circular purse-string suture in the LES to tighten it.

H$_2$ blockers should only be used if the patient has very mild, intermittent symptoms. H$_2$ blockers are not as effective as PPIs. Prokinetic drugs, such as metoclopramide, have an equal efficacy to H$_2$ blockers and less than that of PPIs, and they are rarely used.

All patients should modify their lifestyle to diminish the frequency of GERD symptoms. This means avoiding nicotine, alcohol, caffeine, chocolate, and late-night meals. It also means elevating the head of the bed 6 to 8 inches with blocks to use gravity to help keep the acid in the stomach.

Indication for surgery:
- Refractory side effects with PPIs, e.g., headaches, diarrhea
- No response to PPIs

Barrett Esophagus

Pathogenesis. Barrett esophagus is a complication of long-standing reflux disease. After several years of GERD, the epithelium of the lower esophagus undergoes histologic change from a normal squamous epithelium to a columnar epithelium.

Diagnosis. Patients with Barrett esophagus should have a repeat endoscopy every 2 to 3 years to see whether dysplasia or esophageal cancer has developed. Patients with low-grade dysplasia should undergo repeat endoscopy in 3 to 6 months to see if the lesion has progressed or resolved. Patients with high-grade dysplasia should have a distal esophagectomy or an endoscopic mucosal resection because of its very high rate of progression to invasive esophageal carcinoma. The usual rate of progression to cancer is about 0.5% per year.

Barium studies are typically normal. Endoscopy should be performed if the patient has GERD and if there are alarm symptoms, such as dysphagia, odynophagia, weight loss, anemia, or heme-positive stool. It is not clear when endoscopy should be done when there is a history only of GERD.

Treatment. All patients with Barrett esophagus should receive PPIs.

Peptic Ulcer Disease

Peptic ulcer disease is the term applied to both duodenal ulcers and gastric ulcers. The term is the archaeologic remnant of a misnomer from the early part of the 20th century, in which it was mistakenly believed that the enzyme pepsin caused ulcer disease.

Etiology. Tobacco smoking, alcohol, and the use of steroids by themselves do *not* cause ulcer disease. Tobacco and alcohol use can delay healing and are associated with the development of gastritis, but they do not cause ulcers. The strongest causal relationship for the development of ulcers is the use of NSAIDs, *Helicobacter pylori* infection, cancer of the stomach, Zollinger-Ellison syndrome, Crohn's disease, burns, head trauma, and prolonged intubation and mechanical ventilation.

NSAIDs lead to ulcer formation because they decrease the normal production of the mucous barrier that protects the epithelial cells of the gastric mucosa. Prostaglandins, the major stimulant for mucous production that forms this protective barrier, are inhibited by NSAIDs and hence diminish the protective barrier of the stomach lining. The presumptive mechanism of the formation of stress ulcers from burns and head trauma is that there is an intense vasoconstriction of the vasculature that supplies the gastric mucosa, leading to the sloughing of these cells and ulceration. Steroid use by itself does not lead to peptic ulcer disease and is therefore not a routine indication for stress ulcer prophylaxis.

Parietal cells in the stomach produce acid. The 3 stimulants to the production of acid from the parietal cells are gastrin, acetylcholine, and histamine. Gastrin is produced by G cells in the stomach, and its release is stimulated by distention of the stomach, the presence of amino acids, and vagal stimulation. Vagal stimulation also releases acetylcholine and gastrin-releasing peptide. However, the single most important stimulant to gastrin release is distention of the stomach.

Histamine is released by enterochromaffin-like cells present in the same glandular elements of the stomach that have the parietal and chief cells. Chief cells release pepsinogen, which is converted to pepsin by the acid environment of the gastric lumen. Histamine directly stimulates the parietal cells to both release acid and potentiate the effects of acetylcholine and gastrin on the parietal cells. This is why H_2 blockers such as cimetidine, famotidine, and ranitidine inhibit acid release.

Zollinger-Ellison syndrome is the excessive production and release of gastrin from G cells. Somatostatin is the counterbalance to this system. Somatostatin inhibits the release of gastrin and histamine, as well as having a direct inhibitory effect on the production of acid from the parietal cells. Secretin is released from the S cells of the duodenal lining. The main stimulant to the release of secretin is the presence of acid in the duodenum. Secretin inhibits the production of gastrin, as well as stimulates pancreatic and biliary bicarbonate production and release.

The most common cause of ulcer disease is *Helicobacter pylori* followed by the use of NSAIDs; 80–90% of duodenal ulcers and 70–80% of gastric ulcers are associated with *H. pylori*. Overall, 10–20% of ulcers are idiopathic, and no clear etiology is ever identified.

Clinical Presentation. The most common presentation of ulcer disease is midepigastric pain. There is no definite way to distinguish between duodenal and gastric ulcers simply by symptoms. The only way to be certain is with endoscopy or, occasionally, radiographic studies with barium, such as an upper GI series. Traditionally, gastric ulcers have been associated with pain on eating, and duodenal ulcers were thought to be relieved by eating. Because gastric ulcers were thought to be associated with pain on eating, this more frequently led to weight loss. This description is only a rough approximation, and it is still necessary to perform endoscopy if a definite diagnosis is required.

Tenderness of the abdomen is unusual with ulcer disease. More than 80% are not associated with abdominal tenderness in the absence of a perforation. Nausea and vomiting are occasionally found with both of them.

Diagnosis. Ulcer disease is best diagnosed with upper endoscopy. Barium studies are inferior. In generally healthy patients age <45–55 with epigastric pain, endoscopy can be deferred in favor of a trial of H_2 blockers or proton-pump inhibitors (PPIs). If the symptoms persist, then endoscopy can be performed. In those age >45–55 or those with alarm symptoms (weight loss, anemia, heme-positive stools, or dysphagia), endoscopy should be performed.

The diagnosis of *H. pylori* is based on either serology, urea breath testing, stool antigen testing, or biopsy with histology. Knowing which diagnostic test to perform first for *Helicobacter* is not definitively clear. Serology is the least expensive, is the least invasive, and has a very high degree of sensitivity. This means a negative test for the *Helicobacter* antibody effectively excludes this agent as an etiology of the ulcer disease. The drawback to serology is that it does not reliably distinguish between old disease and new disease and therefore lacks specificity.

In addition, neither serology nor breath testing nor stool antigen tests can exclude the presence of gastric cancer. The advantage of both breath testing and stool antigen detection methods is that they have the same sensitivity as serology and are able to easily distinguish new versus old disease. When *H. pylori* has been treated, both the breath and stool tests readily become negative. This means they can be used to evaluate eradication of the organism post treatment and can test for cure of the infection.

Biopsy with histology is the most sensitive and specific test. Further, it can exclude cancer. Four percent of patients with gastric ulcer disease have cancer. In addition, there is a rapid test on the biopsy, known as a CLO test, that can exclude *Helicobacter*. The CLO is performed to see if the organisms present in the biopsy specimen can produce urease, demonstrating the presence of the bacterium.

Treatment. The treatment of ulcer disease centers largely on the treatment of *H. pylori*. Use a PPI combined with clarithromycin and amoxicillin. Omeprazole, lansoprazole, pantoprazole, rabeprazole, and esomeprazole are all equal in efficacy.

The other 2 choices of antibiotic are tetracycline and metronidazole. Bismuth subsalicylate is not necessary. Regimens that contain PPIs are superior to those that use H_2 blockers, such as ranitidine or cimetidine. The PPI/clarithromycin/amoxicillin regimen should be effective in >90% of patients. Duration of therapy is 10 to 14 days, but sometimes the PPI is continued for a few months in order to heal the gastric mucosa. Repeat endoscopy is essential after treatment for gastric ulcer. The only way to be sure there is no cancer is to document resolution of the ulcer.

In those who fail therapy, a urea breath test should be performed to see if the reason for failure was the inability to eradicate the organism. If the organism was not eradicated, then re-treatment should occur with different antibiotics and the addition of bismuth subsalicylate. In addition, sensitivity testing for the organism should be explored. If the organism was eradicated and the ulcer persists, recurs, or worsens, the patient may need evaluation for Zollinger-Ellison syndrome.

Ordinary ulcers not related to *Helicobacter* can be treated with PPIs alone. Misoprostol is a prostaglandin analog that was developed to prevent the development of NSAID-induced ulcers. It is rarely used because it is not very effective. Cyclooxygenase 1 (COX-1) is the enzyme that produces the prostaglandins that protect the gastric mucosa. COX-2 is the enzyme implicated in the development of pain. COX-2 inhibitors were developed to relieve pain without damaging the gastric lining as much as NSAIDs. COX-2 inhibitors have no effect on platelets.

Indications for surgery in PUD:

- UGI bleeding not amenable to endoscopic procedures
- Perforation
- Refractory ulcers
- Gastric outlet obstruction → can change endoscopic dilation

Gastritis

Etiology. Gastritis is the term applied to describe inflammation, erosion, or damage of the gastric lining that has not developed into an ulcer. Unlike ulcer disease, gastritis can be caused by alcohol, as well as NSAIDs, *Helicobacter*, head trauma, burns, and mechanical ventilation. The type of gastritis from these factors is referred to as type B, which is by far the most common type of gastritis. It is also associated with increased gastric acid production.

Type A gastritis is from atrophy of the gastric mucosa and is associated with autoimmune processes, such as vitamin B_{12} deficiency. Type A is also linked to diminished gastric acid production and achlorhydria. All patients with achlorhydria will have markedly elevated gastrin levels because acid inhibits gastrin release from G cells. MALT (mucosal-associated lymphoid tissue) leads to metaplasia as well as possible dysplasia and then to gastric cancer.

Note

Gastric ulcers must be biopsied to exclude cancer.

Clinical Presentation. Most patients with gastritis present with asymptomatic bleeding. When the gastritis is severe and erosive, patients will have abdominal pain in the same area that patients with ulcer disease feel theirs. Nausea and vomiting may also occur. The bleeding can present either as hematemesis or melena.

Diagnosis and Treatment. The diagnosis and treatment of *Helicobacter* is the same as that for gastritis (described for ulcer disease above). Vitamin B_{12} deficiency and pernicious anemia are initially diagnosed with a low vitamin B_{12} level and an increased methylmalonic acid level. The diagnosis of pernicious anemia is confirmed by the presence of antiparietal cell antibodies and anti-intrinsic factor antibodies. It is treated with B_{12} replacement, as are all cases of vitamin B_{12} deficiency.

Zollinger-Ellison Syndrome

A 42-year-old woman comes to your office with complaints of diarrhea for 6 months. She has stopped all dairy products but there has been no improvement. There is no blood or pus with the stools. She takes maximum doses of omeprazole daily, along with famotidine, and still has ulcer symptoms. She has a mild hypercalcemia. What is the next step in the evaluation of this patient?

Etiology. Zollinger-Ellison syndrome (ZES) is hypergastrinemia caused by cancer of the gastrin-producing cells. There is no known cause for gastrinoma or ZES. Half of these gastrinomas are located in the duodenum, and a quarter are located in the pancreas. A small percentage (<20%) are associated with multiple endocrine neoplasia type 1 (MEN-1) or parathyroid, pituitary, and pancreatic tumors.

Note

The presence of hypercalcemia is the clue to detecting MEN-1. This is because of the hyperparathyroidism.

Clinical Presentation. More than 95% of patients with ZES present with ulcer disease. Less than 1% of people with ulcer disease has an underlying ZES or gastrinoma. How will you recognize the nature of the case in which you should test for gastrin levels to exclude a gastrinoma? ZES presents with ulcers that are recurrent after therapy, multiple in number, and occur in the distal portion of the duodenum or resistant to routine therapy. Routine peptic ulcers usually are <1 cm in size, occur within 2 to 3 cm of the pylorus, are single, and promptly resolve after therapy for *Helicobacter pylori*. Diarrhea occurs in two-thirds of patients. This can be ordinary watery diarrhea, or it can be steatorrhea. Steatorrhea occurs because lipase is inactivated by the large volume of acid passed into the duodenum. Diarrhea may precede the ulcer in 20% of patients. Metastatic disease is evident at the time of diagnosis in 30% of patients at presentation. An additional 20% of patients later develop metastatic disease.

Diagnosis. Although an elevated gastrin level is indicative of ZES, it is critical to remember that all patients on H_2 blockers or PPIs have high gastrin levels. This is because the main stimulus to the suppression of gastrin release is acid. If acid production is suppressed, then gastrin levels go up. To diagnose ZES, the gastrin level must be found elevated while the patient is off antisecretory therapy for several days. Another way to diagnose ZES is to find an elevated gastric acid output while concurrently finding an elevated gastrin level. The secretin stimulation test is positive (abnormal) if there is a rise in gastrin level after the injection of secretin. Normally, secretin should suppress gastrin release. Other causes of increased gastrin are:

- Pernicious anemia
- Chronic gastritis
- Renal failure
- Hyperthyroidism

After confirming a diagnosis of gastrinoma, the most important step is to determine if the lesion is localized or metastatic. Localized lesions can be surgically removed and essentially cured. Metastatic disease can only be suppressed with the use of PPIs. U/S, CT scanning, and MRI have between 60 and 80% sensitivity for the presence of metastatic disease. These tests are specific enough to prove the presence of tumor if they are positive, but not sensitive enough to safely exclude disease if they are negative. A nuclear test, somatostatin-receptor scintigraphy, is 90% sensitive for the detection of metastatic disease. The single most sensitive test is the endoscopic U/S. Typically, both tests are done.

Treatment. Localized disease is surgically resected and metastatic disease is treated with the long-term administration of PPIs simply to block acid production.

Gastroparesis

Pathogenesis. Gastroparesis literally means the presence of a weak stomach. The most common association for gastroparesis is diabetes. Electrolyte problems with potassium, magnesium, and calcium can also weaken the musculature of the bowel wall.

Clinical Presentation. Patients present with early satiety, postprandial nausea, and a general sense of increased abdominal fullness. This is from decreased motility of the stomach and the accumulation of food there. Gastroparesis generally occurs in those presenting with abdominal pain and bloating and who have a long-standing history of diabetes, along with retinopathy, neuropathy, nephropathy, and history of poor glycemic control.

Diagnosis. Although a gastric-emptying study can be done with the ingestion of radioisotope-labeled food, this is rarely necessary. The diagnosis of diabetic gastroparesis is generally obvious as the cause of bloating, vomiting, and nausea in a long-term diabetic after endoscopy excludes other diseases.

Treatment. The treatment of gastroparesis is with agents that will increase motility of the stomach, such as erythromycin or metoclopramide. Erythromycin increases motilin levels.

Dumping Syndrome

Pathogenesis. This is an increasingly rare disorder because of the rarity of the necessity for surgery in the treatment of ulcer disease. It was far more common in the past, when vagotomy and gastric resection were performed to treat severe ulcer disease.

Dumping syndrome is caused by two phenomena. First, there is the rapid release of hypertonic chyme into the duodenum, which acts as an osmotic draw into the duodenum, causing intravascular volume depletion. Next, there is a sudden peak in glucose levels in the blood because of the rapid release of food into the small intestine. This is followed by the rapid release of insulin in response to this high glucose level, which then causes hypoglycemia to develop.

Clinical Presentation. Patients present with sweating, shaking, palpitations, and lightheadedness shortly after a meal.

Treatment. There is no cure for dumping syndrome. The management is to eat multiple, small meals.

Nonulcer Dyspepsia

When all the causes of epigastric pain have been excluded and there is still pain, the diagnosis is functional or nonulcer dyspepsia. There is no specific therapy for nonulcer dyspepsia known to cure the disorder. Antacids of various types from H_2 blockers to liquid antacids to PPIs are tried until something is found to relieve the discomfort. The cause of nonulcer dyspepsia is unknown.

Treatment of *Helicobacter pylori* in nonulcer dyspepsia is of equivocal value. If there is no response to anti-secretory therapy with a PPI, you can try to treat *H. Pylori* by adding clarithromycin and amoxicillin. Treating *H. Pylori* will improve symptoms in another 10–20% of patients.

INFLAMMATORY BOWEL DISEASE

Inflammatory bowel disease (IBD) is a term comprising 2 disease entities: Crohn's disease (CD) and ulcerative colitis (UC). They can be discussed simultaneously because of the large degree of overlap in terms of presentation, testing, and treatment.

- Both CD and UC are idiopathic disorders of the bowel associated with diarrhea, bleeding, weight loss, fever, and abdominal pain.
- Both are most accurately diagnosed with endoscopy and sometimes with barium studies, "string sign" on small bowel follow through after barium meal in CD.
- Both are treated with anti-inflammatory medications, such as mesalamine, azathioprine, and 6-mercaptopurine (6MP).
- Steroids are used for acute exacerbations of both diseases.

Clinical Presentation. IBD presents with fever, diarrhea, weight loss, and, occasionally, abdominal pain and bleeding. The extraintestinal manifestations of IBD are episcleritis, scleritis and iritis, sclerosing cholangitis, joint pains, and skin manifestations, such as pyoderma gangrenosum or erythema nodosum.

Crohn's disease is more likely to be associated with a palpable abdominal mass because CD has granulomas in the bowel wall that are transmural in nature. This can lead to the different loops of bowel being inflamed and sticking together, forming a mass. The abdominal masses of CD can be palpated and cause pain. CD is not necessarily continuous, and one hallmark of the disorder is that there are "skip lesions," or areas of normal tissue in between the areas of disease.

UC is limited exclusively to the large bowel. It is exclusively a mucosal disease, and although it can cause bleeding, it does not result in fistula formation. UC has no skip lesions, no fistula formation, and no oral or perianal involvement. UC is more likely to cause bloody diarrhea.

Both forms of IBD can lead to colon cancer after 8–10 years of involvement of the colon. If the CD does not result in colonic involvement, then it will not lead to cancer. Complications of Crohn's disease are calcium oxalate kidney stones, diarrhea, and cholesterol gallstones.

Diagnosis. IBD is diagnosed with endoscopy and sometimes with barium studies. (CD can result in deficiency of vitamin B_{12}, calcium, vitamin K, and iron because of malabsorption.) Anti–*Saccharomyces cerevisiae* antibodies (ASCA) are associated with CD, and antineutrophil cytoplasmic antibody (ANCA) is associated with UC. If a patient is ASCA positive and ANCA negative, he has a >90% chance of having CD. If the patient is ASCA negative and ANCA positive, he has a >90% chance of having UC.

Prothrombin time may be prolonged in CD because of vitamin K malabsorption. Kidney stones form more often in CD because the fat malabsorption results in a low calcium level and an increased absorption of oxalate, which forms kidney stones.

Note

Sclerosing cholangitis does not correlate to disease activity.

Treatment. Mesalamine derivatives are the mainstay of therapy for IBD in all of its forms. Pentasa is a form of mesalamine released in both the upper and lower bowel; hence, it is used in CD. Asacol is a form of mesalamine released in the large bowel, and it is most useful for UC. Rowasa is used exclusively for rectal disease. Sulfasalazine was used in the past for the same effect. The difficulty with sulfasalazine is that the high load of sulfa delivered causes a number of adverse effects, such as rash, hemolysis, and allergic interstitial nephritis. Sulfasalazine also causes reversible infertility in men and leukopenia by its sulfapyridine group.

Acute exacerbations of IBD are treated with high-dose steroids. Budesonide is a form of steroid that is ideal for IBD. It has a strong local effect when used orally, but is largely cleared by the liver in a first-pass effect. This limits the amount of systemic toxicity. Azathioprine and 6-mercaptopurine are associated with drug-induced pancreatitis, but are still used on a long-term basis to try to keep patients off steroids. Ciprofloxacin and metronidazole are used for CD in those with perianal disease. Infliximab is used for CD in those who form fistulae or have disease refractory to the other forms of therapy. There has been re-activation of tuberculosis with infliximab, and it is important to test for latent tuberculosis with a purified protein derivative (PPD) prior to treatment. If the PPD is positive, then patients should receive isoniazid. The most common side effect of infliximab is arthralgias. Balsalazide and olsalazine are other forms of mesalamine that are only active in the colon and are used occasionally.

Surgery is curative in UC; almost 60% of patients will require surgery within 5 years after diagnosis due to refractory symptoms or severe disease. Surgery is not very effective in CD and disease tends to reoccur at the site of anastomosis.

DIARRHEA

Definition. Diarrhea is either an increased frequency or volume of stool per day; stool can also be defined as diarrhea if the number of stools per day is few, but their consistency is watery.

Pathogenesis. The most common causes of diarrhea are of an infectious, antibiotic-associated, or lactose-intolerance etiology or from irritable bowel or carcinoid syndrome.

Clinical Presentation. The patient is often hypotensive, febrile, and experiencing abdominal pain.

Diagnosis. The first thing to do in the evaluation of diarrhea in terms of direct patient care is to see if there is hypovolemia as defined as hypotension or orthostasis. This is more important than determining the specific etiology because of the chance that the patient may die while waiting for the results to come back.

Treatment. No matter the etiology, if the patient is hypotensive, febrile, and having abdominal pain, he or she should be admitted to the hospital and given IV fluids and antibiotics. The presence of blood in the stool is especially serious and is probably the single strongest indication for the use of antibiotics, such as ciprofloxacin.

Infectious Diarrhea

For all patients, assume that new-onset diarrhea has an infectious etiology. After an infectious cause is excluded, then the other possible causes can be systematically ruled out.

In general, to exclude infection, stool should be evaluated for the presence of white cells or "fecal leukocytes," as well as culture and ova and parasite examination. *Clostridium difficile* toxin and stool *Giardia*-antigen testing are done when there are clues to these diagnoses in the history.

The most common causes of infectious diarrhea are *Campylobacter* and *Salmonella*, especially in patients with sickle cell and achlorhydria. One can only make a definitive determination of the etiology with a stool culture.

Note

As initial steps in management for diarrhea, determining when to admit the patient and when to use IV fluids and antibiotics are more important than determining the precise causative agent.

Clinical presentation

Table 4-1. Clues to the Diagnosis of Infectious Diarrhea Prior to Results of Culture

Causative Agent	Patient Symptoms or History	Additional Comments
Bacillus cereus	Ingestion of refried Chinese food and the spores from *Bacillus* that it contains. Vomiting is prominent. Blood is never present.	Short incubation period (1–6 hours)
Campylobacter	Reactive arthritis, Guillain-Barré syndrome	Most common cause of bacterial gastroenteritis
Cryptosporidia, Isospora	Found in HIV-positive patients with <100/mm³ CD4 cells	—
E. coli 0157:H7	Associated with the ingestion of contaminated hamburger meat. The organism can release a Shiga toxin, provoking hemolytic uremic syndrome.	Hemolytic uremic syndrome happens when the organism dies; that is why antibiotics are contraindicated. Platelet transfusions are also contraindicated, even if the platelet count is low because the new platelets may only make it worse.
Giardia	The ingestion of unfiltered water, as on a camping trip or in the mountains, or in drinking fresh lake water. *Giardia* never gives blood in the stool. There is abdominal fullness, bloating, and gas.	*Giardia* can also simulate celiac disease in terms of causing fat and vitamin malabsorption if it is not eradicated.
Salmonella	Ingestion of chicken and eggs, dairy products	—
Scombroid	Patients who ingest contaminated fish experience vomiting, diarrhea, flushing, and wheezing within minutes of eating it.	Organisms invade, producing and then releasing histamine into the flesh of fish, such as tuna, mahi mahi, and mackerel.
Shigella, Yersinia	No clues strong enough to point to the etiology until the results of the stool culture are known.	*Yersinia* can mimic appendicitis. Also common in people with iron overload, e.g., hemochromatosis.
Vibrio parahaemolyticus	Ingestion of raw shellfish, such as mussels, oysters, and clams	Typically presents as severe systemic gastroenteritis in patients with underlying disease (esp. chronic liver disease)
Vibrio vulnificus	Also in raw shellfish, but has a particularly high incidence in people with underlying liver disease or disorders of iron metabolism. Also associated with the development of skin bullae.	Typically presents as severe systemic gastroenteritis in patients with underlying disease (esp. chronic liver disease)
Viral	Children in day-care centers; the absence of blood and white cells	No systemic manifestation
Staphylococcus aureus	Ingestion of dairy products, eggs, salads. Upper GI symptoms (nausea/vomiting) predominate; rarely diarrhea.	Short incubation period (1–6 hours)
Ciguatera-toxin	2–6 hours after ingestion of large reef fish (grouper, red snapper, and barracuda). Also neurological symptoms → paresthesia, weakness, and reversal of heat and cold.	—

Diagnosis. Stool for fecal leukocytes is the most useful test that can be done immediately. Fecal leukocytes are only found when there has been invasion of the intestinal mucosa, as in dysentery, which is a bacterial infection of the bowel, producing diarrhea and bloody stool.

Invasive organisms need 24 to 36 hours to produce their effect and never give blood in the stool within the first few hours of their ingestion. (The only exception is the protozoan *Entamoeba histolytica*, which can give blood or white cells in stools.) The invasive organisms are *Salmonella, Shigella, Campylobacter, Vibrio parahaemolyticus, Yersinia, Escherichia coli,* and *Vibrio vulnificus* (think people drinking sea water). The most definitive test for these bacterial organisms is a stool culture.

Cryptosporidiosis is diagnosed with a unique test, a modified acid-fast test. The routine ova and parasite examination does not reliably detect cryptosporidiosis.

Giardia is best diagnosed with an ELISA stool antigen test. A single stool antigen test has 90% sensitivity. Three stool ova and parasite examinations have only 80% sensitivity.

Treatment. Most cases of food poisoning and infectious diarrhea will resolve spontaneously and will not need specific antimicrobial therapy. Even when they cause severe disease, as defined by high-volume stools with dehydration, antibiotics generally do not help. Antibiotics are used if there is abdominal pain, blood in the stool, and fever. The decision to use antibiotics is always made prior to knowing the result of the stool culture, so the treatment is always empiric and then modified when the culture results are known. The best empiric therapy for infectious diarrhea is ciprofloxacin or the other fluoroquinolones ± metronidazole.

Scombroid poisoning is treated with antihistamines, such as diphenhydramine. *Giardia* is still treated primarily with metronidazole. A newer agent for *Giardia* is tinidazole, which is effective in a single dose. Cryptosporidiosis is treated with nitazoxanide, although it has limited efficacy. The truly effective therapy for cryptosporidiosis is to raise the CD4 count to >100/mm^3 with antiretrovirals. Nitazoxanide is superior to paromomycin for cryptosporidium.

There is no specific therapy for viral diarrhea. Patients are managed with fluid and electrolyte support until the infection resolves.

Antibiotic-Associated Diarrhea

Pathogenesis. Any antibiotic can lead to diarrhea with *C. difficile*, although clindamycin may have one of the highest frequencies of association.

Clinical Presentation and Diagnosis. If a patient develops diarrhea several days to weeks after using antibiotics, he or she should be evaluated with a stool toxin test for *C. difficile*. The diarrhea may even develop after the use of the antibiotic has stopped.

Treatment. Metronidazole is the drug of choice. If the symptoms resolve and the patient has a recurrence, then he or she should be retreated with metronidazole. Oral vancomycin is only to be used in the very occasional case that does not resolve with metronidazole and there is no response to therapy. IV metronidazole can be used to treat *C. difficile* colitis if the patient is unable to use oral medications. This is not true of vancomycin. IV vancomycin will have no effect in the bowel because it does not pass the bowel wall. Oral vancomycin will have no systemic effect because it also does not pass the bowel wall. Fidaxomicin is not more effective than vancomycin or metronidazole for the first episode. Fidaxomicin seems to decrease the number of episodes of recurrent *C. difficile* colitis.

Note

- TMP/SMX for *Isopora*
- Doxycycline for *Vibrio vulnificus*
- Rifaximin for travelers' diarrhea

Note

Prophylactic antibiotics for traveler's diarrhea is never a correct approach.

Clinical Pearl

Don't confuse diarrhea caused by antibiotics which increase GI motility (e.g., erythromycin) with *C. difficile*-associated diarrhea.

Lactose Intolerance

Pathogenesis. Lactose intolerance is perhaps the single most common potential cause of diarrhea because of the enormously high prevalence of lactase deficiency. This is a disorder so common that the testing and treatment are generally empiric.

Clinical Presentation. The diarrhea produced is associated with gas and bloating, but never has blood or leukocytes in it. Despite the malabsorption of lactose, weight loss does not occur.

Diagnosis and Treatment. A precise diagnosis can be established by finding an increased stool osmolality and increased osmolar gap. The osmolar gap means that the difference between the osmolality measure in the stool and the osmolality calculated from the sodium and potassium levels is >50 mOsm/kg. In other words, the measured stool osmolality is greater than would be expected just by the level of sodium and potassium. The extra osmoles are from lactose. Other causes of an increased stool osmolar gap are magnesium and polyethylene glycol in the stool, also nutrient malabsorption → pancreatic insufficiency, celiac sprue, and bacterial overgrowth.

The routine way to diagnose lactose intolerance is simply to remove milk, cheese, ice cream, and all other dairy products (except yogurt) from the diet and observe for resolution of symptoms, which should occur within 24 to 36 hours. (This is quite different from celiac disease, in which resolution of diarrheal symptoms make take weeks after stopping the ingestion of gluten-containing foods.)

If resolution of symptoms does occur within 24 to 36 hours, then dietary changes are the best therapy. The patient can use lactase supplements.

Irritable Bowel Syndrome

Pathogenesis. Although it is often described at the same time as diarrheal illnesses, irritable bowel syndrome (IBS) is predominantly a pain syndrome of unknown etiology. IBS is an idiopathic disorder in which there is increased frequency of the normal peristaltic and segmentation contractions of the bowel. Pain is often relieved by a bowel movement.

Clinical Presentation. Twenty percent of patients with IBS have constipation only. A large number have diarrhea alone or diarrhea alternating with constipation. Everyone has pain.

No nocturnal symptoms. The majority are women with history of childhood abuse.

Diagnosis. There is no specific diagnostic test for IBS. The physician must first exclude lactose intolerance, inflammatory bowel disease, celiac disease, carcinoid, *Giardia* infection, and anatomic defects of the bowel as the cause.

The diagnostic criteria, called Rome criteria, must occur for at least 3 months:
- Pain relieved by a bowel movement or by a change in bowel habit (e.g., when you develop diarrhea, the pain goes away)
- Fewer symptoms at night
- Diarrhea alternating with constipation

No constitutional signs or symptoms, such as fever, weight loss, anorexia, or anemia.

Treatment. There is no clear definitive therapy for IBS. All patients should be placed on a high-fiber diet in an attempt to increase the bulk of the stool. Those with diarrhea-predominant disease should receive antidiarrheal agents, such as loperamide or diphenoxylate.

Antispasmodic agents are used on a trial-and-error basis until the most effective agent is found. Examples of antispasmodics are hyoscyamine, dicyclomine, and the belladonna alkaloids. The presumptive mechanism of these agents is that they will relax the bowel wall musculature and diminish the pain.

Resistant cases may respond to tricyclic antidepressants. The presumptive mechanism is that the tricyclics are anticholinergic and will relax the bowel. There is also a high frequency of depression in many of these patients, and it is assumed that the tricyclics have an analgesic effect with neuropathic pain.

A newer agent is tegaserod, which is used in constipation-predominant IBS. The major complication of therapy with tegaserod is diarrhea. Another newer agent is alosetron. Alosetron is used in diarrhea-predominant IBS, and it slows motility. Both of these agents work by manipulating serotonin levels in the bowel.

Carcinoid Syndrome

Pathogenesis. Carcinoid syndrome describes tumors of the neuroendocrine system. They are most often located in the appendix and the ileum. Bronchial carcinoids are rare but are highly symptomatic because the serotonin produced from a bronchial carcinoid does not get detoxified in the liver and is released directly into the circulation. With the exception of bronchial carcinoid, carcinoid syndrome by definition implies metastatic disease. Until there is an enormous tumor burden, the liver is able to neutralize all of the serotonin released by the carcinoid in the bowel. This usually does not happen until the metabolic capacity of the liver has been overwhelmed by metastatic disease.

Clinical Presentation. The presentation of carcinoid syndrome is with diarrhea, flushing, tachycardia, and hypotension. A rash may develop from niacin deficiency, which is a direct result of the carcinoid. Serotonin and niacin are both produced from tryptophan. If there is an overproduction of serotonin, it produces a tryptophan deficiency, which leads to a deficiency of niacin. Endocardial fibrosis also occurs because of a constant exposure of the right side of the heart to the serotonin. This leads to tricuspid insufficiency and pulmonic stenosis.

Diagnosis. The diagnosis is confirmed with a urinary 5-hydroxyindolacetic acid level (5-HIAA).

Treatment. Therapy is generally based on controlling the diarrhea with octreotide, which is a somatostatin analog. Very few carcinoids are sufficiently localized to be amenable to surgical resection. If a tumor does happen to be localized, then it should be resected. This is most often possible with bronchial carcinoid. Surgery is also used to relieve obstruction of the bowel.

MALABSORPTION SYNDROMES

Pathogenesis. The major causes of fat malabsorption are celiac disease and chronic pancreatitis, although tropical sprue and Whipple disease are extremely rare but possible causes. What they all have in common is the production of diarrhea characterized as greasy, oily, floating, and fatty, with a particularly foul smell, as if fat were fermenting. This type of diarrhea with fat is referred to as steatorrhea.

All malabsorption syndromes are characterized by weight loss because fat has the highest caloric content of all the foods. In addition, there is malabsorption of the fat-soluble vitamins A, D, E, and K. This can lead to hypocalcemia and easy bruising, as well as prolongation of the prothrombin time.

Iron malabsorption occurs if there is involvement of the duodenum where iron is normally absorbed. Macrocytic anemia results from folate being malabsorbed. Vitamin B_{12} malabsorption is from damage or loss of the mucosal surface of the terminal ileum.

Clinical Presentation. The most common presentation of celiac disease is iron deficiency anemia. The only unique feature of celiac disease is dermatitis herpetiformis. This is a vesicular skin rash on the extensor surfaces of the body seen in approximately 10% of patients. Even without dermatitis herpetiformis, celiac disease is the most likely etiology of fat malabsorption because it is the most common.

Patients with chronic pancreatitis will give a history of repeated episodes of pancreatitis from alcohol or gallstones. Tropical sprue is suspected when there is a history of being in a tropical country. Whipple disease is by far the rarest. In addition to the usual presentation of a fat malabsorption, Whipple disease is characterized by dementia (10%), arthralgias (80%), and ophthalmoplegia.

Diagnosis. Celiac disease is first diagnosed by testing for the presence of antiendomysial and antitransglutaminase antigliadin antibodies. The most accurate test is a small bowel biopsy, which shows flattening of villi. Even if the antibody tests confirm the diagnosis of celiac disease, the bowel biopsy should be done anyway to exclude small bowel lymphoma. And because there is very little that is unique about tropical sprue, it is yet another reason to always do a small bowel biopsy.

Just removing gluten (wheat, rye, and oats) from the diet is not a very accurate way of establishing the diagnosis because the circulating antibodies will continue to be present for weeks after stopping the ingestion of gluten.

Chronic pancreatitis is diagnosed from the history of repeated episodes of pancreatitis and is confirmed by finding calcification of the pancreas on x-ray and CT scan. The most accurate test, although rarely done, is a secretin test, or finding a low trypsin level. Secretin normally causes a voluminous release of bicarbonate and other pancreatic enzymes into the duodenum. If you place a nasogastric tube into the duodenum and inject secretin into the blood, the pancreas will not release bicarbonate or enzymes into the duodenum in a patient with chronic pancreatitis.

D-xylose testing was performed in the past to help distinguish between celiac disease and chronic pancreatitis. D-xylose is a monosaccharide that requires no digestion to be absorbed. If there is no absorption of D-xylose, it means there is a bowel-wall abnormality. D-xylose was absorbed and excreted in chronic pancreatitis, but not in celiac disease, Whipple disease, or tropical sprue, in which there is a bowel-wall abnormality. Antibody testing has largely replaced D-xylose testing. In addition, the presence of the deficiency of iron, folate, and carotene also point to a mucosal defect because they do not need pancreatic enzymes to be absorbed. Vitamin B_{12} is malabsorbed in pancreatic insufficiency and celiac disease. Pancreatic enzymes are necessary to absorb B_{12}. Vitamin K and calcium are malabsorbed because of fat malabsorption.

Tropical sprue and Whipple's disease are diagnosed by finding organisms on a bowel-wall biopsy. The single most sensitive test for Whipple's disease is a polymerase chain reaction (PCR) of the bowel biopsy. A positive *Tropheryma Whippelii* biopsy shows foamy macrophages that are PAS positive.

Treatment. Celiac disease is managed by adhering to a gluten-free diet (no wheat, oats, rye, or barley). Chronic pancreatitis can be managed by orally replacing all the deficient enzymes. Amylase, lipase, and trypsin can all be taken in a single combination pill. Tropical sprue is treated with trimethoprim/sulfamethoxazole or doxycycline for 6 months. Whipple's disease is also treated with trimethoprim/sulfamethoxazole or doxycycline, but it can also be treated with ceftriaxone for 1 year.

DIVERTICULAR DISEASE

Diverticulosis

Pathogenesis. Diverticulosis is so common in older populations in the Western world as to almost be considered simply a normal part of aging rather than a disease. Diverticulosis is presumably caused by a lack of fiber in the diet to give bulk to stool. There is a subsequent rise in intracolonic pressure, leading to outpocketing of the colon. It is prevalent in 50% of persons age >50, with even higher rates in older populations.

Clinical Presentation. Most of the time, these patients are asymptomatic. When they have symptoms, it is of left lower quadrant abdominal pain that can be colicky in nature.

Diagnosis. Diverticulosis is diagnosed with colonoscopy. Endoscopy is superior to barium studies, particularly when bleeding is present. Diverticula are more common on the left in the sigmoid, but bleeding occurs more often from diverticula on the right because of thinner mucosa and more fragile blood vessels. When bleeding occurs from diverticula, it is painless.

Treatment. Diverticulosis by itself is managed only with increasing fiber in the diet with products like Metamucil®, dietary fiber in bran, or bulking agents, such as psyllium husks.

Diverticulitis

Pathogenesis. Diverticulitis is from an infection occurring in one of the diverticula. This occurs more frequently when there is a blockage of the diverticular entrance in the colon from nuts or corn.

Clinical Presentation. Diverticulitis is distinguished from uninfected diverticula by the presence of fever, tenderness, more intense pain, and an elevation of the white blood cell count in the blood.

Diagnosis. Diverticulitis is confirmed by CT scanning. Barium studies and endoscopy are relatively contraindicated in diverticulitis because there is a slightly higher risk of causing perforation. There is no risk of perforation with CT scan.

Treatment. Diverticulitis is treated with antibiotics such as ciprofloxacin and metronidazole. The other choices are ampicillin/sulbactam, piperacillin/tazobactam, or the combination of cefotetan or cefoxitin with gentamicin. Mild disease can be treated with oral antibiotics, such as amoxicillin/clavulanic acid (Augmentin®).

CONSTIPATION

> A 72-year-old woman has a history of upper GI tract bleeding and iron-deficiency anemia, for which she has recently been started on oral ferrous sulfate iron replacement. She also has a history of diabetes with peripheral neuropathy, for which she is on amitriptyline. She has untreated hypothyroidism, but is treated for hypertension with nifedipine. Currently, she has constipation, and when the stool does pass, it is very dark in color, almost black.

Pathogenesis. The most common cause of constipation is generally a lack of dietary fiber and insufficient fluid intake. Calcium-channel blockers, oral ferrous sulfate, hypothyroidism, opiate analgesics, and medications with anticholinergic effects, such as the tricyclic antidepressants, all cause constipation. In the case of the patient described above, the most likely cause of the constipation is the ferrous sulfate.

Clinical Presentation. As written in the case, this patient's stool is dark. This only occurs with bleeding, bismuth subsalicylate ingestion, and iron replacement. However, GI bleeding gives diarrhea and not constipation because blood acts as a cathartic. Blood causes diarrhea, and iron tablets cause constipation.

Treatment. In constipation, the general management is to stop medications that cause constipation and then to make sure the patient is well hydrated. Bulking agents, such as those used to manage diverticular diseases, are also very helpful. Drug treatment of constipation includes milk of magnesia, cascara, bisacodyl, and docusate (Colace®). Enemas can be used for acute and serious constipation. Lactulose and polyethylene glycol (GoLYTELY®) can also be very effective.

COLON CANCER

Pathogenesis. The lifetime risk of colon cancer is >6%. Most cases occur sporadically, which is to say there is no clearly identified etiology. Diets that are high in red meat and fat lead to an increased risk for colon cancer, and smoking also increases the risk for colon cancer.

Clinical Presentation. Patients present with heme-positive, brown stool and chronic anemia when the cancer is in the right side of the colon. Left-sided lesions and cancer of the sigmoid colon are more often associated with symptoms of obstruction and with narrowing of stool caliber. This is because the right side of the colon is wider, and the stool is more liquid in that part of the bowel, making obstruction less likely on the right. Endocarditis by *Streptococcus bovis* and *Clostridium septicum* is often associated with **colon cancer**. Any patient presenting with endocarditis due to one of these organisms requires a GI work-up.

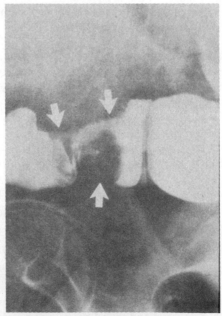

Courtesy of Dr. Conrad Fischer

Figure 4-1. Typical "Apple Core" Lesion Seen in Colonic Carcinoma (Barium Enema)

Diagnosis. Colonoscopy is clearly the most accurate diagnostic test. Sigmoidoscopy will only reach the lesion within the distal 60 cm of the colon. If the lesion is there, then the sensitivity of sigmoidoscopy is equal to colonoscopy. Only 60% of cancer occurs in this distal area. Barium studies are less accurate than colonoscopy. You also cannot biopsy with barium enema.

Treatment. The treatment of colon cancer depends on the stage of disease and the extent of its spread. Cancer that is localized to the mucosa, submucosa, and muscularis layers can easily be resected and cured. However, once the disease has penetrated the serosa and has spread into the surrounding tissues and lymph nodes, surgical resection will not be effective in eradicating the disease. Widespread disease is treated with chemotherapy. The mainstay of chemotherapy for GI malignancies, such as colon cancer, is 5-fluorouracil (5FU). Treatment for a single liver metastatic lesion is surgical resection.

Screening. The standard screening recommendation for colon cancer is annual fecal occult blood testing or colonoscopy every 10 years. Screening should occur in the general population after age 50. The most effective screening method is colonoscopy. False-positive stool guaiac tests can be caused by aspirin, NSAIDs, red meat, and poultry. False-negative tests can be caused by vitamin C. Sigmoidoscopy misses 40% of cancers which are proximal to the sigmoid colon.

If polyps have been found on a previous colonoscopy, then repeat colonoscopy in 3 to 5 years. In those who have a family history of colon cancer, screening should begin at age 40, or 10 years earlier than the family member, whichever is younger.

Hereditary Nonpolyposis Syndrome (Lynch Syndrome)

There are certain families who carry a genetic defect with a high degree of penetrance for causing colon cancer. The genetic defect does not cause polyps, however. By definition, the syndrome consists of having 3 family members in at least 2 generations with colon cancer. As a matter of definition, one of these cases should be premature, which is to say that it occurred in someone age <50. There is a very high incidence of ovarian and endometrial cancer in this syndrome as well. Up to 30% of patients develop endometrial cancer.

Screening. The recommendation for screening this population is to start at age 25 and undergo colonoscopy every 1 to 2 years.

Hereditary Polyposis Syndromes

Familial adenomatous polyposis has a very clear genetic defect. The adenomatous polyposis coli gene (APC) confers 100% penetrance for the development of adenomas by age 35 and of colon cancer by age 50. Polyps can usually be found as early as age 25.

Screening. Flexible sigmoidoscopy for familial adenomatous polyposis should be done every 1 to 2 years beginning at age 12. As soon as polyps are found, a colectomy should be performed, and a new rectum should be made from the terminal ileum.

By contrast, **juvenile polyposis syndrome** confers about a 10% risk of colon cancer. There are only a few dozen polyps, as opposed to the thousands of polyps found in those with familial polyposis. In addition, the polyps of the juvenile polyposis syndrome are hamartomas, not adenomas. Hamartomas confer very little risk of developing into cancer.

Cowden syndrome is another polyposis syndrome with hamartomas that gives only a very slightly increased risk of cancer compared with the general population. These polyposis syndromes can present with rectal bleeding in a child.

Screening. There is no recommendation for increased colon cancer screening with juvenile polyposis.

Note

If an exam question asks, "What do you do if an x-ray finds osteomas as an incidental finding?," the answer would be to perform a colonoscopy.

Other Polyposis and Colon Cancer Syndromes

Gardner syndrome is the association of colon cancer with multiple, soft-tissue tumors, such as osteomas, lipomas, cysts, and fibrosarcomas. The osteomas have a particular predilection for the mandible. The test question may ask, "What would you do if an x-ray finds osteomas as an incidental finding?" The answer would be to do colonoscopy.

Peutz-Jeghers syndrome is the association of hamartomatous polyps in the large and small intestine with hyperpigmented spots. These are melanotic spots on the lips, buccal mucosa, and skin. The risk of cancer is slightly increased above the general population. Most common presentation is with abdominal pain due to intussusception/bowel obstruction.

Turcot syndrome is simply the association of colon cancer with central nervous system malignancies.

Screening. There is no recommendation to perform increased cancer screening in any of these patients. These syndromes are not common enough to warrant a clear recommendation for uniform early screening. There is an association of endocarditis from *Streptococcus bovis* and colon cancer; therefore, if a patient has endocarditis from *S. bovis*, the patient should undergo colonoscopy.

GASTROINTESTINAL BLEEDING

A 72-year-old man with a history of aortic stenosis is brought to the emergency department with red/black stool several times today. His blood pressure is 94/60 mm Hg, and his pulse is 110/min.

What should you do first? The first thing to consider for a patient with GI bleeding is the treatment, not the etiology.

Treatment. The most important step in the **initial management** of severe GI bleeding is to begin fluid resuscitation with normal saline or Ringer's lactate. A complete blood count, prothrombin time, and type and crossmatch should be done, but if the patient is having a high volume bleed, such as in the case described above, you should never wait for the results of the tests to begin fluid resuscitation.

If the prothrombin time is elevated above the control, also give fresh frozen plasma. Vitamin K works too slowly, and if there is liver disease, it will not work at all. Platelets should be transfused if the platelet count <50,000/mm^3 and if the patient is actively bleeding.

A nasogastric tube is only useful to determine the site of bleeding to guide endoscopy. There is no direct therapeutic benefit to nasogastric tube placement. Saline or ice water lavage through the nasogastric tube is of no benefit. If the patient has a history of cirrhosis of the liver, or if there is occult cirrhosis (as found in a long-term alcoholic), octreotide should be added to this initial management plan to decrease portal hypertension.

All of the management described above is more important than performing endoscopy to determine a specific etiology. Fluids, blood, platelets, and plasma are indicated in all forms of severe GI bleeding if there is a coagulopathy. More than 80% of GI bleeding cases will stop spontaneously with appropriate fluid resuscitation, irrespective of the etiology. Endoscopy is performed later to determine the etiology.

Acute Bleeding. For acute bleeding, fluid resuscitation should be performed as described above. The hematocrit should be maintained at ≥30% or above in older patients and those who may have coronary artery disease. Younger patients will form their own reticulocytes and make their own blood over a few days and do not need to be transfused, unless their hematocrit is closer to 20%. Patients with gastritis or the possibility of ulcer disease should be treated with PPIs empirically until a definitive diagnosis can be made. H_2 blockers have no efficacy in acute GI bleeding.

Esophageal varices are treated with octreotide during acute episodes of bleeding in order to lower portal pressure. If this is ineffective, emergency endoscopy should be performed to place bands around the bleeding varices. Sclerotherapy will also stop acutely bleeding varices, but there is a much higher complication rate later on, such as stricture formation. If banding is not effective in stopping an acutely bleeding esophageal varix, then TIPS (transjugular intrahepatic portosystemic shunting) should be performed. A catheter is placed into the jugular vein and guided radiographically through the liver to form a shunt between the systemic circulation in the hepatic vein and the portal circulation through the portal vein. TIPS has largely replaced the need to surgically place the shunt. The most common, long-term complication of TIPS is worsening of hepatic encephalopathy.

A Blakemore tube to tamponade the site of bleeding in the stomach or esophagus is rarely used and is only a temporary bridge to surgery.

Propranolol is a nonselective beta-blocker used in the long-term management of portal hypertension to decrease the frequency of bleeding. Everyone with varices from portal hypertension and cirrhosis should be on a beta-blocker.

Pathogenesis. The most common causes of **upper** GI bleeding are ulcer disease, gastritis, Mallory- Weiss syndrome, esophagitis, and gastric cancer. Variceal bleeding is common in those with portal hypertension from cirrhosis. By definition, upper GI bleeding is defined as bleeding occurring proximal to the ligament of Treitz, which anatomically separates the duodenum from the jejunum. If there is a history of abdominal aortic aneurysm repair in the past 6 months to a year, think about an aortoenteric fistula.

Lower GI bleeding is most commonly caused by diverticulosis, angiodysplasia (also know as AVM or vascular ectasia), hemorrhoids, cancer, and inflammatory bowel disease.

Clinical presentation. Generally, lower GI bleeding presents with red blood in the stool, and upper GI bleeding presents with black stool, or melena.

Upper GI bleeding can also give hematemesis if the volume of bleeding is high enough. About 10% of cases of red blood from the rectum can be from an upper GI source. This can happen if the volume of bleeding is so high that the blood is rapidly transported to the bowel without the time for it to oxidize and turn black. In upper GI bleeding, occult blood–positive brown stool can occur with as little as 5 to 10 mL of blood loss. The same is true of "coffee-ground" emesis. Melena develops when at least 100 mL of blood have been lost.

Orthostasis is defined as a >10-point rise in pulse when the patient goes from the supine to the standing or sitting position. It is also defined as a >20-point drop in systolic blood pressure on a change in position. There should be at least a minute in between the position change and the measurement of the pulse and blood pressure to allow time for the normal autonomic discharge to accommodate to the position change. Orthostasis is when the rise in pulse or drop in blood pressure persists after the position has been changed. It indicates a 15 to 20% blood loss. The measurement of orthostatic changes is not necessary in the patient described in this case because a pulse >100/min or a systolic blood pressure <100/min already indicates a >30% blood loss.

Note

In >80% of cases, GI bleeding will resolve spontaneously with supportive management, irrespective of etiology.

Note

Remember, it's the treatment, not the etiology, that should be considered first when a patient is experiencing GI bleeding.

Note

Lower GI bleeding presents with red blood in the stool, whereas upper GI bleeding presents with black stool or melena.

Diagnosis. Endoscopy is the most accurate test to determine the etiology of both upper and lower GI bleeding. Barium studies are always less accurate. You also cannot biopsy unless endoscopy is performed.

Occasionally, in lower GI bleeding, endoscopy will not reveal the etiology even when there is active bleeding. A nuclear bleeding scan can detect low volume bleeds 0.1–0.5 mL/min. Red cells from the patient are tagged with technetium and reinjected back into the patient. These tagged cells are then detected to determine the site of bleeding.

Angiography is rarely used in the evaluation of lower GI bleeding because it needs a higher volume of blood loss >0.5 mL/min compared with the tagged nuclear scan. Angiography, however, is useful in extremely high-volume bleeding in which so much blood is coming out that endoscopy cannot see the source. It may then be used prior to either embolization of the site of the bleeding or hemicolectomy. Angiography can also help guide the occasional use of a local vasopressin injection in the control of severe lower GI bleeding.

Despite all of these methods, an etiology of GI bleeding cannot be determined in about 5% of patients. This is often because the upper endoscope only goes as far as the ligament of Treitz, and the lower endoscope only reaches just past the ileocecal valve. When both of these modalities are unrevealing, the most likely source of the bleeding is in the small bowel. The small bowel is very difficult to visualize, and barium studies are inaccurate. The newest modality to visualize the small bowel is capsule endoscopy, in which a patient swallows a capsule with an electronic camera that can transmit thousands of images to a receiver near the patient. This will allow anatomic localization of the lesion.

Virtual endoscopy is a CT scan used to try to detect cancer without the need of endoscopy. Virtual endoscopy lacks both sensitivity and specificity and should not be done.

ACUTE PANCREATITIS

Pathogenesis. The majority of pancreatitis is from alcoholism and gallstones. Other causes are as follows:

- Medications such as pentamidine, didanosine (DDI), azathioprine, and sulfa derivatives, like sulfamethoxazole/trimethoprim and thiazide diuretics.
- Hypercalcemia and hypertriglyceridemia can cause it for unclear reasons.
- Endoscopic retrograde cholangiopancreatography (ERCP) causes pancreatitis presumably because of back pressure from injection of the contrast material into the ductal system. Most people who have pancreatic injury from ERCP just have an asymptomatic increase in amylase. Only 2 to 8% of patients actually develop symptomatic pancreatitis.
- Trauma and various viruses, such as mumps.
- Premature activation of trypsinogen into trypsin while still in the pancreas (common pathway of most causes of pancreatitis). This results in autodigestion of the pancreas.

Clinical Presentation. Midepigastric pain with tenderness, nausea, and vomiting has always been the presentation of acute pancreatitis in the majority of cases. The pain of pancreatitis classically radiates straight through to the back. When pancreatitis is extremely severe, it can mimic many of the features of septic shock, such as fever, hypotension, respiratory distress from ARDS, elevation of the white cell count, and a rigid abdomen.

Clinical Pearl

Always consider gallstone pancreatitis and rule it out, even in patients with history of alcohol use.

Diagnosis. The initial tests remain as amylase and lipase. Lipase is more specific to the pancreas than is the amylase. An increased severity of disease and a worse prognosis are indicated by the presence of an elevated white cell count, hypoxia, and elevated glucose, LDH, and AST. The glucose will go up in the most severe forms of pancreatitis because of the loss of both endocrine function and insulin production. Calcium decreases because the malabsorption of fat allows the fat to bind with calcium in the bowel and diminish its absorption. The BUN goes up because of intravascular volume depletion. Hypertriglyceridemia can give a falsely normal amylase level.

The most accurate test to determine the severity of pancreatitis is the CT scan. The CT scan is more accurate than a sonogram is for the presence of inflammation, as well as for detecting necrosis, pseudocysts, abscesses, and the presence of ductal stones. Findings on the CT scan are a more important prognostic indicator than the Ranson criteria. (The Ranson criteria—increased WBC, LDH, AST, BUN, glucose, etc.—were developed before the invention of the CT scan.)

The single most accurate test for the detection of biliary and pancreatic ductal pathology is the ERCP. Urinary assay of trypsinogen activation peptide (TAP) is a new test to predict severity.

Treatment. There is no specific therapy to reverse pancreatitis. The inflammation and autodigestion of the pancreas must resolve on its own over time. For most pancreatitis cases, the management is only supportive, with IV fluids, bowel rest, and pain medication. ERCP is sometimes necessary to remove a stone in the pancreatic duct or to dilate a stricture.

When pancreatitis is very severe, such as when there is >30% necrosis visible on the CT scan, the risk of infected and hemorrhagic pancreatitis markedly increases. For this reason, necrosis on a CT scan is an indication for starting antibiotics, such as imipenem or meropenem, which will diminish both the risk and severity of hemorrhagic and infected pancreatitis. Severe necrosis, particularly when there is a persistent fever, is also an indication to perform a percutaneous needle biopsy of the pancreas. If there is infection of the pancreas in addition to necrosis, urgent surgical debridement is indicated. (This is before the development of an abscess, which does not begin for 4 to 6 weeks after the onset of pancreatitis.)

Pseudocysts develop only 2 to 4 weeks after the episode of pancreatitis. Pseudocysts should be drained if there is pain, fistula formation, and rupture or if the pseudocyst is expanding in size. Asymptomatic pseudocysts do not need to be drained.

Note

Signs of Severe Necrotizing Pancreatitis

- **Cullen sign:** blue discoloration around umbilicus → due to hemoperitoneum

- **Turner's sign:** Bluish purple discoloration of the flanks → tissue catabolism of Hb.

Note

IV fluid intake in large volumes is the most important management of acute pancreatitis.

Other Complications of Pancreatitis

- Ascites (high in amylase)

- Pleural effusion (transudate, ↑ amylase)

- Splenic vein thrombosis (think when there are gastric varices but no esophageal varices)

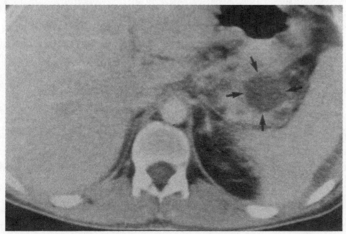

Courtesy of Dr. Conrad Fischer

Figure 4-2. Pancreatic Pseudocyst Seen on CT Scan

LIVER DISEASE AND CIRRHOSIS

Pathogenesis. Cirrhosis develops when there is chronic and severe inflammation of the liver for an extended period of time. The regenerative capacity of the liver is enormous; however, over a long time, fibrosis develops. And when at least 70 to 80% of liver function has been lost, the synthetic capacity of the liver is diminished.

The most common cause of cirrhosis in the United States is alcohol. (However, the most common reason to need a liver transplantation is chronic hepatitis C.) The other causes of cirrhosis are primary biliary cirrhosis, sclerosing cholangitis, alpha-1 antitrypsin deficiency, hemochromatosis, and Wilson disease.

Clinical Presentation/Laboratory Abnormalities. The features common to all forms of cirrhosis, despite the etiology, are a low albumin level, portal hypertension, esophageal varices, ascites, peripheral edema, an elevated prothrombin time, spider angiomata, palmar erythema, asterixis, and sometimes, encephalopathy. Jaundice can develop in any form of cirrhosis or liver disease. The prothrombin time is prolonged because of the loss of ability to synthesize clotting factors. (All of the clotting factors are made in the liver, with the exception of factor VIII and Von Willebrand factor, which are made in the vascular endothelial cells.)

Ascites is the result of portal hypertension. A paracentesis is a sample of the ascitic fluid obtained by needle through the anterior abdominal wall. A paracentesis is used to exclude infection, as well as to determine the etiology of the ascites if it is not clear from the history.

Spontaneous bacterial peritonitis (SBP) is an idiopathic infection of ascites. The Gram stain is rarely positive because the density of microorganisms is so low. Although culture of the fluid is the most specific test, we cannot wait for the results of the culture to make a decision as to whether to give antibiotics. A total white cell count >500/mm^3 or the presence of >250/mm^3 neutrophils are the criteria to determine the presence of infection. Cefotaxime and ceftriaxone are the drugs of choice for SBP and albumin infusion decreases risk of hepatorenal syndrome.

Serum-Ascites Albumin Gradient. Normally, the ascitic fluid albumin level is always less than the serum level. The difference between them is referred to as the serum-ascites albumin gradient, or SAAG. When the albumin level is low in the ascitic fluid, the gradient, or difference between the ascites and the serum, is high. When this gradient, or SAAG, is >1.1, portal hypertension, as from cirrhosis, is generally the cause. When the SAAG is <1.1, it means the ascitic fluid albumin level is high. Cancer and infections generally give a SAAG <1.1.

Treatment. There is no specific therapy to reverse cirrhosis. (A complication to consider is hepatocellular carcinoma.) One can only manage the complications of cirrhosis and treat the underlying causes. Edema and fluid overload in third spaces, such as ascites, are managed with diuretics. The diuretic most useful in cirrhosis is spironolactone. This is because cirrhotics have intravascular volume depletion, which results in a high aldosterone state.

Portal hypertension and varices are managed with propranolol to prevent bleeding. Encephalopathy is managed with neomycin or lactulose, a nonabsorbed disaccharide that bacteria metabolize in the colon, making it more acidic. This converts the NH_3 to NH_4^+, or ammonia to ammonium. Ammonium is not absorbed very well, and this leads to an overall increased excretion of ammonia from the body.

Although vitamin K is often given because of the elevated prothrombin time, it is not effective because the liver is not able to synthesize clotting factors, no matter how much vitamin K is present.

Note

Although a culture of the ascitic fluid is the most specific test for SBP, one cannot wait for the culture results when determining whether to give antibiotics.

Primary Biliary Cirrhosis

Pathogenesis. Primary biliary cirrhosis is an idiopathic autoimmune disorder that occurs more often in middle-aged women. Bilirubin levels do not elevate until the disease is extremely far advanced, which is usually after 5 to 10 years. Primary biliary cirrhosis has a strong association with other autoimmune diseases, such as Sjögren syndrome, rheumatoid arthritis, and scleroderma.

Clinical Presentation. The most common symptoms are fatigue and pruritus. At least a third of patients, however, are asymptomatic but are found to have an elevated alkaline phosphatase level when measured for other reasons. Osteoporosis and hypothyroidism are found in 20 to 30% of patients.

Diagnosis. The transaminases are often normal. The most common abnormality is an elevation of alkaline phosphatase and gamma glutamyl transpeptidase (GGTP). Total IgM levels are also elevated. The most specific blood test is the antimitochondrial antibody.

Biopsy is always the best way to diagnose liver disease. It is the only test more specific than antimitochondrial antibodies.

Treatment. There is no specific therapy for primary biliary cirrhosis. Steroids will not help. Bile acid medication, such as ursodeoxycholic acid and cholestyramine, are used with variable success. Ultraviolet light is recommended to treat the pruritus. Also liver transplant for late stage PBC may also be considered.

Primary Sclerosis Cholangitis

Pathogenesis. This is an idiopathic disorder of the biliary system most commonly associated with inflammatory bowel disease (IBD). Although it is more often found with ulcerative colitis, it can also occur with Crohn's disease. Cancer of the biliary system can develop in 15% of patients from the chronic inflammation.

Clinical Presentation and Diagnosis. The presentation and general laboratory tests are generally the same as those for primary biliary cirrhosis, except that the antimitochondrial antibody test will be negative. The most specific test for primary sclerosis cholangitis is an ERCP or transhepatic cholangiogram. This is the only chronic liver disease in which a liver biopsy is not the most accurate test.

Treatment. Therapy is the same as for primary biliary cirrhosis, with ursodeoxycholic acid. Also, liver transplant may be considered.

Hemochromatosis

Pathogenesis. Hemochromatosis is one of the most common inherited genetic diseases. There is an overabsorption of iron in the duodenum, leading to iron buildup in a number of tissues throughout the body. This leads to chronic hepatic inflammation and fibrosis.

Clinical Presentation. Cirrhosis is the most common finding. Hepatocellular cancer develops in 15 to 20% of patients. Restrictive cardiomyopathy develops in approximately 15% of patients. Arthralgias, skin hyperpigmentation, diabetes, and hypogonadism are also common. *Vibrio vulnificus* and *Yersinia* infections occur with increased frequency because of their avidity for iron.

Diagnosis. Screening for the disorder is by finding an elevated iron level and diminished iron-binding capacity. The ferritin is also elevated. The most accurate test is a liver biopsy and abnormal C282Y gene; MRI can eliminate the need for biopsy if both are present.

Note

Primary sclerosis cholangitis is the only chronic liver disease in which a liver biopsy is not the most accurate test.

Treatment. Phlebotomy is used to remove large amounts of iron from the body—it removes far more iron than does the chelating agents deferoxamine and deferasirox. Deferoxamine and deferasirox are used only in those who cannot undergo phlebotomy.

Wilson Disease

Pathogenesis. Wilson disease is an autosomal recessive disorder leading to the diminished ability to excrete copper from the body. There is also increased copper absorption from the small intestine.

Clinical Presentation. Copper builds up in the liver, brain, and cornea. Basal ganglia dysfunction contributes to the movement disorder that develops. Ten percent of patients have a psychiatric disturbance. Kayser-Fleischer rings are found in the eye on slit-lamp examination. Tremor and Parkinson's occur in one-third of all patients. Fanconi syndrome and type II proximal renal tubular acidosis develop because of copper deposition in the kidney.

Diagnosis. The most specific blood test is a low ceruloplasmin level, but a low ceruloplasmin level alone is not enough. There is also a high urinary copper level. But again, the single most specific test is a liver biopsy, which will demonstrate increased copper deposition in the liver. Occasionally, there is a hemolytic anemia when the copper levels go high and are toxic to the red cells.

Treatment. Penicillamine and trientine are copper chelators. Oral zinc interferes with copper absorption. Liver transplantation is curative, and steroids will not help.

> **Note**
>
> A patient presenting with choreoathetoid movements and psychosis gives the clue to perform the slit-lamp examination. Kayser-Fleischer rings are then found, confirming the diagnosis of Wilson disease.

Alpha-1 Antitrypsin Deficiency

Pathogenesis. This is an autosomal recessive disorder leading to deficient alpha-1 antitrypsin levels.

Clinical Presentation. In addition to cirrhosis, the most prominent finding is emphysema developing at a young age in a nonsmoker.

Diagnosis. Simply find a low level of the enzyme in a person with COPD to confirm the diagnosis.

Treatment. There is no specific therapy for the liver disease. Those with emphysema should receive replacement of the enzyme and stop smoking.

Chronic Hepatitis B and C

Pathogenesis. Hepatitis B and C are transmitted by blood products, needlestick injury, and through sexual contact. Injection drug use is also strongly associated with both viruses.

Clinical Presentation. Most patients are asymptomatic until the disease is very far advanced.

Diagnosis. The persistence of hepatitis B surface antigen >6 months confirms hepatitis B, although it takes years for cirrhosis to develop. Finding an antibody to hepatitis C, and then finding an elevation of the viral load by PCR methods, diagnose chronic hepatitis C. The single most accurate test for both is a liver biopsy.

Treatment. Chronic hepatitis B is treated with interferon, lamivudine, entecavir, telbivudine, or adefovir. Combining these agents does not lead to increased efficacy. Chronic hepatitis C is treated with the combination of pegylated interferon, ribavirin and either boceprevir or telaprevir. The combination has greatly increased efficacy compared with single drug therapy.

The standard of care for hepatitis C is 3 drugs: interferon and ribavirin plus telaprevir or boceprevir.

ACUTE CHEST PAIN/CHEST DISCOMFORT

Chest pain is one of the most common complaints for which a patient comes to the physician's office or the emergency department. Patients presenting with chest pain or chest discomfort may have an underlying cause that is benign and requires only moderate analgesic medication, or they may have a life-threatening condition such as acute myocardial ischemia or aortic dissection that mandates prompt diagnosis and treatment. In the evaluation of chest pain, the focus should be on excluding the more serious conditions.

History

Assessing the setting in which the chest pain occurs is one of the most important aspects of the evaluation. The 26-year-old medical resident with chest pain that occurred after on-call and who is otherwise healthy is unlikely to have cardiovascular disease, no matter the quality or duration of chest pain. Consider the 58-year-old man with type 2 diabetes and dyslipidemia with chest discomfort of any type; now the probability for cardiac-related chest pain increases dramatically.

Overall, the chest pain history is more useful than the physical examination. Important aspects of the history include duration, quality, location, radiation, frequency, alleviating or precipitating factors (especially exercise), and associated symptoms.

- For both stable angina and acute coronary syndromes, the quality of chest pain is described by the patient as "tightness," "heaviness," or "pressure," but symptoms which resemble acute abdomen (pain in the upper abdomen, nausea) are not uncommon. Nausea and vomiting are sometimes the main symptoms in inferoposterior wall ischemia (also, vagal reflexes may cause bradycardia and hypotension, presenting as dizziness or fainting).

- "Sharp" or "knife-like" chest pain and pain which the patient can pinpoint to an "exact area" are less likely to be related to ischemia or infarction, especially if the chest pain is reproduced by changes in position or palpation.

- Myocardial infarction is associated with pain that lasts >20–30 minutes in duration.

- Response of chest pain to nitroglycerin (within a few minutes) is most consistent with transient ischemia or esophageal spasm. Chest pain that worsens with nitroglycerin sometimes occurs with gastroesophageal reflux disease. The response to nitroglycerin is not enough to confirm coronary disease as the cause of chest pain.

- Acute coronary syndromes in women present with atypical symptoms: dyspnea, shortness of breath, fatigue. This may be due to the older age group in which myocardial ischemia and infarction occur in women.

Physical Examination

One of the most important parts of the examination of the chest pain patient is the "initial impression." Diaphoresis, tachypnea, and anxious expression should alert the clinician to a potentially life-threatening process. Tachycardia and tachypnea are both nonspecific but occur in almost all cases of pulmonary embolism.

- Blood pressure should be checked in both arms: a difference of >20 mm Hg systolic suggests aortic dissection and is present in ~70% of cases.

- Hypotension may suggest massive pulmonary embolism or cardiac shock.

- Fever may suggest pneumonia or mediastinitis (esophageal rupture) as the cause of chest pain.

- Evidence of atherosclerosis (corneal lipid rings, narrowed retinal arteries, and pigment and hair changes in the legs) is commonly seen in patients with coronary syndromes.

The chest wall should be inspected for tender areas, respiratory motion, respiratory retractions, or accessory muscle use. If the tender area corresponds to the location of the patient's pain and palpation exactly reproduces the pain, consider musculoskeletal chest pain as the cause of chest pain.

Abnormal heart sounds and new murmurs are commonly found in certain chest pain syndromes. Wide physiologic splitting of the second heart sound (splitting wider with inspiration) can be found in right bundle branch block or in right ventricular infarction. New paradoxical splitting is most often due to left bundle branch block (LBBB), or anterior or lateral infarction. A new fourth heart sound can occur with angina or infarction. An S3 is more likely due to underlying heart failure. A new murmur may be significant: aortic regurgitation occurs in over half of patients with aortic dissection, while mitral regurgitation can occur in patients with angina or infarction and is due to papillary muscle dysfunction.

The lungs should be auscultated for crackles and asymmetrical breath sounds. Asymmetry of breath sounds may be found in patients with spontaneous pneumothorax. Absent lung sounds also may occur in pneumothorax and pleural effusions.

The extremities should be examined for pulses, edema, calf tenderness, and signs of atherosclerotic vessel disease. Absence of pedal pulses may occur in aortic dissection. Any swelling of the legs, especially if unilateral, raises the odds of pulmonary embolism as the cause of chest pain.

Testing

All patients with chest pain should have a 12-lead **electrocardiogram** (ECG) since the **ECG is the single most important test** for the evaluation of the cause of chest pain. The ECG should be done immediately after initial stabilization and taking of vital signs. Most patients with myocardial infarction will have an abnormal initial ECG: 50% with acute MI will have diagnostic findings (ST elevation or Q waves), while 35% will have findings consistent with ischemia (ST depression and/or T wave inversion). In patients presenting with acute chest pain who have **normal ECG**, the chance of acute MI is much less than 10% (in some studies 1–2.6%). An abnormal ECG can be seen in many non-cardiac conditions (pulmonary embolism, electrolyte abnormalities, aortic dissection).

In interpreting the ECG, every effort must be made to obtain previous ECGs, so that the abnormalities can be compared with those on the old tracing. Any ECG finding is assumed to be new unless proven otherwise by an old ECG (if one is available). Also, in patients with acute coronary syndromes, the ECG is the sole test required to select patients for emergency reperfusion.

Serum **cardiac biomarker** determinations play a vital role in the evaluation of patients who present with acute chest pain and in the diagnosis of acute myocardial infarction. Serum markers such as aspartate transaminase, lactate dehydrogenase, and lactate dehydrogenase subforms no longer are used because they lack cardiac specificity and their delayed elevation precludes early diagnosis. Creatine kinase (CK) is found in striated muscle and tissues of the brain, kidney, lung, and GI tract. This widely available marker has low sensitivity and specificity for cardiac damage. Furthermore, CK levels may be elevated in a number of noncardiac conditions, including trauma, seizures, renal insufficiency, hyperthermia, and hyperthyroidism. Currently, the CK marker largely has been replaced by cardiac troponins and CK-MB.

CK-MB isoenzyme: CK-MB is cardiac specific and is useful for the early diagnosis of acute myocardial infarction. CK-MB typically is detectable in the serum 4–6 hours after the onset of ischemia, peaks in 12–24 hours, and normalizes in 2–3 days (*see* Figure 5-1).

Like the CK level, the peak CK-MB level *does not predict infarct size*; however, it can be used to *detect early reinfarction*. Serial CK-MB levels commonly are obtained at admission to the emergency department and are repeated in 6–12 hours.

CK-MB subforms: CK-MB may be further characterized into subforms (or isoforms). CK-MB2 is found in myocardial tissue, and CK-MB1 is found in plasma. The CK-MB subform is not routinely used.

Cardiac troponins: Troponins (T, I, C) are found in striated and cardiac muscle. Because the cardiac and skeletal muscle isoforms of troponin T and I differ, they are known as the "cardiac troponins." They are the *preferred markers* for the diagnosis of myocardial injury. Troponin T and I generally have similar sensitivity and specificity for the detection of myocardial injury. Unlike troponin I levels, troponin T levels may be elevated in patients with renal disease, polymyositis, or dermatomyositis.

The cardiac troponins typically are measured at emergency department admission and repeated in 6–12 hours. Patients with a normal CK-MB level but elevated troponin levels are considered to have sustained *minor myocardial damage,* or microinfarction, whereas patients with elevations of both CK-MB and troponins are considered to have had *acute myocardial infarction*. The cardiac troponins may remain elevated *up to two weeks* after symptom onset, which makes them useful as late markers of recent acute myocardial infarction.

An elevated troponin T or I level is helpful in identifying patients at increased risk for death or the development of acute myocardial infarction. Increased risk is related to the high serum troponin levels. The troponins also can help identify low-risk patients who may be sent home with close follow-up. Those with a normal or nearly normal ECG and a normal troponin I test 6 hours after admission had a very low risk of major cardiac events (0.3%) during the next 30 days.

Myoglobin: Myoglobin levels begin to rise as early as 1–4 hours after the onset of pain. Normal myoglobin at 4 hours has a very high negative predictive value.

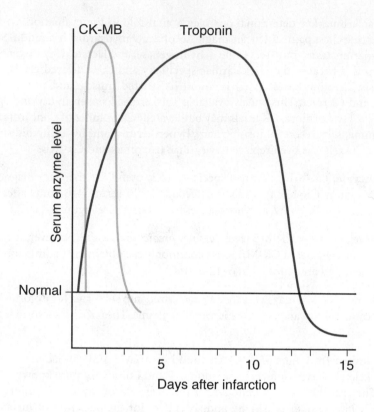

Figure 5-1. Progression of Cardiac Enzyme Serum Levels

A **chest x-ray** should be obtained on patients with chest pain. The x-ray may show pneumo-thorax, pneumomediastinum (such as from esophageal rupture), pleural effusion, or infiltrates. Aortic dissection can cause widening of the mediastinum. Subtle findings such as loss of lung volume or unilateral decrease in vascular markings may suggest pulmonary embolism.

Especially if the clinician suspects a noncardiac diagnosis, other tests may be helpful in the evaluation of patients presenting with acute chest pain. Some of the most common ones used are: arterial blood gases, BNP (see pulmonary and heart failure section), CT angiogram.

Causes of Chest Pain

Aortic Dissection. Pain is sharp, tearing, and extremely severe; typically radiates to back; loss of pulses or aortic insufficiency often develop; mediastinum is widened on chest x-ray; MI may occur if dissection extends into coronary artery; diagnosis confirmed by MRI, CT scan, or transesophageal echocardiogram.

Pulmonary Embolism. Dyspnea, tachycardia, and hypoxemia are prominent; pain is usually pleuritic, especially when pulmonary infarction develops; EKG is usually nonspecific but may show S wave in lead I, Q wave in lead III, or inverted T wave in lead III; diagnosis confirmed by CT angiogram.

Pericarditis. May be preceded by viral illness; pain is sharp, positional, pleuritic, and relieved by leaning forward; pericardial rub often present; diffuse ST elevation occurs without evolution of Q waves; CK level usually normal; responds to anti-inflammatory agents.

Table 5-1. Differential Diagnosis of Conditions Causing Chest Pain

Noncardiovascular Disorders	Differentiating Features
Costochondritis	Pain exacerbated with inspiration; reproduced with chest wall palpitation
Hiatal hernia	Reflux of food; relief with antacids
GERD	Acid reflux; relief with antacids
Peptic ulcer	Epigastric pain worse 3 h after eating
Gallbladder disease	Right upper quadrant abdominal pain and tenderness
Cardiovascular Disorders	**Differentiating Features**
Myocardial infarction	Pain more severe, usually >20 min in duration
Aortic stenosis	Typical systolic ejection murmur
Myocarditis	Pain is usually vague and mild if present
Pericarditis	Pain is sharper, pain worse with lying down and relieved by sitting up
Dissecting aortic aneurysm	Pain is sharp, tearing, often occurs in back
Mitral valve prolapse	Transient pain, midsystolic click murmur, and young female with no risk factors
Pulmonary Disorders	**Differentiating Features**
Pulmonary embolus-infarction	Tachypnea, dyspnea, cough, pleuritic pain, hemoptysis
Pulmonary hypertension	Signs of right ventricle (RV) failure
Pneumothorax	Sudden onset of pain and dyspnea

Myocarditis. May be preceded by viral illness; pain is generally vague and mild if present; total CK and MB fraction of CK (CK-MB) are often elevated; conduction abnormalities and Q waves may occur.

Musculoskeletal Disorders. Most common cause of chest pain. Includes costochondritis, cervical osteoarthritis, radiculitis; pain is atypical, stabbing, localized, may be pleuritic; reproduced by motion or palpation; EKG changes absent.

GI Disorders. Esophageal reflux is often made worse with recumbency or after meals, may be associated with regurgitation and relieved by antacids; episodes of spasm may be brought on by cold liquids, relieved by nitroglycerin, and may closely resemble angina or infarction; diagnosis may be confirmed by upper endoscopy or esophageal manometry. Peptic ulcer disease, pancreatitis, and cholecystitis may occasionally mimic infarction; abdominal tenderness is present, with radiation to back and elevated amylase in pancreatitis; sonography can confirm cholecystitis.

Pneumothorax. Onset abrupt with sharp pleuritic chest pain and dyspnea; breath sounds absent; chest x-ray confirms.

Pleuritis. Pain is sharp and increases on inspiration; friction rub or dullness may be present; other respiratory symptoms and underlying pulmonary infection usually present.

ISCHEMIC HEART DISEASE

Ischemic heart disease (IHD), also known as coronary heart disease, refers to an imbalance in coronary oxygen demand and supply resulting from insufficient blood flow. In nearly all cases, the reduction in blood flow is caused by coronary atherosclerotic disease. When the athero-sclerotic plaque ruptures, there is superimposed thrombus formation that acutely occludes the artery; this is the most common cause of life-threatening acute coronary syndromes.

Rarely, other abnormalities may occur, including coronary artery embolism, coronary artery spasm, coronary arteritis, and coronary artery dissection (*see* section on nonatherosclerotic acute coronary syndromes) that may cause ischemic heart disease in the absence of atheroma formation.

IHD is one of the most prevalent diseases in society, and those affected are likely to die from their disease (though age-specific deaths have declined over the past 30 years). IHD, as part of a systemic process that involves all arteries in the body, is an insidious process that begins in early adulthood with fatty streaks; these lesions progress into plaques and thrombus formation in middle age.

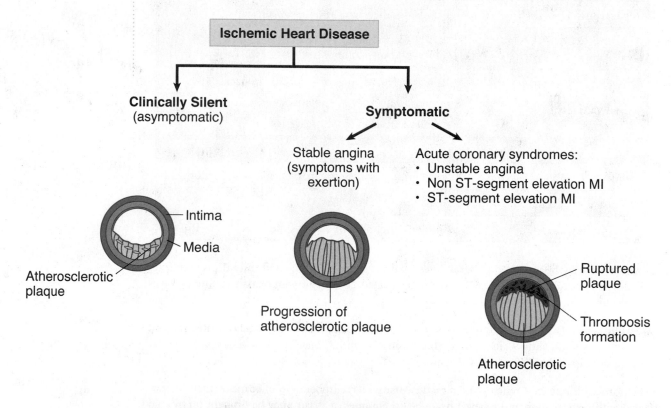

Figure 5-2. Ischemic Heart Disease

The more risk factors a person has, the greater the chance that he will develop heart disease. Also, the greater the level of each risk factor, the greater the risk. For example, a person with total cholesterol 260 mg/dL has a greater risk than someone with total cholesterol 220 mg/dL, even though all people with total cholesterol ≥220 are considered high risk.

Major Modifiable Risk Factors

Elevated cholesterol levels: The risk of IHD rises as blood cholesterol levels increase. The concentrations of lipid fractions, especially low-density lipoprotein (LDL) and high-density lipoprotein (HDL), are also important. LDL cholesterol is the **single most important subgroup** that carries risk for IHD, although there are several other abnormalities that increase coronary risk: low HDL cholesterol, hypertriglyceridemia, increased total-to-HDL-cholesterol ratio and increased lipoprotein A. When other risk factors (such as high blood pressure and tobacco smoke) are present, this risk increases even more.

Proof of the importance of serum cholesterol has come from randomized trials, which showed that reductions in total LDL levels reduce coronary events and mortality.

Tobacco: Cigarette smoking is an important factor for IHD because a smoker's risk of heart attack is >2x that of a nonsmoker. Cigarette smoking also acts with other risk factors (hypertension, dyslipidemia) to greatly increase the risk for IHD.

- Cigar or pipe smokers have a higher risk of death from IHD, though less than cigarette smokers.
- Secondhand smoke or passive smoking increases the risk of heart disease, even for nonsmokers.
- The risk for myocardial infarction in those who quit smoking was reduced to that of nonsmokers within 2 years of cessation; the benefits were seen regardless of how long or how much the patient smoked.

Hypertension (HTN): HTN is a well-established risk factor for increase in risk of myocardial ischemia, stroke, kidney failure, and heart failure. Studies in the general population have shown that the risk for cardiovascular events increases at BP >110/75 mm Hg. Systolic BP is as important as diastolic BP in terms of risk for IHD, especially in older patients.

Treatment of HTN to optimal levels reduces the risk of IHD and all cardiovascular events. In fact, data from recent randomized trials suggest that reducing BP below previously recommended levels is beneficial in high-risk patients.

Physical inactivity and exercise: Inactivity and sedentary lifestyle are risk factors for IHD. Exercise of moderate degree has a protective effect against IHD and cardiovascular events. More vigorous activities are associated with more benefits. Physical activity can help increase HDL cholesterol and control diabetes and obesity, as well as help to lower blood pressure.

Obesity: Patients with increased body fat (elevated body mass index), especially if a lot is in the waist area, are more likely to develop heart IHD and stroke. Excess weight raises blood pressure, blood cholesterol, and triglyceride levels, and it lowers HDL cholesterol levels. It can also increase risk for type 2 diabetes by causing insulin resistance.

Studies have shown that loss of as little as 10–20 lb can significantly reduce the risk of cardiovascular disease.

Diabetes mellitus: Elevated blood glucose levels and insulin resistance are associated with IHD and overall cardiovascular events. All-cause mortality in diabetic patients is comparable to that of all-cause mortality in patients with prior myocardial ischemia; hence, diabetes is now considered an "IHD equivalent." Even when glucose levels are under control, diabetes greatly increases the risk of IHD. Almost 75% of patients with diabetes die of some form of cardiovascular disease.

There is compelling evidence that aggressive treatment of HTN and cholesterol, as well as tight glycemic control, reduces the risk of cardiovascular events in these patients significantly.

Major Uncontrollable Risk Factors

Age: Four out of 5 people who die of IHD are age ≥65. Also, women who develop myocardial ischemia at older ages have a higher mortality than men within the first few weeks of the cardiac event.

Sex: Men have a greater risk of IHD than women, and overall they develop cardiovascular disease earlier in life.

Heredity: Family history is a significant independent risk factor if there is a family history of premature disease (age <55 in male relative and <65 in female relative).

Minor Contributing Factors

Sex hormones: Men have more heart attacks than women before menopause. Several population studies show that the decrease of natural estrogen as women age may contribute to a higher risk of heart disease after menopause.

Stress: Various studies have shown relationship between IHD risk and stress in a person's life. This may be a true association or just a secondary correlation: for example, people under stress may overeat, start smoking, or be less active than people who are not under stress.

Myocardial Ischemia As a Manifestation of IHD

During ischemia, an imbalance occurs between myocardial oxygen supply and demand. Ischemia may manifest in any of the following ways:

- Anginal chest discomfort
- ST-segment deviation on ECG
- Reduced uptake of tracer during myocardial perfusion scanning
- Regional or global impairment of ventricular function

Myocardial ischemia can occur as a result of increased myocardial oxygen demand, reduced myocardial oxygen supply, or both. In the presence of coronary obstruction, an increase of myocardial oxygen requirements caused by exercise, tachycardia, or emotion leads to a transitory imbalance. This condition is frequently termed **"demand ischemia"** and is responsible for most episodes of chronic stable angina.

In other situations, the imbalance is caused by acute reduction of oxygen supply secondary to marked reduction or cessation of coronary flow as a result of platelet aggregates or thrombi. This condition, termed **"supply ischemia,"** is responsible for myocardial infarction (MI) and most episodes of unstable angina (UA). In many circumstances, ischemia results from both an increase in oxygen demand and a reduction in supply.

Angina (Stable Angina)

A 62-year-old man presents with substernal chest pain that occurs with exertion and is relieved by rest. He has been having this on and off for 8 months, and the last episode occurred 3 days ago while he was running to the bus. He has a history of well-controlled diabetes and dyslipidemia. Vital signs, physical examination, and ECG are normal. An exercise stress test shows a 2-mm ST depression.

Stable angina occurs when the myocardium becomes ischemic. This occurs during periods of increased demand for oxygen, such as exercise, or decreased supply, such as hypotension or anemia (*see* demand ischemia, above). Stable angina is typically a substernal pressure lasting 5–15 minutes. It may be accompanied by radiation to the jaw, neck, shoulders, or arms. It is less likely to have the symptoms often associated with MI: sweats, nausea, and shortness of breath. Anginal pain is not typically affected by respiration or by position. Typically, patients with stable angina will have pain after a predictable amount of exertion and will have identical symptoms with each attack.

In certain patients, symptoms other than pain may occur. For example, a profound sense of weakness and breathlessness may be an "angina equivalent." Atypical symptoms are more likely to occur in the elderly and in diabetics.

The physical exam is usually normal. A new S4 may be heard, suggesting a stiff ventricle due to ischemia.

Most patients with angina will have ECG changes **during an attack**. Most commonly, ST segment depression is seen. ST segment elevation occurs in variant angina (Prinzmetal angina) where coronary artery spasm is responsible and rarely during ischemia caused by stable angina (where atherosclerotic disease is responsible).

Diagnosis. The **baseline ECG** is done to exclude previous myocardial ischemia or arrhythmias that would make interpretation of the regular exercise test difficult to interpret.

The **exercise treadmill test (exercise stress test)** is the most useful test in the evaluation of the cause of chronic chest pain when IHD (stable angina) is a consideration. Exercise stress testing provides a controlled environment for observing the effects of increases in the myocardial demand for oxygen.

- *Significant* fixed stenoses of the coronary arteries will result in ECG evidence of ischemia.
- Low-grade stenoses (<50%) may not produce sufficient impairment of blood flow to affect the ECG; in these cases the stress test will be normal.

An exercise stress test is considered positive for myocardial ischemia when large (>2 mm) ST-segment depressions or hypotension (a drop of >10 mm Hg in systolic pressure) occur either alone or in combination. In general, the earlier the angina or ECG abnormalities occur, the more significant they are.

The exercise stress test also allows determination of the severity of IHD and the need for further intervention. For example, severe symptoms (hypotension) early during the course of the exercise test usually occur in patients with triple vessel disease. Other uses of the stress test include assessing the effectiveness of treatment—patients with coronary artery disease who have undergone surgical intervention or are receiving medical therapy have an exercise stress test when they are medically stable and symptom-free. Also, after MI, patients may be candidates for exercise stress testing at a low level of exercise to determine functional capacity and identify any ECG changes or symptoms during exercise.

Exercise stress testing is contraindicated when it may place the patient at increased risk of cardiac instability, as in the setting of aortic dissection, acute myocardial infarction, unstable angina, severe CHF, uncontrolled sustained ventricular arrhythmias, symptomatic supraventricular arrhythmia, significant aortic stenosis, hypertrophic cardiomyopathy, or severe uncontrolled hypertension.

Patients who are unable to exercise or walk should be considered for chemical stress testing, such as dipyridamole (Persantine) or dobutamine stress tests. Presence of baseline ECG abnormalities, such as bundle branch block, left ventricular hypertrophy, or with a pacemaker, may make it more difficult to interpret a patient's test results. Such patients should be evaluated by nuclear stress imaging instead of the exercise stress test. These tests may also be used in patients who are taking digoxin.

In most cases, medications should not be withheld in preparation for an exercise stress test. Certain medications require special consideration since they may invalidate the test results or make them difficult to interpret. Beta blockers may blunt the heart rate during exercise. While patients receiving beta blockers may perform the exercise required for the test, the usual age-adjusted target heart rate may not be a realistic end point for them. The antihypertensive effect of beta blockers, alpha blockers, and nitroglycerin may cause significant hypotension during exercise. Digoxin may depress the ST segments, so if ST-segment depression of 1 mm or more is present on the baseline ECG, the stress test results will be difficult to interpret.

A number of other situations or conditions may reduce the validity of the exercise stress test. Exercise testing in *asymptomatic, young women* yields an increased number of false-positive results, while exercise testing in patients with known CAD may result in an unacceptably high false-negative rate (e.g., a negative stress test in a 64-year-old man with diabetes, hyperlipidemia, and typical stable angina is likely to be a false-negative result).

> A 29-year-old woman has a routine stress test done that shows a 1-mm ST depression. She has no history of chest pain, and she exercises routinely (runs 2–3 miles per day, 3 times per week). Her physical examination is unremarkable.

The **most likely** cause of her abnormal stress test? **False-positive test.**

Other types of stress tests include:

- **Nuclear stress test:** A radioactive substance is injected into the patient and perfusion of heart tissue is visualized. The perfusion pictures are done both at rest and after exercise. An abnormal amount of thallium will be seen in those areas of the heart that have a decreased blood supply. Compared to regular stress tests, the nuclear stress tests have higher sensitivity and specificity (92% sensitivity, 95% specificity vs. 67% sensitivity, 70% specificity). These tests are also not affected by baseline changes in the ECG (LBBB, ST-segment depression at baseline, etc.).

- **Dobutamine or adenosine stress test:** Used in people who are unable to exercise. A drug is given to induce tachycardia, as if the person were exercising.

- **Stress echocardiogram:** Combines a treadmill stress test and an echocardiogram (ECHO). The latter can recognize abnormal movement of the walls of the left ventricle (wall motion abnormalities) that are induced by exercise.

Invasive techniques: Cardiac catheterization is also used in patients with stable angina for (*1*) diagnosis and (*2*) prognosis/risk stratification. Angiography is an appropriate diagnostic test when noninvasive tests are contraindicated or inadequate due to the patient's illness or physical characteristics (e.g., morbid obesity, COPD). Cardiac angiography is also used after conventional stress tests are positive to identify patients that will benefit from stent placement or bypass surgery.

Treatment. For individual episodes of angina, nitroglycerin (NTG) sublingual tablets typically alleviate the pain within 3 minutes. Long-term management is with long-acting nitrates and/or beta blockers. Other medications patients with stable angina should be taking, unless contraindicated, include aspirin and statins (for lipid lowering). Also, modify the risk factors (tobacco cessation, exercise, control of hypertension, etc.).

All patients with stable angina need evaluation of the severity of IHD (cardiac angiography or stress testing, *see* above), and those who will benefit from revascularization (stent or bypass surgery) need to be identified.

Lipid lowering treatment for secondary prevention is important in IHD patients who should be treated aggressively. Most patients will require both pharmacologic and nonpharmacologic interventions to reach target goals. Target goals for hyperlipidemic patients with coronary artery disease include:

- LDL <100 mg/dL
- HDL ≥40 mg/dL
- Triglycerides <150 mg/dL

The optimal LDL-cholesterol goal is considered to be <70 mg/dL for patients considered to be **very high risk**. These are patients with established cardiovascular disease plus diabetes and patients with acute coronary syndromes. Bottom line: almost all patients with chronic stable coronary artery disease will likely need to be on statin therapy, unless contraindicated.

Every effort should be made to ensure that patients with coronary artery disease receive optimal lipid therapy. Statin medications are strongly supported as first-line medications due to compelling evidence of mortality reduction from multiple clinical trials. If patients are intolerant to a statin, consider other statins in reduced doses.

Better medical therapy with aspirin, beta blockers, ACE inhibitors, and statins are decreasing the need for all revascularization procedures.

Coronary bypass graft

- Useful in those with left main coronary disease or 3-vessel disease and left ventricular (LV) dysfunction and low ejection fraction
- Used in those with symptoms despite medical therapy or with severe side effects of medical therapy
- More efficacious in those with diabetes
- More beneficial (although more risky to perform) in those with low ejection fraction

Percutaneous coronary intervention (PCI)

- Stent placement now standard
- Most cases of stable angina do not need PCI
- PCI is most useful in acute coronary syndrome (ACS)

ACUTE CORONARY SYNDROME

Acute coronary syndrome (ACS) is used to describe a range of thrombotic coronary diseases, including unstable angina (UA), non-ST elevation myocardial infarction (NSTEMI), and ST-elevation myocardial infarction (STEMI). Collectively, they represent one of the most common causes of acute medical admission to U.S. hospitals.

The term ACS is clinically useful because the initial presentation and early management of unstable angina, STEMI, and NSTEMI are frequently similar. ACS should be distinguished from stable angina, which develops during exertion and resolves at rest.

ACS is due to coronary vessel atherosclerotic obstruction with superimposed thrombotic occlusion. The natural course of coronary atherosclerotic plaque development and subsequent occlusion does not proceed in a step-wise, uniform manner, gradually progressing to luminal obstruction (and symptoms) over many years. This process is characterized by plaque disruption and mural thrombosis. Angiographic data support the concept that noncritical lesions account for the majority of the ACS. Thus, the pathogenic rate-limiting mechanism of the ACS appears to be acute thrombosis and the resultant obstruction of the coronary lumen.

An operational classification is clinically helpful since it allows the simple distinction of the different types of ACS. In this classification, the ECG is the most important clinical tool. The initial ECG findings, in particular, the presence or absence of ST-segment elevation, will further define the patient's condition and dictate treatment options.

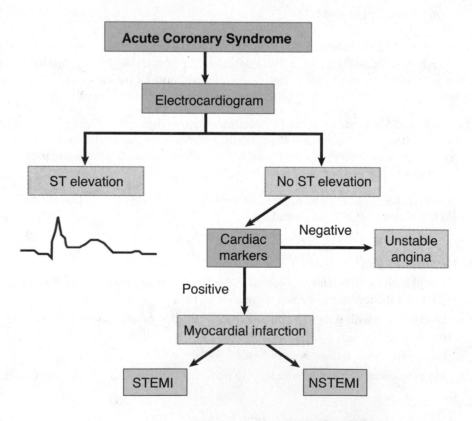

Figure 5-3. Acute Coronary Syndrome

Unstable Angina (UA) and NSTEMI

UA and NSTEMI are closely related in terms of clinical presentation and pathogenesis, but patients with these conditions have widely varying risks. Both are usually caused by atherosclerotic CAD and present an increased risk for death and MI.

- NSTEMI is more severe than UA, and is considered to have occurred if ischemia produces damage detectable by biochemical markers of myocardial injury (troponin I or CK-MB).

- If there are no detectable serum markers of myocardial injury 12–18 hours after symptom onset, the patient should be diagnosed with UA.

- At the time of presentation, UA and NSTEMI may be indistinguishable and can be identically managed.

- Therefore, in establishing the diagnosis of NSTEMI, cardiac troponins (elevated enzymes show evidence of infarction) should be used to distinguish this entity from UA.

Outcomes in UA/NSTEMI are generally better than in STEMI, but certain UA/NSTEMI patients are at high risk for MI or death, and it is important to identify these patients at initial screening because they may require intensive monitoring and management.

Thrombolytic therapy is beneficial in patients with STEMI, but is not effective in UA or NSTEMI and may be harmful.

Unstable angina is sometimes referred to as "crescendo" or "preinfarction" angina. Typically, it is defined as angina of increasing severity, frequency, duration; angina showing increasing resistance to nitrates; or angina occurring at rest. Experts also regard *any new-onset angina* as unstable. Sudden change in the pattern of angina usually means a physical change within the coronary arteries, such as hemorrhage into an atherosclerotic plaque or rupture of a plaque with intermittent thrombus formation.

About 35% of patients with the clinical syndrome of UA will already have coronary thrombosis on catheterization. In fact, untreated UA progresses to MI in 50% of cases, thus the patient with new-onset or unstable angina should be hospitalized for intensive medical treatment.

Most patients with NSTEMI have a normal physical examination. An abnormal ECG, particularly dynamic ST-segment deviation (≥0.5 mm), or new T-wave inversion (≥2 mm), will confirm the diagnosis, but the ECG may be normal or show minor changes in up to 50% of cases.

High-risk features for patients with presumed UA/NSTEMI include:

- Repetitive or prolonged chest pain (>10 min)
- Elevated cardiac biomarkers
- Persistent ECG changes of ST depression ≥0.5 mm or new T-wave inversion
- Hemodynamic instability (SBP <90)
- Sustained ventricular tachycardia
- Syncope
- LV ejection fraction <40%
- Prior angioplasty or prior CABG
- Diabetes
- Chronic kidney disease

General management

Aspirin is recommended (unless contraindicated) in all patients. High-risk patients should be treated with aggressive medical management and arrangements should be made for coronary angiography and possible revascularization, except in those with severe comorbidities. Age alone should not be a barrier to aggressive therapy.

Medical management

Antiplatelet therapy (beyond aspirin): Early treatment should be initiated with aspirin and clopidogrel or prasugrel, with the following considerations:

- Avoid clopidogrel in patients likely to require emergency coronary bypass surgery. Prasugrel and ticagrelor are alternatives to clopidogrel.
- If possible, discontinue clopidogrel 5 days before coronary bypass surgery.
- Use ticagrelor in addition to aspirin for acute coronary syndromes. It is not clearly better than clopidogrel or prasugrel.
- Give heparin along with the recommended antiplatelet therapy for UA/NSTEMI.

Antithrombin therapy: Give unfractionated heparin or subcutaneous enoxaparin until angiography or for 48–72 hours. The enoxaparin dose must be reduced in patients with impaired renal function.

Glycoprotein (GP) IIb/IIIa inhibitors: This class of antithrombotic agents inhibits platelet function by blocking a key receptor involved in platelet aggregation. The use of these agents provides a more comprehensive platelet blockade than the combination of aspirin and heparin.

- These drugs take advantage of the fact that platelets play an important role in the development of ischemic complications that may occur in patients with UA/NSTEMI.
- Tirofiban or eptifibatide is particularly recommended in high-risk patients in whom an invasive strategy is planned.
- Concomitant tirofiban is particularly beneficial and recommended in patients with diabetes.
- Complications include bleeding and thrombocytopenia (occurs with all GP IIb/IIa agents; incidence ranges 1–5.5% in clinical studies; an immune mechanism is likely responsible; all patients receiving parenteral GP IIb/IIa antagonists should be monitored for 24 hours for development of thrombocytopenia).

Other: A beta blocker should be given unless contraindicated. IV nitroglycerin (NTG) can be given for refractory pain.

In patients with diabetes, good glycemic control should be targeted in the hospital and after discharge. This may require considering an insulin-based regimen in hospital.

Invasive management

Early coronary angiography (within 48 hours) and revascularization are recommended in patients with NSTEMI and high-risk features, except in patients with severe comorbidities. Pain or ischemia refractory to medical therapy and high-risk features on early exercise testing can also identify patients suitable for early invasive therapy.

ST Elevation MI

The pain of typical MI (STEMI; in the past referred to as Q wave MI) is substernal, diffuse with a pressure quality. It may radiate to the neck or jaw, shoulders, or arms. Often, the pain is accompanied by additional symptoms, such as dizziness (lightheadedness), nausea or vomiting, diaphoresis, or shortness of breath (dyspnea).

The symptoms of MI last >20 minutes and do not respond completely to nitroglycerin. The duration of the pain is variable. Pain may resolve completely after a few hours or may persist for over a day.

Elderly or diabetic patients are prone to atypical symptoms such as nausea or dyspnea as the sole symptoms of infarction. As many as 20% of MI are "silent"—that is, whatever symptoms were present did not impress the patient enough for them to seek medical care or even to remember the incident.

The exam usually shows the patient to have anxiety and pain. Diaphoresis is often present. Pulse rate may be normal, but often bradycardia is present in inferior infarction. Tachycardia is often seen with large infarctions. Blood pressure is often elevated.

Cardiac exam will usually be normal. Large infarctions may cause signs of ventricular failure or valve dysfunction. A fourth heart sound (S4) is common due to a stiffened ventricle. Mitral regurgitation may occur if papillary muscles malfunction. The second heart sound may be paradoxically split as the left ventricular contraction time increases due to LBBB and weakened left ventricle.

Later in the course of MI, other findings may be present: mild fever, pericardial friction rub, ventral septal defect murmur due to septal rupture, or severe mitral regurgitation due to papillary muscle rupture.

STEMI is defined as clinical symptoms consistent with ACS and ECG features including any of these:

- Persistent ST-segment elevation of ≥1 mm in two contiguous limb leads
- ST-segment elevation of ≥2 mm in two contiguous chest leads
- New LBBB pattern

Initially, you don't need increased cardiac biomarkers (troponin, CPK-MB, etc.) to make the diagnosis of STEMI (although these are usually eventually positive at some point during the course of the disease).

Initial nonspecific management for all patients with possible MI (anyone with a compatible chest pain history) is to keep them on a cardiac monitor. Oxygen therapy and an IV line should be established as quickly as possible. Aspirin should be given unless contraindicated, as early as possible. Nitroglycerin and pain control (morphine) should be given as required.

Patients with STEMI usually have a completely occluded coronary artery with thrombus at the site of a ruptured plaque. This eventually leads to myonecrosis. Restoring coronary patency (emergency reperfusion) as promptly as possible is a key determinant of short-term and long-term outcomes.

Patients with STEMI **who present within 12 hours of the onset of ischemic symptoms** should have a reperfusion strategy implemented promptly. Reperfusion may be obtained with fibrinolytic therapy or percutaneous coronary intervention (PCI).

Patients presenting with NSTEMI will not benefit from thrombolytics.

Note

The strongest indication for PCI is an acute coronary syndrome.

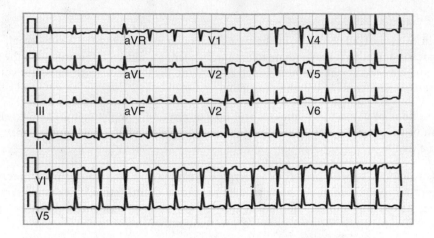

Figure 5-4. Anteroseptal STEMI with Changes in V_1–V_3

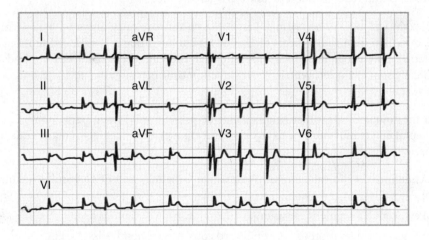

Figure 5-5. Inferior STEMI with Changes in II, III, and aVF

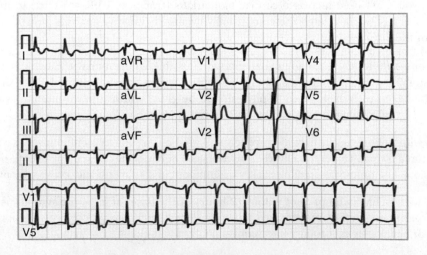

Figure 5-6. NSTEMI Affecting Leads II, III, and aVF

Table 5-2. Localization of STEMI

Area of Infarction	EKG Changes (Q Waves, ST Elevation, T Wave Inversions)	Artery Involved
Inferior	II, III, aVF	Right coronary
Anteroseptal	V_1–V_3	Left anterior descending
Anterior	V_2–V_4	Left anterior descending
Lateral	I, aVL, V_4, V_5, and V_6	Left anterior descending or circumflex
Posterior	V_1–V_2: tall broad initial R wave, ST depression, tall upright T wave; usually occurs in association with inferior or lateral MI	Posterior descending

Table 5-3. Typical Electrocardiographic Evolution of a STEMI

EKG Abnormality	Onset	Disappearance
Hyperacute T waves (tall, peaked T waves in leads facing infarction)	Immediately	6–24 hours
ST-segment elevation	Immediately	1–6 weeks
Q waves longer than 0.04 seconds	One to several days	Years to never
T wave inversion	6–24 hours	Months to years

Emergent reperfusion therapy

The choice of reperfusion therapy is between PCI and thrombolysis therapy. PCI is the best available treatment if provided promptly. PCI improves short-term and long-term outcomes (reduction of deaths and MI) in patients with STEMI presenting within 12 hours when compared with thrombolytic therapy. This benefit over thrombolysis may occur only if the additional time delay associated with PCI is <1 hour. In general, a time delay of 90 minutes from first medical encounter to PCI is the maximum desirable. For patients presenting with STEMI at a facility without PCI access, transfer to another facility capable of performing PCI usually takes too long. Where PCI is delayed or not available, reperfusion with thrombolytic therapy should occur unless contraindicated.

Thrombolytics (Fibrinolytics)

Thrombolytics such as streptokinase or tissue-type plasminogen activator (tPA) restore perfusion to the ischemic area by lysing the clot, thereby reducing infarct size and improving survival.

Thrombolysis benefits patients with all types of ST elevation infarction, but the benefit is several times greater in those with **anterior infarction**. The earlier the treatment is given, the greater the absolute benefit. The greatest benefit is in patients with ST elevation or new left bundle branch block who have had symptoms for <12 hours.

Streptokinase and alteplase are given by IV infusion. Reteplase and tenecteplase can be given by rapid bolus injection. tPA is the most common agent used in the U.S. Prolonged persistence of antibodies to streptokinase may reduce the effectiveness of subsequent treatment; therefore, streptokinase should not be used if used within the previous 12 months in the same patient. Complexity of administration differs among the different thrombolytics: tenecteplase and reteplase are ready in about one minute; for streptokinase or tPA, the typical time from physician order to administration is 12 to 15 minutes.

Bottom line: consider a thrombolytic agent as an alternative to primary PCI in suitable candidates with:

- ST-elevation MI (>1 mm ST elevation in 2 contiguous leads)
- New LBBB

Contraindications to thrombolytic therapy:
Absolute contraindications:

- Active bleeding or bleeding diathesis
- Significant closed head or facial trauma within 3 months
- Suspected aortic dissection
- Prior intracranial hemorrhage
- Ischemic stroke within 3 months

Relative contraindications:

- Recent major surgery (<3 weeks)
- Traumatic or prolonged cardiopulmonary resuscitation
- Recent (within 4 weeks) internal bleeding
- Active peptic ulcer
- Severe, poorly controlled HTN
- Ischemic stroke (<3 months)

Late presentation (>12 hours after symptom onset): Reperfusion therapy with either PCI or fibrinolysis is not routinely recommended in patients who are asymptomatic and hemodynamically stable, and who present >12 hours after symptom onset.

Other interventions may include coronary artery bypass grafting (CABG). CABG surgery may occasionally be more appropriate—particularly in patients who have suitable anatomy and are not candidates for fibrinolysis or PCI. CABG surgery may also be considered in patients with cardiogenic shock or in association with mechanical repair.

Adjuvant therapy used together with reperfusion

Antiplatelet Therapy
Aspirin should be given to all patients with presumed STEMI unless contraindicated, and, in the absence of significant side effects, low-dose therapy should be continued in the long term.

Clopidogrel or prasugrel should be prescribed in addition to aspirin for patients undergoing PCI with a stent. Ticagrelor is an alternative to clopidogrel or prasugrel.

In patients selected for fibrinolytic therapy, clopidogrel should be given in addition to aspirin, unless contraindicated. Note, however, that if it is thought that the patient is likely to require CABG acutely, clopidogrel should be withheld.

Clopidogrel should be continued for at least a month after fibrinolytic therapy, or for up to 9–12 months after stent implantation, depending on the type of stent used.

Antithrombin Therapy
With PCI: Antithrombin therapy should be used in conjunction with PCI. The dose of unfractionated heparin therapy will depend on concomitant use of glycoprotein (GP) IIb/IIIa inhibitors. It may be advisable to give a bolus of heparin while the patient is in transit to the catheterization laboratory.

The role of enoxaparin in acute STEMI in conjunction with PCI remains to be fully determined, but it appears to be safe and effective.

With fibrinolysis: Antithrombin therapy should be used with fibrin-specific fibrinolytic agents.

IV unfractionated heparin should be given as an initial bolus, adjusted to attain the activated partial thromboplastin time (APTT) at 1.5 to 2 times control. IV unfractionated heparin is used when rapid reversal is needed. The half-life is shorter with unfractionated heparin.

Glycoprotein IIb/IIIa Inhibitors
It is reasonable to use abciximab with primary PCI. Epifibatide and tirofiban are the other GPIIb/IIIa inhibitors. Full-dose GP IIb/IIIa inhibitors should be avoided with fibrinolytic therapy as there is evidence of excessive bleeding (including intracranial hemorrhage) with this combination.

The combination of GP IIb/IIIa inhibitors with reduced doses of fibrinolytic therapy is not recommended. There is no significant advantage over full-dose fibrinolytic therapy alone, and the risk of bleeding is increased, particularly in the elderly.

Cardiac surgery

Emergency bypass surgery should be considered in patients with STEMI and: (*1*) failed PCI with persistent pain or hemodynamic instability and coronary anatomy suitable for surgery or (*2*) persistent or recurrent ischemia refractory to medical therapy and suitable anatomy.

Recommended discharge medications after ACS

1. Aspirin: All patients should take daily unless contraindicated.
2. Clopidogrel: There is evidence that clopidogrel or prasugrel should be prescribed for up to 9–12 months after acute myocardial infarction, particularly after stent placement. Clopidogrel may also be prescribed as an alternative when aspirin is contraindicated, or to those intolerant to aspirin, in patients with recurrent cardiac events.
3. B-blocker: These drugs should be prescribed for all patients after an ACS unless contraindicated, and continued indefinitely. Metoprolol and carvedilol particularly should be used in patients after ACS who have heart failure.
4. ACE inhibitors: Should be given in patients with ACS in CHF, left ventricular dysfunction (ejection fraction <40%). Its use should be reviewed later on the course of the patient and discontinued if the heart failure resolves.
5. Statins: Statin therapy should be *initiated in the hospital* in all patients with ACS (the exception is the rare ACS that is not related to atherosclerosis).
6. Nitrates: Long-acting nitrates (isosorbide) should be reserved for the patients with persistent chest pain.
7. Warfarin: It is recommended after ACS *only* for those at high risk of systemic thromboembolism because of atrial fibrillation or mural thrombus.

Note

A mnemonic for remembering issues to consider at the time of discharge is **"ABCDE"** (aspirin and anti-anginals, beta blockers and blood pressure, cholesterol and cigarettes, diet and diabetes, education and exercise).

Secondary prevention through the control or elimination of known risk factors for coronary artery disease (e.g., hyperglycemia in patients with diabetes mellitus, HTN control, tobacco cessation, physical inactivity) also should be part of discharge planning.

> You are asked by your patient, who has a history of ischemic heart disease, about drug treatments that have been shown to decrease mortality in his case. (It doesn't matter if he has stable angina or prior history of acute coronary syndrome.)

Answer: **Lipid lowering agents (statins), ASA, B-blocking agents and CABG in patients with triple vessel disease or left main disease.**

Other testing in ACS

Exercise ECG testing: Increasingly, submaximal testing is performed 4–7 days after infarction. A maximal test can be performed at 3–6 weeks postinfarction. It is used to assess prognosis and to identify those patients with reversible ischemia who should then have an angiogram (if one has not been done) to assess the need for coronary artery bypass graft.

Myocardial perfusion imaging can be performed before hospital discharge to assess the extent of residual ischemia if the patient has not already undergone cardiac catheterization and angiography.

Complications of ACS

Electrical disturbances dysrhythmias

- Bradycardia: sinus, atrioventricular junctional, idioventricular. These are treated acutely with atropine and temporary pacing if severe.
- Premature beats: atrial, ventricular. No treatment is needed for ectopy such as these.
- Tachyarrhythmias (supraventricular): atrial tachycardia, atrial fibrillation, atrial flutter, AV junctional; are seldom caused by ischemia
- Tachyarrhythmias (ventricular): ventricular tachycardia, accelerated idioventricular rhythm, ventricular fibrillation

Conduction Abnormalities
- Atrioventricular nodal: first-, second-, and third-degree block
- Intraventricular: hemiblocks (left anterior, left posterior), bundle branch block, third-degree atrioventricular block

Pump dysfunction
- Contractile dysfunction: left ventricular, right ventricular, and biventricular failure; true ventricular aneurysm; infarct expansion
- Mechanical disruption: acute mitral regurgitation (papillary muscle dysfunction or rupture), ventricular septal rupture, free wall rupture, pseudoaneurysm; treated with emergency surgical repair
- Electromechanical dissociation

Ischemia

- Postinfarction ischemia: ischemia in the infarct and ischemia distant to the infarct
- Early recurrent infarction or infarct extension
- *Postinfarction angina* after thrombolytics or PCI should be treated with *bypass surgery*

Pericarditis—Dressler syndrome (late)

Treated with aspirin, NSAIDs, and later steroids if there is no response.

Thromboembolic

- Mural thrombus with systemic embolism
- Deep vein thrombosis with prolonged immobilization

Sudden cardiac death

Most often due to arrhythmia.

- Ventricular fibrillation (most commonly)
- Ventricular tachycardia

Right ventricular infarction

Accompanies 30% of inferior MIs. It is diagnosed with RV leads and treated with fluids.

Nonatherosclerotic Acute Coronary Syndromes

Although thrombotic complications of the atherosclerotic process account for most cases of acute coronary syndromes, there are a few rare etiologic factors that have been proposed as causes of or contributors to acute coronary occlusion. These causes include coronary artery spasm, spontaneous coronary dissection, coronary artery embolization, coronary arteritis, and hypercoagulability states such as factor V gene mutation, deficiencies of proteins C and S, antithrombin III deficiency, antiphospholipid antibody syndrome, and prothrombin gene mutation.

Prinzmetal angina, or variant angina, is a very uncommon condition in which episodes of severe angina are triggered when one of the major coronary arteries suddenly goes into spasm. These episodes are accompanied by ST-segment elevation on the ECG. Although the spasm almost always terminates spontaneously, Prinzmetal angina may be associated with acute MI, serious ventricular arrhythmias, and sudden death.

As opposed to typical angina, Prinzmetal angina usually occurs during periods of rest, most often at night and in the early morning hours. Frequently, episodes appear in clusters. In men, Prinzmetal angina is often associated with atherosclerosis; in women it is not. Women with Prinzmetal tend to have few risk factors for CAD, though many have a history of migraine headaches (another condition associated with arterial spasm).

Exercise testing and routine coronary angiography usually give normal results. Ergonovine has been used to trigger coronary artery spasm in susceptible patients, confirming the diagnosis. Treatment with calcium channel blockers or nitrates eliminates spasm in most of these patients. Once adequately treated, their prognosis is good.

During an acute episode of pain and ST segment elevation, you cannot tell who has Prinzmetal variant angina and who has an acute ST elevation MI. Therefore, you must initially treat everyone with chest pain and ST elevation as if they were having an acute MI. Prinzmetal angina can be confirmed only after coronary angiography.

Causes of MI without Coronary Atherosclerosis

- Vasculitis
    - Systemic lupus erythematosus
    - Polyarteritis nodosa
    - Takayasu arteritis
    - Mucocutaneous lymph node syndrome (Kawasaki)
- Anomalous origin of coronary artery
- Coronary spasm
    - Variant angina
    - Cocaine abuse
- Coronary artery embolus
    - Atrial myxoma
    - Atrial or ventricular thrombus
- Hypercoagulable states
    - Polycythemia vera
    - Thrombocytosis
    - Factor V Leiden
    - Protein C deficiency
    - Antiphospholipid antibodies

CONGESTIVE HEART FAILURE (CHF)

Case 1:

A 62-year-old man with hypertension and dyslipidemia presents with dyspnea and lower-extremity edema for 2 months. On exam there is jugular venous distention (about 9 cm.), an S3 gallop, and the apical impulse is displaced to the left of the mid-clavicular line at the 6th intercostal space. The chest x-ray shows enlarged cardiac silhouette. The echocardiogram shows a dilated left ventricle with an ejection fraction of 35%.

Case 2:

A 57-year-old man with history of multiple myeloma presents with dyspnea and lower-extremity edema for 2 months. On exam there is jugular venous distention (about 8 cm.), an audible S4, and the apical impulse is non-displaced at the 5th intercostal space. The chest x-ray shows normal cardiac silhouette. The echocardiogram shows a thickened left ventricle with an ejection fraction of 65%.

Heart failure (HF) arises from the inability of the ventricle to efficiently pump blood throughout the circulation. Clinically HF presents with symptoms of breathlessness, exercise intolerance, and fatigue (see below signs and symptoms).

As HF evolves, changes in vascular function, blood volume, and neurohumoral status occur throughout the body. These changes serve as compensatory mechanisms to help maintain cardiac output (primarily by the Frank-Starling mechanism) and arterial blood pressure (by systemic vasoconstriction). However, these compensatory changes over time can worsen cardiac function. Cardiac changes during HF include: increased end-diastolic volume; ventricular dilatation or hypertrophy; decreased stroke volume and cardiac output; reduced ejection fraction (systolic dysfunction) or impaired filling (diastolic dysfunction). Compensatory mechanisms during HF include:

- **Cardiac:** Frank-Starling mechanism, tachycardia, ventricular dilatation;
- **Neuronal:** increased sympathetic adrenergic activity, reduced cardiac vagal activity;
- **Hormonal:** activation of angiotensin-aldosterone system, vasopressin, catecholamines, and natriuretic peptides.

In clinical practice, HF is commonly categorized by whether the abnormality is due to contraction or relaxation of the heart. *Systolic HF* (systolic dysfunction) is due to a loss of contractile strength of the myocardium accompanied by ventricular dilatation. This type of HF is also accompanied by a decrease in normal ventricular emptying (usually ejection fraction <45%). Examples of systolic HF include ischemic cardiomyopathy and dilated cardiomyopathy (Case 1 in this section).

Heart failure with preserved ejection fraction (diastolic dysfunction) occurs when the filling of one or both ventricles is impaired while the emptying capacity is normal (echocardiogram confirms that the ejection fraction is normal). The infiltrative cardiomyopathies (amyloidosis) are typical examples (Case 2 in this section).

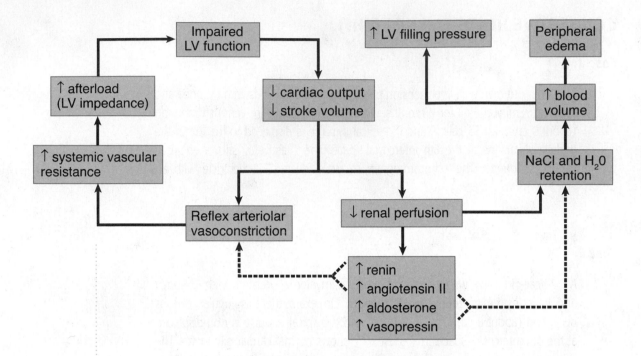

Figure 5-7. Inter-related Cycles in Congestive Heart Failure

Congestive HF indicates a clinical syndrome of dyspnea and fatigue as well as evidence of features of circulatory congestion (peripheral edema, elevated jugular venous pressure [JVP]). In heart failure, intravascular congestion occurs with elevation of left ventricular diastolic and pulmonary venous pressures that eventually causes transudation of fluid from the pulmonary capillaries into the interstitial space. **Pulmonary edema** develops when the rate of fluid accumulation goes above the rate of lymphatic absorption. Pulmonary edema is detected by audible crackles, increased JVP and edema on exam, and chest x-ray findings.

Decompensated HF or exacerbation of HF denotes worsening of symptoms and clinical findings in pre-existing HF. This can be due to precipitating factors such as non-adherance to medication, increase in dietary salt, acute ischemia, tachycardia, or pulmonary infection.

In evaluating patients with HF or worsening of pre-existing HF, it is also important to exclude precipitating factors. Commonly, HF manifests for the first time when a precipitating factor places additional burden on the heart. Such factors include:

- Cardiac ischemia and myocardial infarction
- Infections (especially pulmonary infections)
- Arrhythmias (especially atrial fibrillation)
- Excessive dietary salt (commonly after holiday meals)
- Uncontrolled hypertension (especially after abrupt cessation of anti-hypertensive medication)
- Thyrotoxicosis
- Anemia

HF may occur as a consequence of most causes of heart disease, but ischemic heart disease is responsible for over 70% of all cases in the western world. Other common causes include: hypertensive heart disease, the cardiomyopathies (idiopathic, alcohol related, etc.), and valvular and congenital heart diseases.

Symptoms of HF include:

- Dyspnea (differentiate from pulmonary dyspnea—*See* Table 5-4)
- Orthopnea
- Paroxysmal nocturnal dyspnea
- Fatigue, weakness

Clinical Pearl

In the work-up of patients with new-onset HF, always try to identify potentially reversible causes.

Clinical Pearl

In the work-up of patients with exacerbation of HF, always:

- Check cardiac enzymes to exclude myocardial ischemia or infarction
- Do a chest x-ray to exclude infection

Table 5-4. Most Common Causes of Acute Pulmonary Edema

Ischemia
Arrhythmia
Non-adherence with medication
Dietary indiscretion
Infection

Physical findings in HF:

- Pulmonary rales
- Peripheral edema, ascites
- Hepatomegaly
- Jugular venous distention
- Displaced apical impulse (systolic HF)

The severity of heart failure is commonly classified by using a HF staging system. The New York Heart Association Functional Classification (NYHA staging system) relates symptoms to everyday activities and the patient's quality of life:

- **Class I:** patients have no limitation of activity; they suffer no symptoms from ordinary activities
- **Class II:** patients with slight, mild limitation of activity; they are comfortable with rest or with mild exertion
- **Class III:** patients with marked limitation of activity; they are comfortable only at rest
- **Class IV:** patients are confined to bed or chair; any physical activity brings on discomfort and symptoms occur at rest

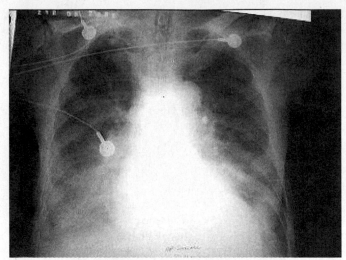

Copyright 2007 Gold Standard Multimedia Inc.

Figure 5-8. Chest X-ray Demonstrating Acute Exacerbation
of Congestive Heart Failure

Diagnosis. Echocardiography is the test-of-choice to confirm the diagnosis of HF and to classify the type (systolic vs. diastolic). With the echocardiogram, the clinician is able to determine ejection fraction and identify valvular heart disease as well as other cardiac anomalies (dilated ventricle, thickened ventricle, etc.).

Chest x-rays are also used to aid in the diagnosis of heart failure. They may show cardiomegaly, vascular redistribution, Kerley B-lines, and interstitial edema.

Electrocardiogram is used to identify ventricular hypertrophy and/or the presence of ischemic heart disease, arrhythmias, or conduction delays which may cause or precipitate HF.

Brain Natriuretic Peptide (BNP) is a polypeptide secreted by the heart in response to excessive stretching of the myocytes. It is a valuable tool in the evaluation of patients with presumed HF or decompensated HF in the acute setting. The BNP is almost always elevated (97% sensitivity) in patients with decompensated HF. Normal BNP excludes CHF as the cause of dyspnea.

Management. The treatment goals in HF are to improve hemodynamics, relieve symptoms (improve quality of life), and prolong survival. Remember, always evaluate for reversible causes at the same time.

Non-pharmacologic treatment includes primarily reduction of salt intake.

For pharmacologic treatment, ACE inhibitors are the basis of therapy and recommended for all patients with HF (especially systolic HF), irrespective of blood pressure status. They improve survival and reduce ventricular hypertrophy—and eventually, symptoms. ACE inhibitors through vasodilation reduce preload and afterload, thereby reducing right atrial, pulmonary arterial, and pulmonary capillary wedge pressures. All ACE inhibitors have been studied and are considered equal in terms of HF treatment. Angiotensin receptor blockers (ARB) are acceptable alternatives if the patient is unable to tolerate ACE inhibitors (cough, angioedema).

Note

BNP is used acutely if the cause of dyspnea is not clear.

Diuretic therapy, especially loop diuretics, is the treatment of choice for the relief of acute pulmonary edema symptoms. Several classes are used but the loop diuretics (furosemide) class is the most commonly used. Thiazide diuretics (hydrochlorothiazide) are useful only in mild HF. Spironolactone and eplerenone (aldosterone antagonists) have been used as add-on therapy to ACE inhibitors in severe heart failure to prolong survival by presumed aldosterone inhibition.

Table 5-5. Vasodilators Used in Congestive Heart Failure

Drug	Site of Action	Route of Administration	Complications
Captopril Enalapril Lisinopril	Arteriolar and venous ACE inhibitor	Oral	Rash, nonproductive cough, proteinuria, renal failure, taste disturbance, agranulo-cytosis, hypotension
Nitroprusside	Arteriolar and venous	IV	Thiocyanate toxicity, methemoglobinemia
Nitroglycerin	Venous (arteriolar at high doses IV)	SL, IV, cutaneous ointment, or patch	Headache, postural hypotension, methemoglobinemia
Isosorbide dinitrate	Venous	Oral or SL	Headache, postural hypotension
Hydralazine	Arteriolar	Oral	Positive ANA, SLE-like syndrome (10–20% if >400 mg/d) drug fever, rash

Chronic adrenergic activation has been implicated in the pathogenesis of HF and thus β-**adrenergic blocking** agents are an important part of HF therapy. Along with ACE inhibitors, beta blockers have been demonstrated to decrease mortality, reduce hospitalizations, improve functional class, and improve ejection fraction in several large-scale, randomized, placebo-controlled trials.

Start patients on beta blockers after stabilization of symptoms with diuretic and ACE inhibitor therapy, irrespective of blood pressure status. The beta blockers carvedilol and metoprolol have been demonstrated in trials.

Note

Bottom line

ACE inhibitor (any one will do) and a diuretic are considered first line for all patients with HF. Once the patient is stable, add carvedilol or metoprolol. Don't substitute β-blockers in HF since not all β-blockers have the same efficacy.

Table 5-6. Commonly Used Diuretics in Heart Failure

Drug	Site of Action	Complications
Thiazides (inhibits NaCl cotransport); used mostly for treatment of hypertension • Hydrochlorothiazide • Chlorothiazide	Distal tubule	Hyponatremia, hypokalemia, hypercalcemia, metabolic alkalosis, hyperuricemia, allergy, agranulocytosis, leukopenia, pancreatitis, glucose intolerance
Indapamide	Distal tube (direct vasodilator)	As above, but hypokalemia and lipid abnormalities less common
Loop diuretics (inhibitors Na/K, 2Cl cotransport); most commonly used diuretics in heart failure • Furosemide • Ethacrynic acid • Bumetanide	Loop of Henle	Hyponatremia, hypokalemia, hypocalcemia, metabolic alkalosis, hyperuricemia, interstitial nephritis, ototoxicity, thrombocytopenia, agranulocytosis, leukopenia
Potassium-sparing diuretics • Spironolactone (aldosterone antagonist)	Distal tubule	Hyperkalemia, gynecomastia (spironolactone only)

Other vasodilators, such as a combination of hydralazine and isosorbide, may be used when ACE inhibitors and ARBs are not tolerated or contraindicated (renal failure). There is a reduction in death and a decrease in hospitalization when a combination of hydralazine and isosorbide is used.

In severe HF and especially if there is no improvement of symptoms while the patient is on standard therapy (diuretic, ACE inhibitor, and beta blocker), the **addition of spironolactone** may be of benefit. The addition of spironolactone in patients with severe CHF significantly reduces (about 30% relative risk) death and hospitalizations among treated patients. Spironolactone is used in patients with NYHA class III-IV. Once the patient is started on spironolactone, serum potassium levels have to be monitored closely.

Eplerenone is an alternative to spironolactone that does not cause gynecomastia.

The addition of inotropic agents to patients with severe HF improves symptoms and quality of life and reduces hospitalizations but does not improve survival. The most commonly used inotropic agent is **digitalis**. Digitalis inhibits Na+/K+ - ATPase pump which results in increased intracellular concentration of Na+ and decreased exchanges of intracellular Ca2+. The end result is an increase in intracellular concentration of Ca2+ which results in improved cardiac contractility.

Cardiac glycosides work by inhibition of Na^+/K^+-ATPase pump, which results in:
- Increased intracellular concentration of Na^+
- Decreased exchange of intracellular Ca^{2+} for extracellular Na^+
- The end result is an increase in the intracellular concentration of Ca^{2+}, which gives the (+) inotropic effect characteristic of glycosides

Note

Agents which lower mortality in systolic dysfunction
- ACE (ARB)
- Beta blockers
- Spironolactone (or eplerenone)

Remember that K^+ and digitalis compete for myocardium binding sites. Hyperkalemia will decrease digitalis activity, whereas hypokalemia results in toxicity.

Digitalis will increase both the force and the velocity of the myocardial contraction. It will also promote a more complete emptying of the ventricles.

It is used for the treatment of:

- CHF
- Atrial fibrillation/flutter
- Paroxysmal atrial tachycardia/SVT

Conditions which predispose to digitalis toxicity are:

- Renal insufficiency
- Electrolyte disturbances (hypokalemia, hypercalcemia, hypomagnesemia)
- Advanced age
- Sinoatrial and atrioventricular block
- Thyroid disease, especially hypothyroidism

Note

Agents which improve heart failure symptoms but do not reduce mortality:

- Digoxin
- Diuretics

Table 5-7. Drug Interactions Associated with Digoxin

Drug	Effect*	Mechanism
Quinidine	Increase	Decreases renal clearance of digoxin
Verapamil, diltiazem	Increase	Decreases renal clearance of digoxin
Cholestyramine, colestipol	Decrease	Binds digoxin in GI tract; interferes with enterohepatic circulation
Spironolactone	Increase	Inhibits tubular secretion of digoxin
Thiazides, furosemide	Increase	Diuretic-induced hypokalemia and/or bumetanide hypomagnesemia potentiates digitalis action

*Increase indicates enhances digitalis effect; decreases diminishes digitalis effect.

Toxic Effects of Digitalis

- Nausea and vomiting
- Gynecomastia
- Blurred vision
- Yellow halo around objects
- Arrhythmias—commonly paroxysmal atrial tachycardia (PAT) with block, PVCs (premature ventricular contractions), and bradycardia

Treatment for Intoxication

- Stop drug
- Lidocaine and phenytoin (for arrhythmia)
- Digibind only for acute overdose

Sympathomimetic amines (dopamine, doputamine) and phosphodiesterase inhibitors (amrinone, milrinone) are sometimes used in the management of severe **acute** HF (hospitalized patients). They must be administered by IV infusion and need continuous monitoring of the blood pressure and cardiac rhythm.

Monitoring of patients with HF includes calculation of fluid intake and excretion (in the hospital) as well as monitoring body weight (in the out-patient setting).

In refractory HF (defined as progression of HF despite standard treatment), the patient may be considered for: biventricular pacing, implantable defibrillator, and heart transplantation.

Medical Devices for Systolic Dysfunction

The automatic implantable cardioverter/defibrillator (AICD) is a standard therapy for ischemic dilated cardiomyopathy. Since the most common cause of death in CHF is an arrhythmia, it is logical that a device which interrupts arrhythmia will lower mortality. A biventricular pacemaker will "resynchronize" the heart when there is dilated cardiomyopathy and a QRS >120 mSec. When there is a wide QRS, the 2 ventricles do not beat or depolarize in synchrony. When you put a biventricular pacemaker into the heart, this will "resynchronize" the 2 ventricles, resulting in an immediate decrease in symptoms.

When do I answer AICD?

- Dilated cardiomyopathy with a persistent ejection fraction <35%

When do I answer biventricular pacemaker?

- Dilated cardiomyopathy with a QRS wider than 120 mSec

Summary of therapy for dilated cardiomyopathy

The following classes of medications lower mortality:
- ACE inhibitor or ARBs; use one or the other, not both
- Beta blockers
- Spironolactone (or eplerenone)
- AICD
- Biventricular pacemaker (if QRS >120 mSec)

ACE inhibitors are a class effect; there is no difference in efficacy between the drugs. There is no benefit to adding an ARB to an ACE inhibitor. With beta blockers, not all the drugs are equal; those that benefit mortality in CHF are metoprolol, carvedilol, and bisoprolol. Biventricular pacemakers and cardiac resynchronization therapy also have implantable defibrillator function.

Clinical Pearl

Diastolic HF may worsen when diuretics and vasodilators are used excessively. The goal in diastolic HF is to slow the heart rate with beta blockers and calcium channel blockers (verapamil, diltiazem) in order to allow adequate diastolic filling.

Pulmonary Edema

Pulmonary edema is considered a medical emergency and requires hospitalization. It leads to impaired gas exchange and may cause respiratory failure. There are non-cardiogenic causes of pulmonary edema but in this section we will discuss only cardiogenic pulmonary edema. Cardiogenic pulmonary edema is caused by an acute increase in left ventricular pressure due to ventricular dysfunction which leads to fluid accumulation in the pulmonary interstitium.

Signs and Symptoms
- Increased respiratory rate
- Cough with expectoration (pink frothy sputum)
- Cyanosis
- Nocturnal dyspnea
- Rales, rhonchi, wheezing

Chest X-ray Findings
- Prominent pulmonary vessels
- Effusions
- Enlarged cardiac silhouette
- Kerley B lines

EKG is used to determine if an arrhythmia is contributing to the development of the pulmonary edema.

Treatment
- Oxygen
- Diuretic therapy (furosemide) reduces preload
- Morphine sulfate; side effects include respiratory depression and rarely hypotension
- Sitting the patient upright
- Nitroglycerin to reduce preload
- Digoxin if in atrial fibrillation
- IV ACE inhibitors

VALVULAR HEART DISEASE

Mitral Stenosis

Definition. Most common lesion caused by rheumatic fever consisting of thickened mitral valve leaflets, fused commissures, and chordae tendineae. May result in right ventricular failure.

Etiology. Two-thirds of patients with mitral stenosis are women.
- Usually due to abnormalities of the mitral leaflets
- Most cases are secondary to rheumatic fever
- Rarely due to a congenital defect

Pathogenesis

- Mitral valve stenosis impedes left ventricular filling
- Increased left atrial pressure is referred to the lungs, causing pulmonary congestion
- Forward cardiac output becomes reduced, secondary pulmonary vasoconstriction occurs, and eventually right ventricular failure results

Clinical Symptoms. Usually manifest slowly over years.

- Dyspnea
- Orthopnea
- Paroxysmal nocturnal dyspnea
- Fatigue
- Wasting
- Hemoptysis (due to rupture of pulmonary vessels)
- Systemic embolism (due to stagnation of blood in an enlarged left atrium)
- Hoarseness (due to impingement of an enlarged left atrium on the recurrent laryngeal nerve)
- Right-sided heart failure
    - Hepatomegaly
    - Ascites
    - Peripheral edema

Physical Signs

- Atrial fibrillation (irregular cardiac rhythm)
- Pulmonary rales
- Decreased pulse pressure
- Loud S_1
- Opening snap following S_2
- Diastolic rumble (low-pitched apical murmur)
- Sternal lift (due to right ventricular enlargement)

Diagnosis

EKG

- May show signs of right ventricular hypertrophy
- May show left and right atrial abnormalities
- Atrial fibrillation often occurs

Chest X-ray

- Large left atrium (indicated by a double-density right heart border, posterior displacement of esophagus, and elevated left mainstem bronchus), straightening of the left heart border
- May show signs of pulmonary hypertension, including Kerley B lines and increased vascular markings
- Large pulmonary artery

Echocardiography

- Shows thickening of mitral valve leaflets and a reduction in the excursion and area of the valve leaflets
- May also show left atrial enlargement

Treatment

Medical Therapy

- Diuretics and salt-restricted diet
- Digitalis to control the ventricular rate in patients with AF
- Anticoagulants in patients with AF
- Balloon valvulotomy is the standard of care for MS

Surgical Management

- Indicated when patient remains symptomatic (functional class III) despite medical therapy
- Mitral commissurotomy or valve replacement, if balloon dilation fails
- Pulmonary hypertension is not a contraindication for surgery

Mitral Regurgitation

Definition. Backflow of blood from the left ventricle into the left atrium, due to inadequate functioning (insufficiency) of the mitral valve. Most commonly from ischemia.

Etiology. Due to abnormalities of the mitral leaflets, annulus, and chordae tendinea.

- Common causes are hypertension, CHF, ischemic heart disease, rheumatic fever, and any cause of dilation of the left ventricle
- Occurs more commonly in men

Table 5-8. Acute versus Chronic Etiologies of Mitral Valve Regurgitation

Acute	Chronic
• Rupture chordae tendineae (permits prolapse of a portion of a mitral valve leaflet into the left atrium) • Papillary muscle rupture • Endocarditis (may lead to valvular destruction) • Trauma	• Rheumatic heart disease (causing scarring and retraction of valve and leaflets) • Papillary muscle dysfunction • Mitral valve prolapse (click-murmur syndrome, Barlow syndrome, floppy mitral valve) • Endocarditis • Calcification of the mitral valve annulus • Accompanying hypertrophic obstructive cardiomyopathy • Congenital endocardial cushion defect, corrected transposition • Endocardial fibroelastosis • Severe left ventricular dilatation

Pathogenesis

- A portion of the left ventricular stroke volume is pumped backward into the left atrium instead of forward into the aorta, resulting in increased left atrial pressure and decreased forward cardiac output.
- Volume overload occurs, increasing preload.
- Afterload is decreased as the left ventricle empties part of its contents into the relatively low-pressure left atrium.
- This helps to compensate for the regurgitation by augmenting ejection fraction.
- Left ventricular dysfunction occurs after prolonged compensation.

Clinical Manifestations

Left ventricular failure is manifested by:

- Dyspnea
- Orthopnea
- Paroxysmal nocturnal dyspnea

Severe and chronic mitral regurgitation lead to right-sided failure presenting with:

- Edema
- Ascites
- Anorexia
- Fatigue

May also have pulmonary hypertension as a late finding.

Physical Signs

- Hyperdynamic and displaced (downward and to the left) left ventricular impulse
- Carotid upstroke diminished in volume but brisk
- Holosystolic apical murmur radiating to the axilla and often accompanied by a thrill
- S_3 heard with a soft S_1 and widely split S_2
- Distended neck veins when severe or acute

Diagnosis

- EKG shows signs of left ventricular hypertrophy and left atrial enlargement.
- Chest x-ray shows cardiac enlargement, with vascular congestion when the regurgitation has led to heart failure.
- Echocardiography: The mitral valve can prolapse into the left atrium during systole in cases of a ruptured chordae or mitral valve prolapse. Regardless of the cause, left atrial and left ventricular enlargement occurs if the condition is chronic.
- Catheterization is the single most accurate test.

Treatment. With medical therapy, the goal is to relieve symptoms by increasing forward cardiac output and reducing pulmonary venous hypertension.

- ARBs or hydralazine
- Arteriolar vasodilators (ACE inhibitors)
- Digitalis
- Diuretics

With surgery, mitral valve replacement is used. Guidelines for selecting patients with mitral regurgitation for operation:

- With significantly limiting symptoms and severe mitral regurgitation, surgery is usually indicated. The risk of surgery rises in chronic heart failure.
- In patients with regurgitation who have few or no symptoms, surgery should be deferred. Their condition may remain stable for years.
- Surgery is indicated when symptoms persist despite optimal medical management.
- Criterion is an ejection fraction <60% or left ventricular end systolic diameter >40 mm.
- Repair is preferable to replacement.

Mitral Valve Prolapse

Definition. The most common congenital valvular abnormality typically seen in young women and associated with connective tissue disease (e.g., Marfan or idiopathic).

Presentation. Most patients are asymptomatic. Lightheadedness, palpitations, syncope, and chest pain may occur. These symptoms are often due to arrhythmias, which may occur.

Auscultation

- Mid-to-late systolic click and a late systolic murmur at the cardiac apex
- Worsens with Valsalva or standing
- Improves with squatting or leg raise

Complications (all very rare)

- Serious arrhythmias
- Sudden death
- CHF
- Bacterial endocarditis (but does not mean routine dental prophylaxis is indicated)
- Calcifications of valve
- Transient cerebral ischemic attacks

Laboratory

Two-Dimensional/Doppler Echocardiography: Marked systolic displacement of mitral leaflets with coaptation point at or on the left atrial side of the annulus; moderate systolic displacement of the leaflets with at least moderate mitral regurgitation.

Treatment. No specific treatment is needed in the majority of cases.

Medical Management: Beta blocker for chest pain and palpitations

Surgical Management: Mitral valve replacement, rarely

Aortic Stenosis

Etiology

- Calcification and degeneration of a congenitally normal valve; more common in the elderly population. This is the most common cause.
- Calcification and fibrosis of a congenitally bicuspid aortic valve.
- Rheumatic valvular disease: If the aortic valve is affected by the rheumatic fever, the mitral valve is also invariably affected.

Pathophysiology

Aortic stenosis results in elevation of left ventricular systolic pressure, and the resultant left ventricular hypertrophy maintains cardiac output without dilation of the ventricular cavity. Therefore, the stroke volume is normal until the late stages of the disease.

Forceful atrial contraction augments filling at the thick, noncompliant ventricle and generates a prominent S_4 gallop that elevates the left ventricular end-diastolic pressure.

Left ventricular hypertrophy and high intramyocardial wall tension account for the increased oxygen demands and, along with decreased diastolic coronary blood flow, account for the occurrence of angina pectoris.

As the myocardium fails, mean left ventricular diastolic pressure increases, and symptoms of pulmonary congestion ensue.

Clinical Manifestations

- Classic symptoms are angina, syncope, and dyspnea from CHF
- Pulsus tardus et parvus
- Carotid thrill
- Systolic ejection murmur in aortic area, usually with thrill, harsh quality, radiates to carotids
- S_4 gallop
- A_2 decreased, S_2 single or paradoxically split
- Aortic ejection click

Diagnosis

- EKG will often show left ventricular hypertrophy.
- Chest x-ray may present with calcification, cardiomegaly, and pulmonary congestion.
- Echocardiography shows thick aortic valve leaflets with decreased excursion and LVH.

Treatment

- Endocarditis prophylaxis is no longer recommended.
- Surgery (valve replacement) is advised when symptoms develop, which is when the valve area is reduced below 0.8 cm^2 (normal aortic orifice, 2.5–3 cm^2). Generally, if patient has symptoms from stenosis, surgery is the treatment of choice.
- Balloon valvuloplasty may be useful in those too ill to tolerate surgery.

Clinical Pearl

Look for AS in older patients presenting with syncope related to exertion.

Table 5-9. Differential Diagnosis of Aortic Valve Stenosis

Disease Entity	Differentiating Features
Aortic valve sclerosis of the elderly, without stenosis	• Systolic murmur does not peak late • Carotids do not have delayed upstrokes • No left ventricular hypertrophy by EKG • Echocardiographic visualization of excursion of valve leaflets usually normal or mildly reduced, but valves may not be visualized • No hemodynamically significant aortic valve gradient by cardiac catheterization
Hypertrophic obstructive cardiomyopathy	• Brisk bifid carotid upstrokes • Murmur usually does not radiate into neck • Characteristic change in murmur with various maneuvers • Pseudoinfarct pattern (large septal Q waves) on EKG • Characteristic echocardiographic features
Mitral regurgitation	• Murmur is holosystolic and radiates to axilla and not carotids • Carotid upstroke may be normal • Dilated left ventricle • Aortic valve normal on echocardiogram unless there is associated aortic valve disease
Pulmonic stenosis	• Murmur does not radiate into neck; loudest along the left sternal border; increases with inspiration • Physical examination, chest x-ray, and EKG may reveal enlarged right ventricle • Echocardiogram reveals right ventricular enlargement and hypertrophy

Note: All of the above have a systolic murmur that can be confused with aortic stenosis.

Table 5-10. Effect of Various Maneuvers on Systolic Murmurs

	Valsalva	Phenylephrine Handgrip	Squatting	Amyl Nitrite	Leg Raising
Aortic stenosis	Decrease	Decrease	Increase or decrease	Increase	Increase
Hypertrophic obstructive cardiomyopathy	Increase	Decrease	Decrease	Increase	Decrease
Ventricular septal defect	Decrease	Increase	No change	Decrease	Increase
Mitral regurgitation	Decrease	Increase	Increase	Decrease	Increase

Aortic Regurgitation

Etiology. Systemic hypertension and ischemic heart disease are the most common causes of aortic regurgitation.

- It may occur after infectious endocarditis.
- Conditions that may affect the ascending aorta and cause aortic regurgitation:
  - Syphilis
  - Ankylosing spondylitis
  - Marfan syndrome
  - Rheumatic fever
  - Aortic dissection
  - Aortic trauma

Pathophysiology

Aortic regurgitation results in a volume overload of the left ventricle.

- The ventricle compensates by increasing its end-diastolic volume according to the Frank-Starling mechanism.
- The left ventricular dilation is thought to overstretch the myofibrils, leading to less actin–myosin interaction and decreased contractility.
- In acute severe aortic regurgitation, the left ventricle has not had the opportunity to dilate, its compliance is relatively high, and the aortic regurgitation therefore leads to very high left ventricular end-diastolic pressure.

If mitral regurgitation ensues, the elevated left ventricular diastolic pressure is reflected back to the pulmonary vasculature, and acute pulmonary edema may occur.

Acute aortic regurgitation results in a lower cardiac output, narrower aortic pulse pressure, and a smaller left ventricle than does chronic aortic regurgitation.

Aortic diastolic pressure decreases in chronic aortic regurgitation because of both the regurgitation of blood into the left ventricle and a compensatory decrease in systemic vascular resistance to maintain forward cardiac flow to the periphery. The increased pulse pressure in chronic aortic regurgitation is due to the large stroke volume, causing increased systolic and decreased diastolic pressure.

Clinical Manifestations

- Dyspnea is the most common complaint.
- Diastolic decrescendo murmur is the most typical.
- Systolic flow murmur
- Duroziez sign: Systolic and/or diastolic thrill or murmur heard over the femoral arteries
- S_3 in early left ventricular decompensation
- Austin-Flint murmur
- Remember: Aortic regurgitation can cause 3 different murmurs.

Diagnosis

- **EKG:** LV hypertrophy often with volume overload pattern (narrow deep Q waves in left precordial leads)
- **Chest x-ray:** LV and aortic dilation
- **Echocardiography:** Dilated LV and aorta; left ventricular volume overload; fluttering of anterior mitral valve leaflet

Treatment. Endocarditis prophylaxis is no longer recommended.
- Salt restriction, diuretics, after load reduction (e.g., ACE inhibitors)
- Aortic valve replacement when symptoms worsen or ejection fraction decreases.
- Vasodilators such as an ACE, ARB, or nifedipine are the standard of care.
- Perform surgery when the ejection fraction is <55% or left ventricular systolic diameter is >55 mm.

MYOCARDIAL DISEASE

Cardiomyopathy

Definition. A disease involving the heart muscle itself.

Classification. Cardiomyopathies can be classified according to morphologic and hemodynamic characteristics.

Table 5-11. Morphologic and Hemodynamic Characteristics of Cardiomyopathies

	Dilated	Hypertrophic	Restrictive
	Biventricular dilatation	Marked hypertrophy of left ventricle and occasionally of right ventricle; can have disproportionate hypertrophy of septum	Reduced ventricular compliance; usually caused by infiltration of myocardium (e.g., by amyloid, hemosiderin, or glycogen deposits)
Cardiac output	↓	Normal or ↓	Normal to ↓
Stroke volume	↓	Normal or ↑	Normal or ↓
Ventricular filling pressure	↑	Normal or ↑	↑
Chamber size	↑	Normal or ↓	Normal or ↑
Ejection fraction	↓	↑	Normal to ↓
Diastolic compliance	Normal	↓	↓
Other findings	May have associated functional mitral or tricuspid regurgitation.	Obstruction may develop between interventricular septum and septal leaflet of mitral valve.	Characteristic ventricular pressure tracing that resembles those recorded in constrictive pericarditis, with early diastolic dip-and-plateau configuration

Dilated (congestive) cardiomyopathy

Characterized by diminished myocardial contractility, usually involving both ventricles; most common cause for heart transplants.

Etiologies of Dilated (Congestive) Cardiomyopathy

- Idiopathic: most common
- Alcoholic
- Peripartum
- Postmyocarditis due to infectious agents (viral, parasitic, mycobacterial, Rickettsiae)
- Toxins (cobalt, lead, arsenic)
- Doxorubicin hydrochloride, cyclophosphamide, vincristine
- Metabolic: chronic hypophosphatemia, hypokalemia, hypocalcemia, uremia

Clinical Manifestations. Symptoms and signs of left and right ventricular failure. Typical symptoms of systolic dysfunction.

Diagnosis

- X-ray: cardiomegaly with pulmonary congestion
- EKG: sinus tachycardia, arrhythmias, conduction disturbances
- Echo (key diagnostic study): dilated left ventricle, generalized decreased wall motion, mitral valve regurgitation
- Catheterization: dilated hypocontractile ventricle, mitral regurgitation

Differential diagnosis

- Valvular heart disease (e.g., regurgitant valve lesions)
- Coronary artery disease (ischemic cardiomyopathy)
- Hypertensive heart disease

Treatment. Patients are treated as those with systolic heart failure. ACE, beta blockers, and spironolactone lower mortality. Diuretics and digoxin decrease symptoms. Implantable defibrillator may decrease risk of sudden death when the ejection fraction is <35%.

Hypertrophic Obstructive Cardiomyopathy

Etiology. Although hypertrophic cardiomyopathy can apparently develop sporadically, it is hereditary in >60% of cases and is transmitted as an autosomal dominant trait.

- An abnormality on chromosome 14 has been identified in the familial form of the disease.
- The distinctive hallmark of the disease is unexplained myocardial hypertrophy, usually with thickening of the *interventricular septum.*

Pathophysiology

- As a result of the hypertrophy, left ventricular compliance is reduced, but systolic performance is not depressed.
- Diastolic dysfunction is characteristic, resulting in decreased compliance and/or inability for the heart to relax.
- The heart is hypercontractile, and systole occurs with striking rapidity.
- Ejection fractions are often 80–90% (normal is 60%, ±5%), and the left ventricle may be virtually obliterated in systole.
- The ability to provoke obstruction or to increase/decrease already existing obstruction is influenced by the factors found in Table 5-12.

Table 5-12. Factors That Modify Obstruction in Hypertrophic Obstructive Cardiomyopathy

Increase Obstruction		Decrease Obstruction	
Mechanism	**Physiologic or Pharmacologic Factors**	**Mechanism**	**Physiologic or Pharmacologic Factors**
Increase in contractility	• Tachycardia • Digitalis glycosides • β-adrenergic stimulation (e.g., epinephrine, exercise) • Premature beats	Decrease in contractility	• β-adrenergic blockade • Heavy sedation and general anesthesia • Calcium channel blockers, disopyramide, and other drugs that depress myocardial function
Reduction in preload	• Valsalva maneuver • Decrease in intravascular volume • Standing • Nitroglycerin • Vasodilator drugs • Tachycardia	Increase in preload	• Intravascular volume expansion • Squatting • Bradycardia • β-adrenergic blockade
Reduction in afterload	• Hypovolemia • Nitroglycerin and related drugs • Vasodilator drugs	Increase in afterload	• Intravascular volume expansion • Squatting • α-adrenergic stimulation (e.g., phenylephrine) • Handgrip

Clinical Manifestations

- Dyspnea, angina, presyncope, syncope with exertion, and palpitations
- Large jugular A wave, bifid carotid pulse, palpable S_4 gallop, systolic murmur and thrill, mitral regurgitation murmur
- Sudden death can sometimes be the first manifestation.

Diagnosis

- EKG: left ventricular hypertrophy, pseudo Q waves (often seen V_1–V_3), ventricular arrhythmias
- **Echocardiogram** is the mainstay of diagnosis. It typically shows hypertrophy, systolic anterior motion of mitral valve, and midsystolic closure of aortic valve

Treatment

- Beta-blockers
- Calcium channel blockers
- Disopyramide, occasionally
- Use implantable defribillator if there is syncope
- Surgery in severe cases—septoplasty

Restrictive Cardiomyopathy

Least common of the causes of cardiomyopathy. Myocardial disorder characterized by rigid noncompliant ventricular walls.

Etiologies

- Infiltrative
  - Sarcoidosis; amyloidosis
  - Hemochromatosis
  - Neoplasia
- Scleroderma
- Radiation

Pathophysiology. The myocardium is rigid and noncompliant, impeding ventricular filling and raising cardiac filling pressures from abnormal diastolic function. Systolic performance is often reduced, but the overriding problem is impaired diastolic filling, which produces a clinical and hemodynamic picture that mimics constrictive pericarditis.

Clinical Manifestations

- Dyspnea, exercise, intolerance, weakness
- Elevated jugular venous pressure, edema, hepatomegaly, ascites, S_4 and S_3 gallop, Kussmaul sign

Diagnosis

- X-ray: mild cardiomegaly, pulmonary congestion
- EKG: low voltage, conduction disturbances, Q waves
- Echo: characteristic myocardial texture in amyloidosis with thickening of all cardiac structures
- Catheterization: square root sign; elevated left- and right-sided filling pressures

Treatment. There is no good therapy; ultimately results in death from CHF or arrhythmias; consider heart transplantation.

PERICARDIAL DISEASE

Acute Pericarditis

Definition. Inflammation of the pericardial lining around the heart.

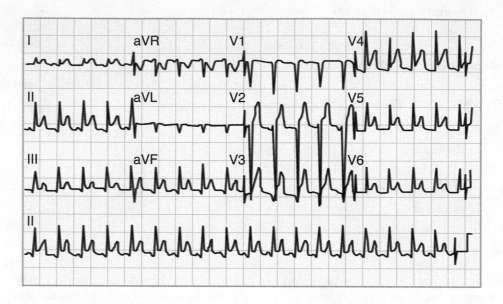

Figure 5-9. Acute Pericarditis with Diffuse ST Segment Elevation

Etiology

- Idiopathic
- Infections (viral)
- Vasculitis—connective tissue disease group
- Disorders of metabolism
- Neoplasms
- Trauma
- Inflammation—uremia

Clinical Manifestations. Chest pain, often localized substernally or to the left of the sternum, is usually worsened by lying down, coughing, and deep inspiration (which helps in the differential diagnosis with MI) and is relieved by sitting up and leaning forward.

Pericardial friction rub (diagnostic of pericarditis) is a scratchy, high-pitched sound that has 1 to 3 components corresponding to atrial systole, ventricular systole, and early diastolic ventricular filling. The ventricular systole component is present more consistently. The rub is often transient and is best heard with the diaphragm of the stethoscope as the patient sits forward at forced-end expiration.

Diagnosis. EKG may be diagnostic and reveals a diffuse ST-segment elevation with upright T waves at the onset of chest pain. PR segment depression is very specific.

Differential Diagnosis. The diffuseness of the ST-segment elevation, absence of reciprocal leads, and absence of the development of Q waves distinguish the characteristic pattern of acute pericarditis from the pattern seen in acute MI.

Treatment of the patient with acute pericarditis involves treating its etiology. In idiopathic pericarditis, treatment with anti-inflammatory medications (NSAIDs, aspirin, corticosteroids) is appropriate. Adding colchicine to an NSAID decreases recurrence.

Pericardial Effusion

Etiology. Fluid may accumulate in the pericardial cavity in virtually all forms of pericardial disease. The fluid may be a transudate, as are the serous cavity effusions that develop in patients with CHF, overhydration, or hypoproteinemia. More often, however, the pericardial effusion is an exudate, reflecting the presence of pericardial injury.

- Serosanguineous pericardial fluid is a classic sign in tuberculosis and neoplastic diseases.
- Frank blood in the pericardial space may occur in cases of aortic aneurysm or aortic dissection.
- Hemopericardium may also be produced by closed or penetrating trauma, rupture of the heart in acute MI, and bleeding caused by coagulation defects.
- When fluid accumulates slowly, the pericardium expands to accommodate it. When fluid accumulates rapidly, however, it compresses the heart and inhibits cardiac filling (cardiac tamponade).

Diagnosis. Echocardiography is the most effective laboratory technique available. The presence of pericardial fluid is recorded as a relatively echo-free space between the posterior pericardium and the posterior left ventricular epicardium in patients with small effusions. In patients with large effusions, the heart may swing freely within the pericardial sac, and this motion may be associated with electrical alternans.

Chest x-ray may show a "water-bottle" configuration of the cardiac silhouette.

Treatment

- Fluid aspiration
- Management of acute pericarditis etiology

Cardiac tamponade

Definition. A life-threatening condition in which a pericardial effusion has developed so rapidly or has become so large that it compresses the heart.

Etiology

- Neoplasia
- Idiopathic (usually viral) pericarditis
- Nonviral infection
  - Tuberculous
  - Suppurative

- Intrapericardial hemorrhage with or without pericarditis
- Wounds, including surgery of
  - Chest
  - Heart
  - Pericardium
- Postpericardiotomy syndrome
- Uremia
- Mediastinal and juxtamediastinal radiation therapy
- Vasculitis–connective tissue disease group

Clinical Manifestations

- Most patients with cardiac tamponade complain of dyspnea, fatigue, and orthopnea.
- Pulsus paradoxus, characterized by a decrease in systolic blood pressure >10 mm Hg with normal inspiration, frequently is present. The paradoxical pulse often can be noted by marked weakening or disappearance of a peripheral pulse during inspiration. Paradoxical pulse is not diagnostic of cardial tamponade and can occur in chronic lung disease, acute asthma, severe CHF, and in some cases of hypovolemic shock.
- Neck vein distension with clear lung
- Shock (hypotension)
- Decreased heart sounds

Diagnosis. Clinical manifestations followed by echocardiography and cardiac catheterization, which confirms that left and right atrial pressures are equal.

Treatment

- Pericardiocentesis
- Subxiphoid surgical drainage

Constrictive Pericarditis

Definition. The diffuse thickening of the pericardium in reaction to prior inflammation, which results in reduced distensibility of the cardiac chambers.

- Cardiac output is limited and filling pressures are increased to match the external constrictive force placed on the heart by the pericardium.
- The fundamental hemodynamic abnormality is abnormal diastolic filling.

Etiologies

- Idiopathic, unknown
- Following open-heart surgery
- Following thoracic radiation
- Postviral infection

Clinical Manifestations

- Most patients complain of dyspnea on exertion due to limited cardiac output.
- Orthopnea occurs in about 50% of patients.

- Symptoms and signs related to systemic venous hypertension frequently are reported and include ascites, edema, jaundice, hepatic tenderness, and hepatomegaly (manifestations of right-side failure).
- Jugular venous distension that increases with inspiration (Kussmaul sign)
- Heart sounds are distant, and an early diastolic apical sound, or "pericardial knock," is often present and can be confused with an S_3 gallop.

Diagnosis

- EKG: Findings include low-voltage and nonspecific T-wave changes.
- Chest x-ray: The heart usually is normal in size.
- Chest CT or MRI: Shows thickened pericardium; pericardial calcifications may be seen in tuberculous constriction.
- Cardiac catheterization: A marked "y" descent is present in the right atrial pressure tracing. Left and right ventricular pressure tracings demonstrate a characteristic "dip and plateau" or "square root" sign. There is equalization of end-diastolic pressures in all 4 chambers and the pulmonary artery.

Differential Diagnosis

- It is sometimes difficult to distinguish from restrictive cardiomyopathy. Left ventricular ejection fraction is more likely to be decreased in patients with restrictive cardiomyopathy.
- Computed tomography is the procedure of choice to demonstrate the thickened pericardium.

Treatment. Patients may be treated conservatively at first with mild sodium restriction and diuretics. Pericardiectomy may be needed.

RATE AND RHYTHM DISTURBANCES

Disorders of Sinus Node Function

Sinus bradycardia
Ventricular complexes are normal width, evenly spaced, rate <60/min.

Etiology

- Excessive vagal tone causes:
  - Acute MI, particularly diaphragmatic
  - Carotid sinus pressure
  - Vomiting
  - Valsalva maneuver
  - Phenothiazines
  - Digitalis glycosides
- Depression of the sinus node automaticity:
  - Beta-adrenergic blocking agents
  - Calcium blocking drugs

- Marathon running and swimming
- Hypothyroidism
- Normal variant

Treatment
- None necessary in the absence of symptoms
- Atropine acutely if symptoms are present
- Pacemaker if symptoms and bradycardia persist despite atropine

Atrioventricular (AV) block

May be classified in two ways:

- Anatomical, based on the site of block as determined by His bundle electrocardiography.
- Clinical, based on the routine ECG. The 3 classic clinical types are first-, second-, and third-degree (or complete) AV block.

First-Degree AV Block
Definition. Pulse rate (PR) interval >0.20 s at a heart rate of 70 beats/min.

Etiology
- Degenerative changes in the AV conduction system caused by:
  - Aging
  - Digitalis
  - Exaggerated vagal tone
  - Ischemia (diaphragmatic infarction)
  - Inflammation (myocarditis, acute rheumatic fever)
- Cardiomyopathies

Second-Degree AV Block
See Table 5-13.

Table 5-13. Type I versus Type II Second-Degree AV Block

	Type I (Mobitz I, Wenckebach)	Type II (Mobitz II)
	Mobitz Type I Progressive prolongation of the PR interval until a P wave is completely blocked and a ventricular beat is dropped. PR interval of the next conducted beat is shorter than preceding PR interval.	Mobitz Type II Blocked beat occurs suddenly and is not preceded by a change in duration of the PR interval. Patient is equipped with a pacemaker, which cuts in to sustain a regular ventricular rhythm.
Site of block	Usually AV nodal (supra-Hisian)	Infranodal (intra- or infra-Hisian)
QRS complex	Usually normal in width	Usually wide (bundle branch block) with infra-Hisian block; narrow with intra-Hisian block
Causes	Degenerative changes in AV node; diaphragmatic myocardial infarct; digitalis toxicity; myocarditis; rheumatic fever; increased vagal tone	Extensive anterior myocardial infarct; degenerative changes in His-Purkinje system; massive calcification of mitral or aortic valve anulus
EKG	• PR interval lengthens progressively until ventricular beat is dropped • PR interval shortens after dropped beat • RR interval lengthens progressively up to the dropped beat	• PR interval is usually normal in duration and constant in length; • if PR interval is prolonged, the duration of prolongation is fixed • Blocked beats occur suddenly without progressive lengthening of the PR interval • RR interval of conducted beats is constant or a multiple of a basic RR interval cycle length
Effect of carotid sinus pressure	May increase degree of block	No effect
Effect of atropine	Frequently shortens PR interval and increases AV conduction	No effect
Consequences of progression to complete heart block	Escape focus usually junctional; narrow QRS complex; rate >45 beats/min; Adams-Stoke attacks uncommon	Escape focus infrajunctional (usually ventricular) wide QRS complex; rate <45 beats/min; Adams-Stoke attacks common
		Junctional escape may be present with intra-Hisian block

Third-Degree (Complete) AV Block

In third-degree, or complete, heart block, all atrial beats are blocked, and the ventricles are driven by an escape focus distal to the site of block.

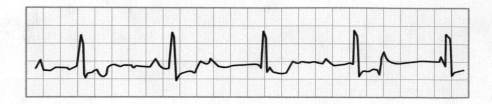

Figure 5-10. Third-Degree AV Block

Etiology

- Most common cause in adults is simple fibrous degenerative changes in the conduction system that results from aging (Lenègre disease)
- Inferior or posterior infarction
- Infectious and inflammatory processes, such as abscesses, tubercles, tumors, infiltrative disease of the myocardium, sarcoid nodules, and gummas, myocarditis, and rheumatic fever
- Drugs like digitalis
- Ankylosing spondylitis

Clinical Manifestations

- Symptoms are associated with Adams-Stoke attacks and occasionally CHF.
- Adams-Stoke attacks are caused by either sudden asystole or the development of ventricular tachyarrhythmias, such as transient ventricular tachycardia or ventricular fibrillation, that lead to circulatory arrest.
- The bradycardia associated with complete heart block may lead to congestive heart block in patients with myocardial disease.

Treatment. Pacing.

Supraventricular arrhythmias

Sinus tachycardia is defined as a normal rhythm with a rate of >100 beats/minute. In sinus tachycardia, the ventricular complexes are of normal width, evenly spaced, and a P-wave precedes a QRS complex. It usually represents a physiologic response to fever, hypotension, volume depletion, anxiety, and pain. Other causes include thyrotoxicosis, anemia, and some drugs.

Transient sinus tachycardia is occasionally the result of a rebound phenomenon following the discontinuation of beta-adrenergic blocking drugs.

Paroxysmal supraventricular tachycardia is a group of ectopic tachyarrhythmias characterized by sudden onset and abrupt termination. They are usually initiated by a supraventricular premature beat (includes paroxysmal atrial tachycardia)

- 80% are caused by re-entry, mainly in the AV node.
- Manifests as an absolutely regular rhythm at a rate 130–220 beats/min (average 160).
- Initial therapy consists of maneuvers aimed at increasing vagal tone, particularly right carotid sinus massage. Carotid sinus massage is followed by adenosine.
- IV adenosine is effective in >90% of cases.
- IV propranolol or esmolol, verapamil
- IV digitalis
- Synchronized external cardioversion if patient is unstable

Multifocal atrial tachycardia is characterized by an irregular supraventricular rhythm, at rates 100–200 beats/min.

- The morphology of the P waves (at least 3 different P wave forms) varies from beat to beat, as does the PR interval. Each QRS complex, however, is preceded by a P wave.
- Generally seen in elderly patients or those with chronic lung disease who are experiencing respiratory failure
- Use diltiazem, verapamil, or digoxin; avoid beta blockers because of lung disease

Atrial flutter generally presents as an absolutely regular rhythm with a ventricular rate of 125–150 beats/min and an atrial rate of 250–300 beats/min (i.e., 2:1 block).

It has been associated with:

- Chronic obstructive lung disease
- Pulmonary embolism
- Thyrotoxicosis
- Mitral valve disease
- Alcohol
- Atrial flutter may occur as a paroxysmal arrhythmia in persons with normal heart.
- Therapy is cardioversion if hemodynamically unstable (e.g., hypotension), digitalis, verapamil, diltiazem, and beta-blockers.

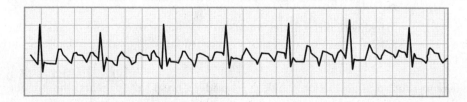

Figure 5-11. Atrial Flutter

Atrial Fibrillation

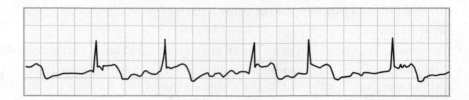

Figure 5-12. Atrial Fibrillation

Atrial fibrillation (AF) is the most common sustained cardiac rhythm disturbance. AF is associated with heart disease but also occurs with no detectable disease. Thromboembolic events occur with AF and can cause significant morbidity and mortality.

AF is a supraventricular tachyarrhythmia characterized by uncoordinated atrial activation with subsequent decline of atrial function. On the ECG, there is replacement of consistent P waves by fibrillatory waves that vary in size, shape, and timing, associated with an irregular, frequently rapid ventricular response (irregularly, irregular). The ventricular response to AF depends on electrophysiologic properties of the AV node, the level of vagal and sympathetic tone, and the action of drugs. Extremely rapid rates (>200 bpm) suggest the presence of an accessory pathway (W-P-W syndrome), which may manifest as AF. The rate of ischemic stroke among patients with nonrheumatic AF averages 5% per year, which is 2–7 times the rate for people without AF.

- The CHADS score is a clinical prediction rule for estimating the risk of stroke in patients with atrial fibrillation. It is used to determine whether treatment is required with anticoagulation or antiplatelet therapy.
- A high CHADS score corresponds to a greater risk of stroke (**C** for CHF; **H** for hypertension; **A** for age over 75; **D** for diabetes; **S** for prior stroke or TIA).
- Each condition receives 1 point except prior stroke, which gets 2.

CHADS Score	Treatment
0	Give aspirin
1	Give aspirin or warfarin
≥2	Give warfarin

When AF is compared with atrial flutter, atrial flutter is found to be more organized than AF, with a sawtooth pattern of regular atrial activation called flutter (f) waves on the ECG, particularly visible in leads II, III, and aVF.

The diagnosis of atrial fibrillation should be considered in elderly patients who present with complaints of shortness of breath, dizziness, or palpitations. The arrhythmia should also be suspected in patients with acute fatigue or exacerbation of CHF. In some patients, atrial fibrillation may be identified on the basis of an irregularly irregular pulse or an ECG obtained for the evaluation of another condition.

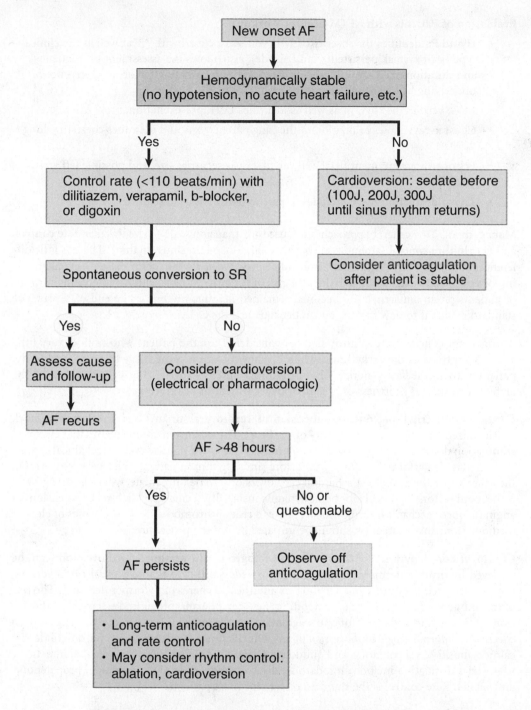

Figure 5-13. Management of Atrial Fibrillation (AF)

Cardiac conditions commonly associated with the development of AF include rheumatic mitral valve disease, coronary artery disease, CHF, and hypertension (cause atrial structures to dilate). Noncardiac conditions that can predispose patients to develop atrial fibrillation include hyperthyroidism, hypoxemia, and alcohol intoxication.

Evaluation of Patients with AF (Minimum Workup):

- **H and P:** identifies the severity of symptoms associated with AF as well as the clinical type (paroxysmal, persistent, first episode); also allows the assessment of frequency and duration of AF, as well as identification of precipitating factors and presence of underlying heart or lung disease.
- **ECG:** verifies the rhythm as well as identifies LVH, pre-excitation, prior MI.
- **Chest x-ray:** allows evaluation of the lung parenchyma and identifies coexisting lung disease.
- **Echocardiogram:** identifies LVH, valvular disease, atrial size, and possible left atrial thrombus.
- **Thyroid function tests:** excludes hyperthyroidism as a cause of AF.

Management. Two general approaches are used for managing AF: (*1*) ventricular **rate control**, and (*2*) **rhythm control** (attempts to convert to and maintain sinus rhythm). There is little difference in mortality between rate control and *pharmacologic* rhythm control. Studies confirm the importance of anticoagulation to reduce the risk of stroke in patients with AF. Interestingly, <25% of patients on an antiarrhythmic regimen remained in sinus rhythm at the end of 1 year. The standard of care is to slow the rate and anticoagulate if the CHADS score is >1.

As a general concept, rate control alone is considered for the patient who notices very little of the symptoms of the arrhythmia, while rhythm control is more likely to be applied to the patient who immediately notices the arrhythmia and is experiencing consequences of the arrhythmia, such as shortness of breath, or development of heart failure.

Cardioversion (rhythm control)—mechanical cardioversion: Involves an electrical shock synchronized with the intrinsic activity of the heart. The synchronization ensures that electrical stimulation does not occur during the vulnerable phase of the cardiac cycle. Mechanical cardioversion may be performed electively to restore sinus rhythm in patients with persistent AF. On the other hand, the need for mechanical cardioversion can be immediate, when the arrhythmia is the main factor responsible for hemodynamic instability (acute heart failure, hypotension, or angina). Since mechanical cardioversion carries a risk of thromboembolism, in cases of elective cardioversion, anticoagulation should be initiated before the procedure.

Cardioversion (rhythm control)—pharmacologic cardioversion: Cardioversion can be achieved by drugs. Pharmacologic cardioversion is less effective than electrical cardioversion, but the latter requires conscious sedation or anesthesia, whereas the former does not. The risk of thromboembolism or stroke does not differ between pharmacologic and electrical cardioversion. Thus, recommendations for anticoagulation are the same for both methods. Drugs proven *effective for pharmacologic cardioversion* of atrial fibrillation include: amiodarone, dofetilide, flecainide, ibutilide, propafenone, and quinidine. Drugs used to *maintain sinus rhythm* in patients with atrial fibrillation include amiodarone, disopyramide, dofetilide, flecainide, propafenone, and sotalol. Rate control is the standard of care for most patients.

Catheter ablation of AF foci is sometimes used as one of the nonpharmacologic therapies for eradicating AF. The techniques evolved with the demonstration that most AF is initiated by ectopic beats from focal areas that may be targeted for ablation. These foci arise more commonly from the 4 pulmonary veins. Thus, techniques have focused on the identification and elimination of these foci.

Note

Routine rhythm control for atrial fibrillation is not indicated. It is an exception.

Ventricular **rate control** to achieve a rate of <100–110 beats/min is one of the first steps in managing AF. Beta blockers, calcium channel blockers, and digoxin are the drugs most commonly used for rate control. These agents *do not* convert atrial fibrillation to sinus rhythm and should not be used for that purpose. Beta blockers and calcium channel blockers are effective in reducing the heart rate at rest and during exercise in patients with AF. Digoxin, because of the inotropic effects, is the drug of choice in patients with coexisting systolic heart failure. Factors that should guide drug selection include the patient's medical condition and the presence of concomitant heart failure. The following drugs are recommended for their demonstrated efficacy in rate control at rest and during exercise: diltiazem, atenolol, metoprolol, and verapamil.

Other key points: Rate control with chronic anticoagulation is the recommended strategy for the majority of patients with chronic AF. Rhythm control has not been shown to be superior to rate control (with chronic anticoagulation) in reducing morbidity and mortality.

Control the heart rate, then anticoagulate. Use aspirin for those with CHADS 0 or 1, and dabigatran, rivaroxaban, or warfarin for CHADS 2 or more. Heparin is not necessary prior to starting oral anticoagulants.

Patients with AF should receive chronic anticoagulation with dabigatran, rivaroxaban, or adjusted-dose warfarin, unless they have a specific contraindication.

Initial management: The goals are hemodynamic stabilization, ventricular rate control, and prevention of embolic complications. When AF does not terminate spontaneously, the ventricular rate should be treated to slow ventricular response and anticoagulation started.

Pre-excitation syndrome

Wolff-Parkinson-White Syndrome (WPW)

- Pre-excitation has been defined as a condition in which all or some portion of the ventricle is activated by atrial impulses earlier than if the impulses were to reach the ventricles by way of the normal cardiac conduction pathways. This is achieved by the use of accessory pathways (Kent bundle).
- Classically, the EKG shows a short PR interval followed by a wide QRS complex with a slurred initial deflection, or delta wave, that represents early ventricular activation.
- WPW is associated with:
  - Paroxysmal supraventricular arrhythmias alternating with ventricular arrhythmias
  - Atrial fibrillation and flutter

Treatment

- If the patient is hemodynamically unstable, then immediate electrical cardioversion is indicated (synchronized cardioversion).
- If the patient is hemodynamically stable, then procainamide is the best medication. Avoid digoxin, and calcium-channel blockers; these medications can inhibit conduction in the normal conduction pathway. This will potentially increase the likelihood of developing ventricular or supraventricular tachycardia. If conduction is inhibited in the normal pathway, this will increase conduction in the aberrant conduction pathway.
- Ablation is used as definitive treatment.

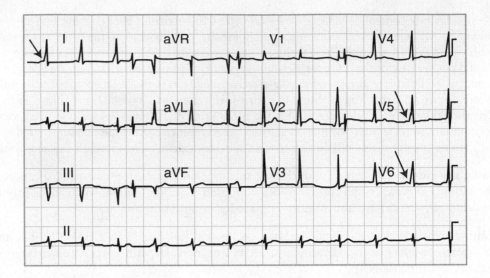

Figure 5-14. Wolff-Parkinson-White Syndrome

Ventricular arrhythmias

Ventricular Tachycardia (VT) is defined as 3 or more consecutive beats of ventricular origin at a rate >120 beats/min. QRS complexes are wide and often bizarre.

Etiology

- Particularly after an acute MI
- Cardiomyopathies and rarely seen in patients with mitral valve prolapse
- Metabolic derangements, such as hypokalemia, hypercalcemia, hypomagnesemia, and hypoxia
- Digitalis toxicity and thioridazine drugs

Clinical Manifestations

- Patients with VT often present with concomitant hypotension, CHF, syncope, or cardiac arrest.
- Independent and asynchronous atrial and ventricular contractions produce the following signs. These signs are absent when atrial fibrillation is present.
  - Variation in systolic blood pressure, as measured peripherally
  - Variation in the intensity of the heart sounds
  - Intermittent cannon A waves in the jugular venous pulses caused by the simultaneous contraction of the atrium and the ventricles
  - Extra heart sounds
- Because of asynchronous activation of the right and left ventricles, the first and second sounds are widely split.

Diagnosis and differential diagnosis: *See* Table 5-14.

Table 5-14. QRS Complex

Wide (≥0.12 s)		Narrow (≤0.12 s)	
Regular	**Irregular**	**Regular**	**Irregular**
Ventricular tachycardia	Atrial fibrillation (rarely)	Sinus tachycardia	Atrial fibrillation
Supraventricular tachycardia (aberration)		Paroxysmal supraventricular tachycardia	Multifocal atrial tachycardia
Wolff-Parkinson-White syndrome		Atrial flutter	

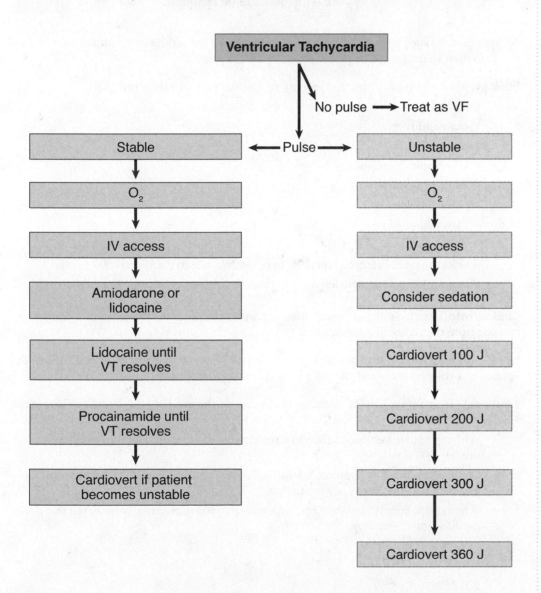

Figure 5-15. Management of VT

Torsade de Pointes

Definition. Characterized by undulating rotations of the QRS complexes around the electro-cardiographic baseline.

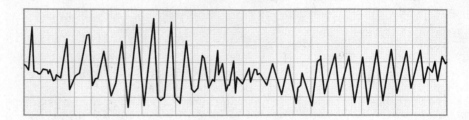

Figure 5-16. Torsade de Pointes

Arrhythmias initiated by a ventricular premature beat in the setting of abnormal ventricular repolarization characterized by prolongation of the QT interval.

Etiology. Antiarrhythmic drugs that prolong ventricular repolarization include:

- Quinidine
- Procainamide
- Disopyramide
- Psychotropic drugs, such as:
  – Phenothiazines
  – Thioridazine
  – Tricyclics
  – Lithium
  – Electrolyte imbalances, especially hypokalemia and hypomagnesemia
  – Central nervous system lesions, such as subarachnoid or intracerebral hemorrhage

Clinical manifestations. Patients with long QT interval are prone to recurrent dizziness or syncope from the ventricular tachycardia.

Sudden auditory stimuli, such as the ringing of the telephone at night, may initiate Torsade de Pointes in a vulnerable individual with a long QT interval syndrome.

Treatment. Treat the underlying disorder. In the case of the antiarrhythmics, use a drug such as lidocaine.

- With electrolyte imbalance disorders, repletion with potassium and magnesium is needed.
- Cardiac pacing or an isoproterenol infusion may suppress episodes of tachycardia and may be useful for emergency treatments.
- If hemodynamically unstable (e.g., hypotension), consider cardioversion, but this dys-rhythmia often reoccurs.

Ventricular Fibrillation

See the Emergency Medicine section.

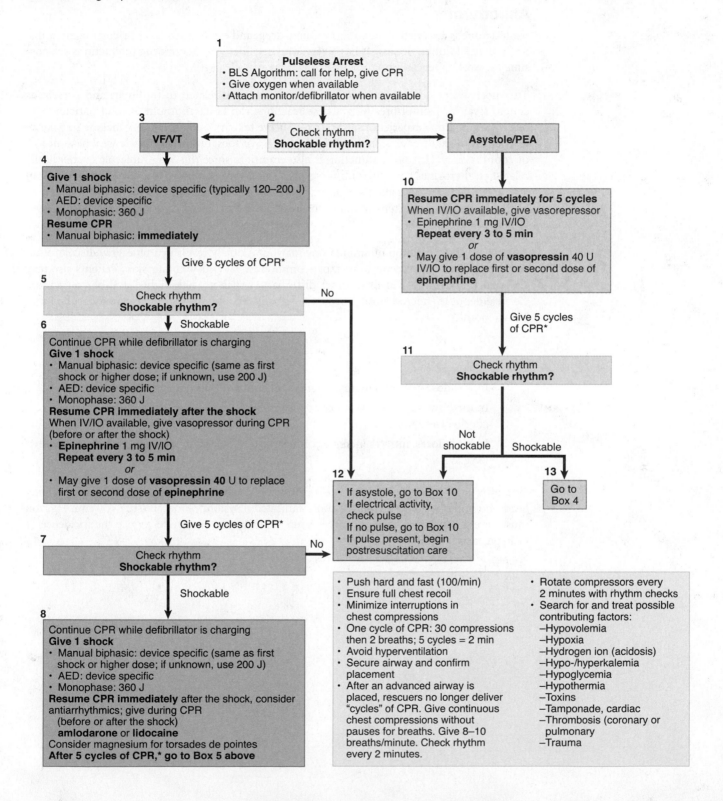

1

Pulseless Arrest
• BLS Algorithm: call for help, give CPR
• Give oxygen when available
• Attach monitor/defibrillator when available

2

Check rhythm
Shockable rhythm?

3

VF/VT

9

Asystole/PEA

4

Give 1 shock
• Manual biphasic: device specific (typically 120–200 J)
• AED: device specific
• Monophasic: 360 J
Resume CPR
• Manual biphasic: **immediately**

Give 5 cycles of CPR*

5

Check rhythm
Shockable rhythm?

No

6

Continue CPR while defibrillator is charging
Give 1 shock
• Manual biphasic: device specific (same as first shock or higher dose; if unknown, use 200 J)
• AED: device specific
• Monophase: 360 J
Resume CPR immediately after the shock
When IV/IO available, give vasopressor during CPR (before or after the shock)
• **Epinephrine** 1 mg IV/IO
  Repeat every 3 to 5 min
    or
• May give 1 dose of **vasopressin 40** U to replace first or second dose of **epinephrine**

Give 5 cycles of CPR*

7

Check rhythm
Shockable rhythm?

No

Shockable

8

Continue CPR while defibrillator is charging
Give 1 shock
• Manual biphasic: device specific (same as first shock or higher dose; if unknown, use 200 J)
• AED: device specific
• Monophase: 360 J
Resume CPR immediately after the shock, consider antiarrhythmics; give during CPR
(before or after the shock)
  amiodarone or **lidocaine**
Consider magnesium for torsades de pointes
After 5 cycles of CPR,* go to Box 5 above

10

Resume CPR immediately for 5 cycles
When IV/IO available, give vasorepressor
• Epinephrine 1 mg IV/IO
  Repeat every 3 to 5 min
    or
• May give 1 dose of **vasopressin** 40 U IV/IO to replace first or second dose of **epinephrine**

Give 5 cycles of CPR*

11

Check rhythm
Shockable rhythm?

Not shockable

Shockable

12

• If asystole, go to Box 10
• If electrical activity, check pulse
  If no pulse, go to Box 10
• If pulse present, begin postresuscitation care

13

Go to Box 4

• Push hard and fast (100/min)
• Ensure full chest recoil
• Minimize interruptions in chest compressions
• One cycle of CPR: 30 compressions then 2 breaths; 5 cycles = 2 min
• Avoid hyperventilation
• Secure airway and confirm placement
• After an advanced airway is placed, rescuers no longer deliver "cycles" of CPR. Give continuous chest compressions without pauses for breaths. Give 8–10 breaths/minute. Check rhythm every 2 minutes.

• Rotate compressors every 2 minutes with rhythm checks
• Search for and treat possible contributing factors:
  –Hypovolemia
  –Hypoxia
  –Hydrogen ion (acidosis)
  –Hypo-/hyperkalemia
  –Hypoglycemia
  –Hypothermia
  –Toxins
  –Tamponade, cardiac
  –Thrombosis (coronary or pulmonary)
  –Trauma

Figure 5-17. ACLS Pulseless Arrest Algorithm

DRUGS USED TO TREAT CARDIOVASCULAR DISEASE

Amiodarone

Amiodarone is a very effective antiarrhythmic drug, and can be used in ventricular tachycardia, AF, and atrial flutter. Because it has a very long half-life (>50 days), drug interactions are possible for weeks after discontinuation.

The most severe side effects of amiodarone therapy are related to the lungs and present as cough, fever, or painful breathing. These reactions can be fatal. About 20% of patients who receive amiodarone experience some form of nerve toxicity. Symptoms may include imbalance or changes in gait, tremor, numbness in the fingers or toes, dizziness, muscle weakness, or loss of coordination. Thyroid dysfunction is also common, since the drug molecule is chemically related to thyroxine. Hypothyroidism seems to be more common, but hyperthyroidism can also occur. Since many patients experience an exaggerated response to the harmful effects of sunlight, avoidance of extensive sun exposure and the use of protective clothing should be used to help prevent this.

Long-term administration of amiodarone may occasionally result in a blue-gray discoloration of the skin. This effect seems to be more common in patients with fair skin. Patients also may experience visual impairment or other disturbances such as "halo lights" and blurred vision. Corneal deposits (microdeposits) occur in virtually all patients who receive amiodarone for at least 6 months.

Nitrates

- In **low doses**, nitrates increase venous dilation and subsequently reduce preload.
- In **medium doses**, nitrates increase arteriolar dilatation and subsequently decrease afterload and preload.
- In **high doses**, nitrates increase coronary artery dilatation and subsequently increase oxygen supply.

Side effects: Vasodilation can lead to orthostatic hypotension, reflex tachycardia, throbbing headache, and blushing. Nitrates are contraindicated if systolic blood pressure <90 mm Hg. You must have a window-free period of >8 hours with nitrate therapy to reduce the incidence of tachyphylaxis.

Antiarrhythmic Drugs

Table 5-15. Antiarrhythmic Drugs

Drug	Adverse Effects
Disopyramide	Anticholinergic effects; hypotension; heart failure; heart block; tachyarrhythmia
Lidocaine	CNS (drowsiness, agitation, seizures); heart block
Phenytoin	CNS (ataxia, nystagmus, drowsiness); hypotension and heart block with rapid IV injection
Procainamide	Lupus-like syndrome; GI; rash; hypotension; aggravation of arrhythmia; blood dyscrasias
Quinidine	Aggravation of arrhythmias ("quinidine syncope"); thrombocytopenia; fever, rash; cinchonism; GI symptoms; digoxin-quinidine interaction (elevation of digoxin levels)
β-adrenergic blocking agents	Heart block; hypotension; asthma; hypoglycemia; lethargy; impotence
Verapamil	CHF, asystole, constipation
Adenosine	Transient dyspnea, noncardiac chest pain, rarely hypotension
Mexiletine	Lidocaine-like drug; local anesthetic
Tocainide	Lidocaine-like drug
Amiodarone	Very long half-life (20–40 d); may increase digoxin level; may worsen existing cardiac conduction disturbances; may prolong Coumadin effect
Encainide	Negative inotropism; QRS and PR prolongation
Flecainide	Negative inotropism; QRS and PR prolongation
Propafenone	Negative inotropism; QRS and PR prolongation

Beta Blockers

- Decrease heart rate, blood pressure, and contractility, which decrease myocardial oxygen requirement
- Contraindicated in presence of severe asthma in about one-third of patients
- Nonselective beta blockers may mask hypoglycemic symptoms in insulin-dependent diabetics
- Shown to improve survival after an acute MI and in CHF

Adverse effects of beta blockade therapy are as follows:

- Fatigue, insomnia
- Mental depression
- Adverse effects on lipid panel
- Hallucinations
- Raynaud phenomenon
- Bronchoconstriction
- Mask signs and symptoms of insulin-induced hypoglycemia
- Sexual dysfunction

**Table 5-16. Pharmacologic Properties of Select
β-Blocking Agents**

Generic Name (Trade Name)	Cardio-Selective
Metoprolol (Lopressor)	Yes
Atenolol (Tenormin)	Yes
Propanolol (Inderal)	No
Nadolol (Corgard)	No
Timolol (Blocadren)	No
Pindolol (Visken)	No
Acebutolol (Sectral)	Yes
Labetalol (Normodyne or Trandate)	No
Esmolol (IV)	Yes

Nebivolol is a unique beta blocker; it is a beta-1 specific blocker that increases nitric oxide and thus does not cause erectile dysfunction.

Calcium Channel Blockers

Calcium channel blockers work by producing decreases in preload and afterload. They may be harmful in the postinfarction period, especially if the patient has left ventricular failure. Their efficacy in angina is very limited—there is no mortality benefit.

Adverse effects of calcium channel blockers are as follows:

Cardiac
- CHF
- Reflex tachycardia
- Hypotension
- Lightheadedness
- AV block

Noncardiac
- Flushing
- Headache
- Weakness
- Constipation
- Nasal congestion
- Wheezing
- Peripheral edema
- Gingival hyperplasia

Hematology 6

ANEMIA

Definition. A hematocrit (Hct) <41% in men or <36% in women, or a hemoglobin <13.5 gm/dL in men or <12 gm/dL in women.

Etiology. Anemias are most easily classified according to their cell size.

- **Microcytic anemia** means a low mean corpuscular volume (MCV) <80. These are most commonly a result of iron deficiency, anemia of chronic disease, thalassemia, sideroblastosis, and lead poisoning. Anemia of chronic disease can be either microcytic or normocytic.

- **Macrocytic anemia** is characterized by an elevated MCV >100. This is most commonly from vitamin B_{12} or folic acid deficiency but can also result from the toxic effects of alcohol, liver disease, or chemotherapeutic agents such as methotrexate or medications such as zidovudine (AZT) or phenytoin.

- **Normocytic anemia** is characterized by a normal MCV. This can be from an early form of the conditions described above, as well as most forms of hemolysis and aplastic anemia.

Clinical Presentation. The predominant symptoms of anemia are based on the severity of the anemia rather than the specific etiology. Early symptoms include fatigue, tiredness, and poor exercise tolerance. As the anemia worsens, the patient develops dyspnea on exertion and light-headedness. Eventually, confusion and altered mental status may develop as oxygen delivery to the brain decreases. Death from anemia is most often from decreased oxygen delivery to the heart, resulting in the development of myocardial ischemia.

The severity of symptoms is profoundly related to the underlying condition of the patient. A healthy young patient may have no symptoms at all with hematocrit 27–29%, whereas an older patient with heart disease may develop dyspnea or anginal symptoms with the same hematocrit.

Diagnosis. Once a diagnosis of anemia is determined based on a low hematocrit or hemoglobin, the first step is to determine the MCV. Iron studies, reticulocyte count, peripheral smear, red cell distribution of width (RDW), Coombs test, vitamin B_{12}, folate levels, and even occasionally a bone marrow biopsy may be necessary to determine a specific etiology. The tests ordered depend on the specifics of the case presented.

Treatment. Besides blood transfusion, treatment cannot be generalized. Packed RBCs are used to maintain a hematocrit >25–30%. This is based on the underlying condition of the patient. A healthy young patient can have transfusion withheld until the hematocrit is in the low 20%s. An older patient with coronary artery disease will need to be maintained when hematocrit >30%. The hematocrit should rise approximately 3 points for every unit of packed RBCs given. Whole blood is rarely, if ever, used.

MICROCYTIC ANEMIA

Iron Deficiency Anemia

Definition. An anemia with diminished red blood cell production and an MCV <80 characterized by hypochromic cells and low levels of stored iron in the body.

Etiology. Iron deficiency anemia is almost always caused by blood loss from the body. The most common type of blood loss is GI or menstrual. Iron absorption is tightly regulated in the body. A man requires about 1 mg per day and a woman about 2–3 mg per day on average. It is difficult for the body to increase the level of iron absorption. If there is even a modest increase in blood loss—occult blood in the stool, a heavier menstrual flow, or an increased demand such as during pregnancy—the body is poorly equipped to increase its level of absorption to exceed 3–4 mg per day. Other etiologies are increased urinary loss of blood, malabsorption, hemolysis, and poor oral intake.

Clinical Presentation. Mild anemia may result in absent or very limited symptoms. As the hematocrit approaches 30%, symptoms of fatigue and poor exercise tolerance may develop. As the hematocrit lowers to 25%, tachycardia, palpitations, dyspnea on exertion, and pallor develop. Older patients and those with coronary artery disease may become dyspneic at higher levels of hematocrit. More severe anemia results in lightheadedness, confusion, syncope, and chest pain. A systolic ejection murmur ("flow" murmur) may develop in any patient with moderately severe anemia. These symptoms are not specific for iron deficiency anemia and may develop with any form of anemia provided it is sufficiently severe.

Symptoms specific to iron deficiency are very rare and cannot be relied upon to determine the diagnosis. These include brittle nails, spoon shaped nails, glossitis, and pica. Iron deficiency anemia as a specific diagnosis is determined by laboratory findings, not symptoms.

> **Clinical Pearl**
>
> In early iron deficiency, serum iron may be normal. (Ferritin is low and TIBC is elevated.)

Diagnosis. A low serum ferritin <10 ng/mL is the most characteristic finding of iron deficiency anemia. Low ferritin has good specificity (>99%) but poor sensitivity (60%) because the ferritin level may be falsely elevated because it is an acute phase reactant and may be elevated in other inflammatory states or with malignancy. MCV is low in individuals with anemia except in very early cases. The serum iron is low and the total iron binding capacity is high. The RDW and platelet count are elevated. The most specific test, although rarely necessary, is a bone marrow biopsy looking for stainable iron stores. The reticulocyte count should be low. Platelet levels rise in iron deficiency.

Treatment. Oral therapy with ferrous sulfate tablets is the most common method of therapy. Oral therapy should be continued until Hb and Ht have normalized and an additional 2-3 months to "restore" iron stores. With replacement of iron, a brisk increase in reticulocytes will be seen 2 weeks into treatment. Parenteral iron is used in patients with malabsorption, kidney disease, or an intolerance to oral therapy. Blood transfusion is the most effective method of delivering iron but, of course, is not a standard method of correcting iron deficiency anemia.

Anemia of Chronic Disease

Definition. A defect in the ability to make use of iron sequestered in stores within the reticuloendothelial system. It can be either microcytic or normocytic.

Etiology. Anemia can accompany virtually any chronic inflammatory, infectious, or neoplastic condition.

Clinical Presentation. The symptoms are based on the severity of the anemia as described above. The only other symptoms are based on the specifics of the underlying disease.

Diagnosis. The serum ferritin level is normal or elevated. The serum iron level and total iron binding capacity (TIBC) are both low. The reticulocyte count is low.

Treatment. Correct the underlying disease. Iron supplementation and erythropoietin will not help, except in renal disease and anemia caused by chemotherapy or radiation therapy for malignancies.

Sideroblastic Anemia

Definition. A microcytic anemia caused by a disorder in the synthesis of hemoglobin characterized by trapped iron in the mitochondria of nucleated RBCs.

Etiology. There are both hereditary as well as acquired forms. The hereditary form is from either a defect in aminolevulinic acid synthase or an abnormality in vitamin B_6 metabolism. Acquired forms are from drugs such as chloramphenicol, isoniazid, or alcohol. Lead poisoning can cause sideroblastic anemia as well. There is an association with myelodysplastic syndromes and refractory anemia. These can progress to acute myelogenous leukemia in a small percentage of patients.

Clinical Presentation. The symptoms are related to the severity of the anemia as described above. There is no specific presenting finding that will be sufficiently suggestive of sideroblastic anemia to allow a diagnosis without significant laboratory evaluation.

Diagnosis. The serum ferritin level is elevated. Transferrin saturation is very high, and therefore the TIBC is very low. The serum iron level is high. The most specific test is a Prussian Blue stain of RBCs in the marrow that will reveal the ringed sideroblasts. (Marrow reticuloendothelial iron is strikingly increased.) Sideroblastic anemia is the only microcytic anemia in which serum iron is elevated.

Treatment. Remove the offending drug as appropriate. Some patients, especially those with INH-associated sideroblastic anemia, will respond to pyridoxine therapy 2-4 mg per day. Occasionally, sideroblastic anemia may be severe enough to warrant transfusion. In refractory cases, BMT may be considered.

> **Clinical Pearl**
>
> Both iron deficiency and anemia of chronic disease may have decreased serum iron.

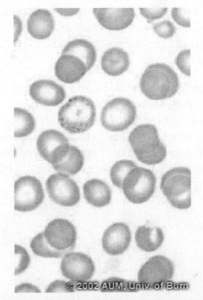

© 2002 AUM. Univ. of Bum

Copyright 2007 Gold Standard Multimedia Inc.

Figure 6-1. Basophilic Stippling, a Feature of Lead Poisoning and Other Diseases

Thalassemia

Definition. The hereditary underproduction of either the alpha or beta globin chains of the hemoglobin molecule resulting in a hypochromic, microcytic anemia.

Etiology. Gene deletion results in variable levels of disease. There are 4 genes coding for the alpha chain of hemoglobin. There can be deletions of 1, 2, 3, or all 4 genes. Beta thalassemia can be mutated in either one or two genes. Alpha thalassemia is more common in Asian populations. Beta thalassemia is more common in Mediterranean populations.

Clinical Presentation. The presentation is dependent on the number of abnormal genes. In alpha thalassemia, 1 gene deleted yields a normal patient. The CBC is normal, the hemoglobin level is normal, and the MCV is normal. Individuals with 2 genes deleted have a mild anemia with hematocrits ranging from 30–40% with a strikingly low MCV. Those with 3 genes deleted have more profound anemia with hematocrits 22–32% as well as the very low MCV. Four-gene-deleted alpha thalassemia patients die in utero secondary to gamma chain tetrads called hemoglobin Barts.

In beta thalassemia trait there is a mild anemia with marked microcytosis (low MCV). Patients with beta thalassemia major are homozygous for mutations of both genes coding for the beta hemoglobin gene. These patients with beta thalassemia major, also known as Cooley anemia, become severely symptomatic starting at 6 months of age when the body would normally switch from fetal hemoglobin to adult hemoglobin. They are severely symptomatic with growth failure, hepatosplenomegaly, jaundice, and bony deformities secondary to extramedullary hematopoiesis. They are later symptomatic from hemochromatosis, cirrhosis, and CHF from chronic anemia and transfusion dependence.

Diagnosis. Clues to the diagnosis of thalassemia trait is a mild anemia with a profound microcytosis. Beta thalassemia major has the severe symptoms, large spleen, and bone abnormalities described above. Both forms of thalassemia are diagnosed by having a microcytic anemia with normal iron studies. Hemoglobin electrophoresis tells which type of thalassemia is present. In beta thalassemia, there is an increased level of hemoglobin F and hemoglobin A_2. In beta thalassemia major, the hemoglobin is as low as 3–4 g/dL. Those with alpha thalassemia will have normal amounts of hemoglobins F and A_2. Tetrads of beta chains are called hemoglobin H. Hemoglobin H is present in alpha thalassemia with 3 of 4 genes deleted. Target cells are present in all forms of thalassemia trait and thalassemia major. The RDW is normal in all forms because all of the cells are of the same size.

Treatment. Thalassemia traits of both the alpha and beta types do not require specific treatment. Beta thalassemia major patients require blood transfusions once or twice a month. The chronic transfusions lead to iron overload, which requires treatment with deferasirox. Oral deferasirox is the standard of care. This is easier to give than deferoxamine, which requires a subcutaneous pump. Splenectomy eliminates a major area of hemolysis and therefore helps reduce transfusion requirements. A small number of patients can be treated with a bone marrow transplantation.

MACROCYTIC ANEMIA

A 72-year-old alcoholic man comes to the office with several weeks of memory loss and tingling in his feet. He has a hematocrit of 32% with an MCV of 110.

Vitamin B$_{12}$ (Cyanocobalamine) Deficiency

Definition. Decreased absorption or intake of vitamin B$_{12}$ resulting in hematologic and/or neurologic abnormalities.

Etiology. The most common cause of B$_{12}$ deficiency is pernicious anemia, which is a disorder resulting in decreased intrinsic factor production due to autoimmune destruction of parietal cells. The incidence of pernicious anemia increases with age. Gastrectomy and atrophic gastritis can also decrease intrinsic factor production. Various forms of malabsorption such as sprue, regional enteritis, and blind loop syndrome can block absorption of vitamin B$_{12}$. Pancreatic insufficiency can result in the inability to absorb the vitamin. Rarely, tapeworm infection with *Diphyllobothrium latum* can decrease absorption. Decreased intake is unusual and requires several years to produce disease.

Clinical Presentation. The manifestations of vitamin B$_{12}$ deficiency vary with the severity of the anemia. As such, you cannot specifically determine that a patient has B$_{12}$ deficiency only from the symptoms of anemia. Neurologic manifestations may involve almost any level of the neurologic system. Patients may have peripheral neuropathy, position sense abnormality, vibratory, psychiatric, autonomic, motor, cranial nerve, bowel, bladder, and sexual dysfunction. Glossitis, diarrhea, and abdominal pain may occur. You may have either the hematologic or neurologic deficits individually or combined.

Diagnosis. Anemia with macrocytosis (increased MCV). A smaller number of patients may have the neurologic deficits alone. The WBCs have hypersegmented neutrophils with a mean lobe count >4. The red cells are characterized by macro-ovalocytes. Although macrocytosis can occur with hemolysis, liver disease, and myelodysplasia, these give *round* macrocytes. B$_{12}$ and folate deficiency give oval macrocytes. The hematologic pattern of vitamin B$_{12}$ deficiency is indistinguishable from folate deficiency. The reticulocyte count is reduced, although the bone marrow is hypercellular. Pancytopenia may occur. An elevated LDH, bilirubin, and iron level may occur and are due to mild hemolysis of immature erythrocytes.

The most specific test is a low B$_{12}$ level. Antibodies to intrinsic factor and parietal cells confirm the etiology as pernicious anemia. The Schilling test is rarely used to determine the etiology of vitamin B$_{12}$ deficiency. It is not necessary if the patient has a low B$_{12}$ level combined with the presence of antibodies to intrinsic factor. An elevated methylmalonic acid level occurs with B$_{12}$ deficiency and is useful if the B$_{12}$ level is equivocal.

Treatment. Replace the vitamin B$_{12}$ lifelong. Options available for treating clinical vitamin B12 deficiency include **oral (daily)** and **parenteral (monthly intramuscular or subcutaneous)** preparations. Parenteral route is recommended for patients with neurologic manifestations of B12 deficiency. IV dosing is not recommended because that would result in most of the vitamin being lost in the urine.

Response of vitamin B12 deficiency anemia to treatment is usually rapid, with reticulocytosis occurring within 2–5 days and hematocrit normalizing within weeks. Treatment with cobalamin effectively halts progression of the deficiency process but **might not fully reverse more**

advanced neurologic effects. If the underlying cause of the vitamin B12 deficiency is treatable (e.g., fish tapeworm infection or bacterial overgrowth), then treatment should include addressing the underlying etiology.

Patients who have vitamin B12 deficiency with associated megaloblastic anemia might experience severe **hypokalemia** and fluid overload early in treatment due to increased erythropoiesis, cellular uptake of potassium, and increased blood volume. Once treated for a vitamin B12 deficiency due to pernicious anemia or other irreversible problems with absorption, patients need to continue some form of cobalamin therapy **lifelong**.

Folic acid replacement can correct the hematoligic abnormalities of B_{12} deficiency, but not the neurologic abnormalities.

Folic Acid Deficiency

Definition. Deficiency in folic acid levels leading to anemia.

Etiology. Folic acid deficiency is almost always due to some form of decreased dietary intake. Occasionally, increased requirements from pregnancy, skin loss in diseases like eczema, or increased loss from dialysis and certain anticonvulsants such as phenytoin may occur. Alcoholics have decreased folate intake.

Clinical Presentation. Entirely dependent on the severity of the anemia. As described above.

Diagnosis. The hematologic presentation of folic acid deficiency is identical to B_{12} deficiency. The diagnosis is based on a low red-blood-cell, folic-acid level.

Treatment. Replace folic acid, almost always orally.

HEMOLYTIC ANEMIA

Definition. Hemolytic anemias are caused by decreased red blood cell survival from increased destruction of the cells. The destruction may be either in the blood vessels (intravascular) or outside the vessels (extravascular), which generally means inside the spleen.

Etiology. Hemolytic anemias may either be chronic, as in sickle cell disease, paroxysmal nocturnal hemoglobinuria, and hereditary spherocytosis, or acute, such as in drug-induced hemolysis, autoimmune hemolysis, or glucose 6-phosphate dehydrogenase deficiency.

Clinical Presentation. The usual symptoms of anemia are present based on the severity of the disease, not necessarily the etiology. Fatigue and weakness occur with mild disease. Dyspnea and later confusion occur with more severe disease. The major difference between hemolytic anemia and the micro- and macrocytic anemias is that hemolysis is more often the etiology when the onset is sudden. This is, of course, provided that simple blood loss has been excluded. Hemolysis is often associated with jaundice and dark urine as well. Specific findings associated with each disease are described below. Fever, chills, chest pain, tachycardia, and backache may occur if the intravascular hemolysis is particularly rapid.

Diagnosis. Patients with hemolytic anemias generally have a normal MCV, but the MCV may be slightly elevated because reticulocytes are somewhat larger than older cells. The reticulocyte count is elevated. The LDH and indirect bilirubin are elevated. Bilirubin levels above 4 are unusual with hemolysis alone. The peripheral smear may aid in the specific diagnosis, and the haptoglobin may be low with intravascular hemolysis. Hemoglobin may be present in the urine when intravascular hemolysis is sudden and severe because free hemoglobin spills into the urine. There should not be bilirubin in the urine because indirect bilirubin is bound to albumin and should not filter through the glomerulus. Hemosiderin is a metabolic product of hemoglobin. Hemosiderin may be present in the urine if the hemolysis is severe and lasts for several days.

Treatment. Transfusion is needed as in all forms of anemia when the hematocrit becomes low. Hydration is, in general, useful to help prevent toxicity to the kidney tubule from the free hemoglobin. Specific therapy is discussed with each disease below.

Sickle Cell Disease

Definition. A hereditary form of chronic hemolysis ranging from asymptomatic to severe, overwhelming crisis. It is characterized by irreversibly sickled cells and recurrent painful crises.

Etiology. Sickle cell disease is an autosomal recessive hereditary disease. Hemoglobin S is due to a substitution of a valine for glutamic acid as the sixth amino acid of the beta globin chain. The heterozygous form (trait) is present in 8% of the African-American population, and the homozygous form (disease) is present in 1 in 400 African-Americans. Almost all of those with the trait are asymptomatic. A sickle cell acute painful crisis can be precipitated by hypoxia, dehydration, acidosis, infection, and fever. However, the crisis may occur without the presence of these factors. Sickle cell crisis is most often not associated with an increase in hemolysis or drop in hematocrit. When increased hemolysis occurs, another etiology such as concomitant glucose 6 phosphate dehydrogenase deficiency (G6PD) or acute splenic sequestration in a child should be considered. Sudden drops in hematocrit may also be caused by Parvovirus B_{19} infection or folate deficiency. This drop in hematocrit is from acute aplasia (decrease in cell production), not hemolysis.

Clinical Presentation. Chronic manifestations include renal concentrating defects (isosthenuria), hematuria, ulcerations of the skin of the legs, bilirubin gallstones, aseptic necrosis of the femoral head, osteomyelitis, retinopathy, recurrent infections from *Pneumococcus* or *Haemophilus*, growth retardation, and splenomegaly followed in adulthood by autosplenectomy. The acute painful crisis consists of back, rib, chest, and leg pain. Occasionally some patients will have very severe and life-threatening manifestations of sickling. These include the acute chest syndrome consisting of severe chest pain, fever, leukocytosis, hypoxia, and infiltrates on the chest x-ray. The acute chest syndrome is indistinguishable from pneumonia. Stroke and TIA may also occur. Priapism can occur from infarction of the prostatic plexus of veins. Blindness and even myocardial infarction and cardiomyopathy may also occur. Pregnant patients experience increased rates of spontaneous abortion and low birth weight. Sickle trait gives a normal hematologic picture with no anemia and a normal MCV. The only significant manifestation of trait is the renal concentrating defect presenting with isosthenuria. Sickle trait also increases the frequency of UTI. Those with trait will rarely develop the acute pain crisis under conditions of profound hypoxia and acidosis.

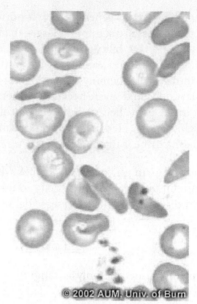

Copyright 2007 Gold Standard Multimedia Inc.

Figure 6-2. Sickle Cells Noted on a Peripheral Blood Smear

Diagnosis. Patients with sickle cell disease typically have a mild to moderate anemia with a normal MCV. The reticulocyte count should always be elevated in the 10–20% range unless they have folate deficiency or Parvovirus B_{19} aplastic crisis. LDH and bilirubin are elevated as in all types of hemolytic anemias. The hemoglobin electrophoresis is the most specific test. The peripheral smear shows sickled cells. The sickle prep (or Sickledex) is a quick screening test used to diagnose evidence of sickle cell trait and cannot distinguish between trait and homozygous disease. The urinalysis usually has blood present, although it is often microscopic. The white blood cell count is often elevated in the 10,000–20,000 range, although this can also indicate the presence of infection.

Treatment. An acute sickle cell pain crisis is treated with fluids, analgesics, and oxygen. Antibiotics are given with infection or even to patients with fever and leukocytosis even if a definite site of infection has not been documented. Ceftriaxone is the preferred agent because it covers *Pneumococcus* and *Haemophilus* influenza. Severe or life-threatening manifestations such as acute chest syndrome, CNS manifestations, priapism, and acute cardiac manifestations are managed with red blood cell transfusions if the hematocrit is low, and **exchange transfusion** if the hematocrit is high. Chronic management includes folic acid replacement and vaccinations against *Pneumococcus* and influenza. **Hydroxyurea** is used to decrease the frequency of the vaso-occlusive pain crisis. Bone marrow transplantation can be curative but should still be considered experimental at this time.

Autoimmune, Cold Agglutinin, and Drug-Induced Hemolytic Anemia

Definition. Various forms of acquired hemolytic anemias resulting from the production of IgG, IgM, or activation of complement C_3 against the red cell membrane. They are often sudden and idiopathic. The lysis can be either extravascular or intravascular but is far more often extravascular. This is based on the fact that the destruction of the cells most often occurs through macrophages in the spleen or by Kupfer cells in the liver.

Etiology. Autoimmune destruction is often idiopathic. Known causes of autoimmune destruction are from antibodies produced in relationship to various forms of leukemia, especially chronic lymphocytic leukemia, viral infections, lymphoma, collagen vascular diseases like lupus, or in relationship to drugs. The most common drugs are the penicillins, cephalosporins, sulfa drugs, quinidine, alphamethyldopa, procainamide, rifampin, and thiazides.

Ulcerative colitis can also lead to autoimmune hemolytic anemia. Cold agglutinin disease is an IgM antibody produced against the red cell in association with malignancies such as lymphoma or Waldenstrom macroglobulinemia and infections such as Mycoplasma or mononucleosis. Cold agglutinin destruction occurs predominantly in the liver. Liver-mediated destruction is not affected by steroids. Up to 50% of patients do not have an associated underlying disorder.

Clinical Presentation. Symptoms are generally related to the severity of the anemia, not the etiology. The onset may be very sudden resulting in fever, syncope, congestive failure, and hemoglobinuria. Mild splenomegaly is present when the disease has been occurring long enough for the time it takes for the spleen to enlarge. The drug history is often the clue with drug-induced varieties. Cold agglutinin disease results in cyanosis of the ears, nose, fingers, and toes. Weakness, pallor, jaundice, and dark urine may occur as it can in all forms of hemolysis of sufficient severity.

Diagnosis. Autoimmune hemolysis gives a normocytic anemia, reticulocytosis, increased LDH, absent or decreased haptoglobin, and increased indirect bilirubin, as can all forms of hemolysis. The Coombs test is the specific test that diagnoses autoimmune, cold agglutinin, and often even drug-induced hemolysis. Spherocytes are often present on the smear.

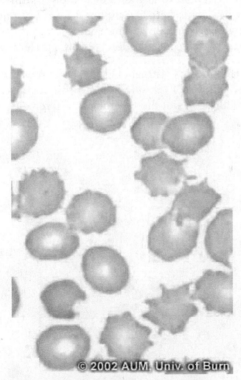

© 2002 AUM. Univ. of Burn

Copyright 2007 Gold Standard Multimedia Inc.

Figure 6-3. Acanthocytes, a Feature of Several Hematologic and Systemic Diseases

Treatment. Mild disease often occurs, which needs no treatment. Stop the offending drug. More severe autoimmune hemolysis is treated with steroids first. Splenectomy is done for those unresponsive to steroids. Cold agglutinin disease is primarily managed with avoiding the cold. Most cases of cold agglutinin disease are mild, but in those who have severe disease despite conservative measures, azathioprine, cyclosporine, or cyclophosphamide can be used. Rituximab is also useful. This is an anti-CD20 antibody. Steroids and splenectomy don't work well with cold agglutinin disease because the destruction occurs in the liver. You need to control the lymphocytes which control the production of IgM.

Hereditary Spherocytosis

Definition. A chronic mild hemolysis with spherocytes, jaundice, and splenomegaly from a defect in the red cell membrane.

Etiology. An autosomal dominant disorder where the loss of spectrin in the red cell membrane results in the formation of the red cell as a sphere, rather than a more flexible and durable biconcave disc. Hemolysis occurs because the spheres are not able to pass the narrow passages in the spleen.

Clinical Presentation. A chronic disorder with mild to moderate symptoms of anemia. Because the hemolysis occurs in the spleen, there is often splenomegaly and jaundice. Severe anemia occasionally occurs from folate deficiency or Parvovirus B_{19} infection such as in sickle cell disease. Bilirubin stones often occur, leading to cholecystitis, often at a young age.

Diagnosis. A normal to slightly decreased MCV anemia with the elevated LDH; indirect bilirubin and reticulocyte count similar to any kind of hemolysis. Although spherocytes may be present with autoimmune hemolysis, hereditary spherocytosis has a negative Coombs test. The cells have increased sensitivity to lysis in hypotonic solutions known as an osmotic fragility test. The mean corpuscular hemoglobin concentration (MCHC) is elevated.

Treatment. Most patients require no treatment beyond folate replacement chronically. In those with more severe anemia, removal of the spleen will eliminate the site of the hemolysis. The symptoms and jaundice will resolve but the spherocytes will remain.

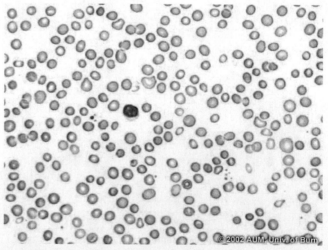

Copyright 2007 Gold Standard Multimedia Inc.

Figure 6-4. Features of Hereditary Spherocytosis Seen on Peripheral Blood Smear

Paroxysmal Nocturnal Hemoglobinuria (PNH)

Definition. A red cell membrane defect leading to intermittent dark urine and venous thrombosis and a chronic form of hemolysis.

Etiology. A red cell membrane defect in phosphatidyl inositol glycan A (PIG-A) allows increased binding of complement to the red cell leading to increased intravascular hemolysis. It is a clonal stem-cell disorder and therefore can develop into aplastic anemia and leukemia as well. The cells are more susceptible to lysis by complement in an acid environment. Everyone becomes a little acidotic at night because of a relative hypoventilation.

Clinical Presentation. In addition to symptoms of anemia, these patients characteristically present with dark urine from intravascular hemolysis. **Thrombosis** of major venous structures, particularly the hepatic vein (Budd-Chiari syndrome), is a common cause of death in these patients. The hemoglobinuria is most commonly in the first morning urine because the hemolysis occurs more often when patients develop a mild acidosis at night.

Diagnosis. Besides the usual lab findings of hemolysis, such as an increased LDH, bilirubin, and reticulocyte count, these patients have brisk intravascular hemolysis and therefore have a low haptoglobin and hemoglobin in the urine. Hemosiderinuria occurs when the capacity of renal tubular cells to absorb and metabolize the hemoglobin is overwhelmed, and the sloughed off iron-laden cells are found in the urine. The gold standard test is flow cytometry for CD55 and CD59 on white and red cells. In PNH, levels are low or absent.

Treatment. Iron replacement can be necessary if the degree of urinary blood loss is severe. Corticosteroids are helpful when the disease is severe for unclear reasons. Thromboses are treated with anticoagulation. Eculizumab inhibits complement effect on red cells. It is a costly drug but its use is increasing.

Glucose-6-Phosphate Dehydrogenase (G6PD) Deficiency

Definition. The hereditary deficiency of an enzyme for producing the reducing capacity necessary for neutralizing oxidant stress to the red cell resulting in acute hemolysis.

Etiology. Various forms of oxidant stress result in sudden hemolysis. The most common type of oxidant stress is actually from infections, not drugs. The most commonly implicated drugs are sulfa drugs, primiquine, dapsone, quinidine, and nitrofurantoin.

Clinical Presentation. Patients are normal until exposed to the stress. A sudden, severe, intravascular hemolysis can occur including jaundice, dark urine, weakness, and tachycardia. The history of recent drug ingestion is the main clue to the diagnosis.

Diagnosis. The usual findings of an intravascular hemolysis include high LDH, bilirubin, and reticulocyte count with a normal MCV, low haptoglobin, and hemoglobinuria. Heinz bodies are precipitated hemoglobin inclusions seen in red cells. Bite cells are seen on smear indicating the removal of the Heinz bodies. The definitive test is the G6PD level, which can be falsely normal immediately after an episode of hemolysis. Hence, the level is best tested about 1 week after the event.

Treatment. There is no specific therapy beyond hydration and transfusion if the hemolysis is severe. The main therapy is to avoid oxidant stress in the future.

Note

Decay accelerating factor (DAF) is also known as CD55 and CD59. DAF are the main proteins that protect RBCs from complement destruction.

APLASTIC ANEMIA

Definition. Failure of all 3 cell lines produced in the bone marrow, resulting in anemia, leukopenia, and thrombocytopenia (pancytopenia). The marrow is essentially empty with the absence of precursor cells.

Etiology. Although there are many things that can cause bone marrow failure, the most common cause of true aplastic anemia is rarely precisely determined. Radiation, toxins such as benzene, drugs such as nonsteroidal anti-inflammatory agents, choramphenicol, alcohol, and chemotherapeutic alkylating agents can all cause aplastic anemia. Infiltration of the marrow with infections such as tuberculosis or cancer such as lymphoma can cause pancytopenia, but this is not truly aplastic anemia. Aplastic anemia can also be caused by infections such as hepatitis, HIV, CMV, Epstein-Barr virus, or Parovirus B19 in immunocompromised patients.

Clinical Presentation. Patients most commonly present with bleeding from the thrombocytopenia, but may present with a combination of the findings associated with deficiencies in all 3 cell lines. Fatigue from anemia and infections from neutropenia may also occur. The clinical presentation may give a clue to the presence of pancytopenia but is not sufficient to determine a true aplastic anemia by clinical manifestations alone. The absence of a classical association such as benzene, radiation, or chloramphenicol would most certainly not exclude a diagnosis of aplastic anemia. The most common single etiology is idiopathic.

Diagnosis. Pancytopenia on a CBC is the first test. A bone marrow biopsy confirms the diagnosis when alternative etiologies for a pancytopenia are not present. In other words, the marrow is empty of almost all precursor cells as well as evidence of primary or metastatic cancer, infection, or fibrosis. The marrow is hypoplastic and fat filled with no abnormal cells seen.

Treatment. Bone marrow transplantation should be carried out whenever the patient is young and healthy enough to withstand the procedure and there is a donor available. Allogeneic transplant can cure up to 80–90% of patients under 50. When a bone marrow transplantation is not possible, immunosuppressive agents should be tried. This is a combination of antithymocyte globulin, cyclosporine, and prednisone. These agents can lead to remission in 60–70% of patients. It is believed that T lymphocytes are primarily causal in the bone marrow failure, so drugs are used to decrease the T-cell response.

ACUTE LEUKEMIA

Definition. The rapid onset of bone marrow failure from the derangement of the pluripotent stem cell resulting in the relentless destruction of the normal production of the entire bone marrow. The blood cells lose the ability to mature and function normally.

Etiology. Most cases of acute leukemia arise with no apparent cause. There are several well known associations with the development of acute leukemia that are sometimes present. These include radiation exposure, benzene, chemotherapeutic agents such as melphalan and etoposide, as well as some retroviruses. Genetic disorders such as Down syndrome and Klinefelter can result in an increased incidence of leukemia. Myelodysplasia and sideroblastic anemia can also develop into acute leukemia.

Clinical Presentation. The most common presentation results from the effects of the leukemic blast cells crowding out the normal marrow cells, resulting in symptoms of bone marrow failure (even if total WBC count is elevated or normal). Fatigue from anemia is the most common presenting complaint. Bleeding from thrombocytopenia occurs. Infection from the underproduction or abnormal function of WBCs also occurs.

Acute lymphocytic leukemia (ALL) is more common in children and acute myelogenous leukemia (AML) is more common in adults, but they are indistinguishable clinically. ALL is more often associated with infiltration of other organs, but AML can do it as well. Enlargement of the liver, spleen, and lymph nodes and bone pain are common at presentation. Disseminated intravascular coagulation (DIC) is associated with M3 promyelocytic leukemia. CNS involvement resembling meningitis is present at the time of initial diagnosis in about 5% of patients. CNS involvement is most characteristic of M4 and M5 monocytic leukemia. Rarely, a syndrome of "leucostasis" can occur when the white cell count is extremely elevated. This results from sludging of the leukemic cell in the vasculature, resulting in headache, dyspnea, confusion, and brain hemorrhage.

Diagnosis. The CBC is the first clue to the diagnosis. Depression of all 3 cell lines is common at presentation. WBC can be low, normal, or elevated. Thrombocytopenia and anemia are usual. Many other disorders can present as pancytopenia similar to leukemia such as aplastic anemia, infections involving the marrow, metastatic cancer involving the marrow, vitamin B_{12} deficiency, SLE, hypersplenism, and myelofibrosis. None of these will have leukemic blasts circulating in the peripheral blood, however. A bone marrow biopsy showing >20% blasts confirms the diagnosis of acute leukemia. The presence of blasts tells you the patient has acute leukemia, but blast analysis cannot be relied upon to always tell which type is present. AML is characterized by the presence of Auer rods, myeloperoxidase, and esterase. ALL is characterized by the presence of the common ALL antigen (CALLA) and terminal deoxynucleotidyl transferase (TdT). Auer rods are most specific for M3. Ultimately, the diagnosis rests upon the use of monoclonal antibodies, which recognize specific types of leukemia as well as the expression of specific CD antigens on the surfaces of the cells. Nonspecific findings that are also present are hyperuricemia and an increased level of LDH.

Treatment. Chemotherapy is used initially in all patients to induce a remission. Inducing a remission means a removal of over 99.9% of the leukemic cells in the body and the elimination of peripheral blasts in circulation. This is followed by further rounds of chemotherapy to "consolidate" the leukemia further. After chemotherapy, adults with AML or ALL should be referred for allogeneic bone marrow transplantation. The initial chemotherapy for AML is cytosine arabinoside (AraC) and either daunorubicin or idarubicin. The initial chemotherapy for ALL is daunorubicin, vincristine, and prednisone. Promyelocytic leukemia is managed with the addition of the **vitamin A derivative all-trans-retinoic acid** (ATRA). Leucostasis events are managed with leukapheresis in addition to the chemotherapy.

ALL patients must also undergo prophylaxis of the central nervous system to prevent relapse there. The best agent for this is intrathecal methotrexate.

CHRONIC LEUKEMIA

Chronic Myelogenous Leukemia (CML)

Definition. A chronic myeloproliferative disorder characterized by the massive overproduction of myeloid cells. These cells retain most of their function until later in the course of the disease.

Etiology. Although the Philadelphia chromosome is characteristic of the disease, the cause of the production of this chromosome is unknown. It is a clonal disorder of myelocytes. The Philadelphia chromosome is a translocation between chromosomes 9 and 22, resulting in a gene producing an enzyme with tyrosine kinase activity. Five percent of cases are Philadelphia chromosome negative.

Note

CML can be confused with a leukemoid reaction. They are distinguishable based upon the leukocyte alkaline phosphatase score.

Clinical Presentation. A markedly elevated white blood cell count can be found on routine blood count. The most common symptoms are fatigue, night sweats, and low-grade fever. Abdominal pain from massive enlargement of the spleen is common. Bone pain from infiltration with white cells can occur. Enlarged lymph nodes are rare. Infection and bleeding are uncommon because these white cells retain the majority of their function. Rarely, a leukostasis reaction can occur from extremely elevated amounts of white cells being produced in the range of 200,000–500,000/mm^3. The white cells then clog up the vasculature, resulting in dyspnea, blurry vision, priapism, thrombosis, and stroke.

Diagnosis. The main feature of the disease is an elevated white blood cell count consisting predominantly of neutrophils with a left shift. Blasts are either absent or present in very small amounts (<5%). The leukocyte alkaline phosphatase score (LAP) is diminished. Basophilia is characteristic of CML and *all* myeloproliferative disorders such as polycythenia vera. Although the B$_{12}$ level is often elevated, this would not be enough to establish the diagnosis. The Philadelphia chromosome is a far more specific test for CML and should be done in a patient with a markedly elevated white cell count. A low LAP score is not as important as the PCR for Bcr/Abl. The platelet count can also be markedly elevated.

Treatment. The best initial therapy for CML is imatinib, which is also known by the manufacturer's name, Gleevec®. Imatinib is a direct inhibitor of the tyrosine kinase produced by the Philadelphia chromosome. There is nearly a 90% hematologic response to imatinib, and as many as 60 to 70% of patients may lose the Philadelphia chromosome. The milder the disease, the greater the degree of hematologic response. Bone marrow transplantation is no longer the clear first choice as therapy for CML. This is because of the extraordinary response to imatinib, as well as the high mortality associated with the bone marrow transplantation itself. If imatinib fails, then the therapy is bone marrow transplantation.

Chronic Lymphocytic Leukemia (CLL)

Definition. Massive overproduction of mature, but still leukemic, lymphocytes usually from the monoclonal production of B lymphocytes.

Etiology. The etiology of CLL is unknown.

Clinical Presentation. CLL can often present as an asymptomatic elevation of white cells found on routine evaluation of patients or during investigations for other problems. Patients are exclusively older with 90% being age >50. When patients do have symptoms, they are often nonspecific—fatigue, lethargy, and uncomfortable enlargement of lymph nodes. Infiltration of other parts of the reticuloendothelial system such as the spleen, liver, and bone marrow also occurs. Infection and bleeding are unusual presentations of the disease. Staging for CLL is as follows:

- **Stage 0: lymphocytosis alone**
- **Stage 1: lymphadenopathy**
- **Stage 2: splenomegaly**
- **Stage 3: anemia**
- **Stage 4: thrombocytopenia**

Staging is important because the survival of untreated stage 0 and stage 1 disease is 10–12 years even without treatment. The survival of stage 3 and stage 4 disease is 1–2 years. CLL can be associated with various autoimmune phenomena such as thrombocytopenia and autoimmune hemolytic anemia.

Diagnosis. CLL is strongly suspected when an older patient has a marked elevation in the white cell count with a marked lymphocytic predominance in the range of 80–98% lymphocytes. The marrow is often infiltrated with the leukemic lymphocytes. CD19 is an antigen strongly associated with CLL. The cell count is usually elevated in the range of 30,000–50,000, but may go as high as 150,000. "Smudge cells" seen on a smear are characteristic of CLL.

Treatment. Early stage CLL with only an elevated white cell count or enlargement of lymph nodes is not treated. However, patients with symptomatic disease always need to be treated. Those with more advanced-stage disease should receive initial therapy with fludarabine. Fludarabine has greater efficacy than chlorambucil and should be considered the drug of choice. Autoimmune hemolysis and thrombocytopenia are treated with prednisone. Rituximab is used in those patients who express CD20, especially with autoimmune ITP or hemolytic anemias.

Myelodysplasic Syndrome (MDS)

MDS is an idiopathic disorder that is considered "pre-leukemic," in that a number of people go on to develop acute myelogenous leukemia (AML). MDS is probably from a genetic defect. The most common defect is 5q deletion or "5q–." Patients are usually elderly and present with a pancytopenia, elevated MCV, fatigue, infections, and/or bleeding because of the low cell counts. There is a small number of blasts from 1–20% and, in fact, it is the percentage of blasts present that tells how "close" a person is to AML.

Most patients die of infection or bleeding before they develop AML. This is because the disorder is slowly progressive and older patients "wear out" so to speak from cytopenias, more often than not going into the "blast phase" that characterizes AML. By definition, you must exclude B_{12} and folate deficiency because the disorder is so similar.

CBC and bone marrow are indispensible. You may find a bi-lobed neutrophil called a Pelger-Huet cell which is characteristic. Genetic testing for the 5q– is essential.

Treatment is periodic transfusions and control of the infections as they arise. Disease-specific therapy consists of the TNF inhibitor lenalidomide or thalidomide. Azacitidine or decitabine is useful when the 5q- is present. Some patients who are young enough with a match can undergo bone marrow transplantation.

Polycythemia Vera

Definition. A disorder of red cell production. Red cells are produced in excessive amounts in the absence of hypoxia or increased erythropoietin levels.

Clinical Presentation. Patients present with:
- Markedly elevated hematocrit
- Splenomegaly
- Sometimes elevation of the platelet and white cell counts
- Thromobosis
- "Plethora" or redness and fullness of the face

Diagnosis. Diagnose with a high hematocrit in the absence of hypoxia, carbon monoxide poisoning, or elevated erythropoietin level. The most specific test is the Janus Kinase or JAK-2. Treat with phlebotomy.

Essential Thrombocythemia

Essential thrombocythemia is a type of platelet cancer. The platelet is over a million. There is either thrombosis or bleeding. The most specific test is JAK-2. Treat with hydroxyurea and sometimes anagrelide.

PLASMA CELL DISORDERS

Multiple Myeloma

Definition. A clonal abnormality of plasma cells resulting in their overproduction replacing the bone marrow as well as the production of large quantities of functionless immunoglobulins. The disease is characterized by various systemic manifestations such as bone, kidney, and infectious complications.

Etiology. The cause of multiple myeloma is unknown.

Clinical Presentation. Bone pain is the most common clinical manifestation. This is most commonly in the back and the ribs, secondary to pathologic fractures. Radiculopathy from the compression of spinal nerve roots is also common. Infection particularly with encapsulated organisms such as *Pneumococcus* and *Haemophilus* is common. Renal failure and anemia are common. The symptoms of hypercalcemia such as polyuria, polydipsia, and altered mental status may occur. Weakness, fatigue, and pallor are common. Rarely, symptoms of a hyperviscosity syndrome such as blurry vision, confusion, and mucosal bleeding may occur.

Diagnosis. Although a normochromic, normocytic anemia is the most common laboratory finding, this is not specific for myeloma. A protein electrophoresis with a markedly elevated monoclonal immunoglobulin spike is present in almost all cases. This is most commonly IgG but may be IgA, IgD, or rarely a combination of two of these. Plain x-ray of the skeletal system and skull will reveal the punched-out lytic lesion caused by the overproduction of osteoclast activating factor from the plasma cells. Serum B_2 microglobulin is elevated in 75% of patients. Hypercalcemia from the destruction of bone is common, as is an elevation in the BUN and creatinine from the damage to the kidney from the immunoglobulins, Bence-Jones protein, calcium, and hyperuricemia. A bone marrow biopsy with >10% plasma cells confirms a diagnosis of multiple myeloma. Bence-Jones protein is often not detected by a standard protein test on a urinalysis, which mainly is meant to detect albumin. A specific test for Bence-Jones protein involving acidification of the urine is required. Increased gamma globulin levels will increase the total protein and decrease the albumin level.

Treatment. Younger patients (age <70) should be treated with **autologous bone marrow transplantation** in an attempt to cure the disease. Older patients should receive a combination of melphalan and prednisone. Patients who are candidates for transplants should receive thalidomide (or lenalidomide) and dexamethasone. Patients who are not candidates for transplants should receive melphalon, prednisone, and thalidomide. Hypercalcemia is treated initially with hydration and loop diuretics and then with bisphosphonates such as pamidronate.

Bortezomib is a proteasome inhibitor useful for relapsed myeloma or in combination with the other medications. It can be combined with steroids, melphalan, or lenalidomide (thalidomide).

Monoclonal Gammopathy of Uncertain Significance (MGUS)

Definition. The overproduction of a particular immunoglobulin by plasma cells without the systemic manifestations of myeloma such as bone lesions, renal failure, anemia, and hypercalcemia.

Etiology. The cause of MGUS is unknown. MGUS is a very common abnormality present in 1% of all patients age >50 and in 3% of those age >70. Some patients with MGUS may progress to multiple myeloma.

Clinical Presentation. Patients with MGUS have no symptoms. It is found on routine blood testing for other reasons.

Diagnosis. An elevated monoclonal immunoglobulin spike of serum protein electrophoresis (SPEP) in amounts lower than found in myeloma. The creatinine, calcium, and hemoglobin levels are normal. An elevated total serum protein is the clue to the diagnosis. There are no lytic bone lesions, and the bone marrow has <5% plasma cells. The beta-2 microglobulin level will be normal in most patients.

Treatment. Treatment is neither effective nor necessary.

LYMPHOMA

> A 32-year-old woman comes to the office with a neck mass for the last several weeks. She also has fever, weight loss, and sweats.

Hodgkin Disease

Definition. A neoplastic transformation of lymphocytes particularly in the lymph node. It is characterized by the presence of Reed-Sternberg cells on histology which spreads in an orderly, centripetal fashion to contiguous areas of lymph nodes.

Etiology. Although there is a clear increase in Hodgkin disease among relatives of those with the disease, there are no clear environmental or infectious etiologies for the disorder.

Hodgkin disease has bimodal age distribution—one peak in the 20s and 60s.

Clinical Presentation. Enlarged, painless, rubbery, nonerythematous, nontender lymph nodes are the hallmark of the disease. Patients may also develop what are labeled "B" symptoms, which are drenching night sweats, 10% weight loss, and fevers. Although pruritus is common in the disease, it is not one of the "B" symptoms. Cervical, supraclavicular, and axillary lymphadenopathy are the most common initial signs of disease. Lymphadenopathy may develop anywhere in the body, however. Extralymphatic sites such as splenic involvement, skin, gastric, lung, CNS, or any other organ may possibly be involved. Extralymphatic involvement is more common with non-Hodgkin lymphoma.

Staging is as follows:

Stage I: One lymphatic group or single extra lymphatic site.

Stage II: Two lymphatic groups or extra lymphatic sites on the same side of the diaphragm.

Stage III: Involvement of lymphatic groups on both sides of the diaphragm or involvement of any extralymphatic organ contiguous to the primary nodal site.

Stage IV: Widespread disease with involvement of diffuse extralymphatic sites such as the bone marrow or liver.

The staging is the same for both Hodgkin as well as non-Hodgkin lymphoma. In Hodgkin lymphoma, staging is the single most important predictor of outcomes.

Diagnosis. An excisional lymph node biopsy is the essential first step in determining the diagnosis. After the initial diagnosis is determined by the biopsy, the most important step is to determine the extent of disease because the stage will determine the nature of the therapy, i.e., radiation versus chemotherapy. Chest x-ray or chest CT, abdominal CT, or MRI is used to determine if the disease is localized to the supraclavicular area. Lymphangiography and laparotomy are no longer routinely used for staging. CT scan is sensitive enough to detect any involved lymph nodes. A bone marrow biopsy is used to definitively determine if the disease is truly localized.

Size alone is insufficient to determine the content of some enlarged nodes. PET scan can also be used for that purpose.

Other labs tests that are often abnormal, but don't directly alter the stage of the disease, include a CBC looking for anemia as well as increased white cell or platelet count. Eosinophilia is common. An elevated LDH level indicates an adverse prognosis. The ESR is useful prognostically. Elevated liver function tests help determine the need for liver biopsy.

Treatment. Therapy is entirely based on the stage of the disease. Localized disease such as stage IA and IIA is managed predominantly with radiation. In the early stages (IA, IIA), adjunct chemotherapy may be used with radiation. All patients with evidence of "B" symptoms as well as stage III or stage IV disease are managed with chemotherapy. The most effective combination chemotherapeutic regimen for Hodgkin disease is ABVD (adriamycin [doxorubicin], bleomycin, vinblastine, and dacarbazine). ABVD is superior to MOPP (meclorethamine, oncovin [vincristine], prednisone, and procarbazine) because ABVD has fewer adverse effects such as permanent sterility, secondary cancer formation, leukemia, aplastic anemia, and peripheral neuropathy.

Hodgkin disease has several histologic subtypes. Lymphocyte-predominant has the best prognosis, and lymphocyte-depleted has the worst prognosis. The histologic subtype does not alter anything described above. The lab tests, staging, and treatments are the same.

Non-Hodgkin Lymphoma (NHL)

Definition. The neoplastic transformation of both the B and T cell lineages of lymphatic cells. NHL causes the accumulation of neoplastic cells in both the lymph nodes as well as more often diffusely in extralymphatic organs and the bloodstream. The Reed-Sternberg cell is absent.

Note

Adverse Prognostic Factors

- Large mediastinal lymphadenopathy
- Age >40
- "B" symptoms
- ↑ ESR

Etiology. There are a number of infectious and autoimmune disorders associated with the development of NHL. Their absence, however, by no means excludes the presence of NHL. Infections such as HIV, hepatitis C, Epstein-Barr, HTLV-I, and *Helicobacter pylori* predispose to the development of NHL. HIV and Epstein-Barr are both more often associated with Burkitt lymphoma. HIV can also be associated with immunoblastic lymphoma. The main point of knowing this is that they are both high-grade lymphomas with an aggressive progression of disease.

Clinical Presentation. Enlarged, painless, rubbery, nonerythematous, nontender lymph nodes are the hallmark of the disease. Patients may also develop what are labeled "B" symptoms, which are drenching night sweats, 10% weight loss, and fevers. Although pruritus is common in the disease, it is not one of the "B" symptoms. In this sense, NHL is the same as Hodgkin disease. The difference is that Hodgkin disease is localized to cervical and supraclavicular nodes 80–90% of the time, whereas NHL is localized only 10–20% of the time. NHL is far more likely to involve extralymphatic sites as well as to have blood involvement similar to chronic lymphocytic leukemia. CNS involvement is also more common with NHL. HIV-positive patients often have CNS involvement.

The staging system for NHL is the same as that for Hodgkin disease as described above.

Diagnosis. The diagnosis of NHL rests initially on an excisional lymph node biopsy. After this, the most important step is to determine the stage of the disease to determine therapy. Although this is quite similar to that described above for Hodgkin disease, there are several significant differences because NHL is far more likely to be widespread at initial presentation. Lymphangiography is never necessary, and staging laparotomy is rarely needed. The bone marrow biopsy is more central as an initial staging tool. Because the presence of marrow involvement means the patient has Stage IV disease and therefore needs combination chemotherapy, further invasive testing such as the laparotomy is not necessary. As with Hodgkin disease anemia, leukopenia, eosinophilia, high LDH, and high ESR often accompany the disease. PET scanning is highly sensitive and specific for nodal and extranodal sites but not for bone marrow disease.

Treatment. As with Hodgkin disease, local disease such as stage IA and stage IIA are treated predominantly with radiation, and all those with "B" symptoms as well as stages III and IV receive combination chemotherapy. Given the frequency of more widespread disease with NHL, however, this means few NHL patients are treated with radiation alone. The initial chemotherapeutic regimen for NHL is still CHOP (cyclophosphamide, hydroxy-adriamycin, oncovin [vincristine], prednisone). More elaborate chemotherapeutic regimens for NHL, of which there are many, are beyond the scope of what is necessary to know for the Step 2 exam.

CNS lymphoma is often treated with radiation, possibly in addition to CHOP. Relapses of NHL can be controlled with autologous bone marrow transplantation. Knowing each of the histologic subtypes of NHL is not necessary for the USMLE Step 2 exam. Some patients with NHL express CD20 antigen in greater amounts. When this occurs, monoclonal antibody rituximab should be used. Rituximab is an anti-CD20 antibody that has limited toxicity and adds survival benefit to the use of CHOP. Thus, R-CHOP would then become first-line therapy. Prior to using R-CHOP, always test completely for hepatitis B and C, as rituximab can cause fulminant liver injury in those with active hepatitis B or C disease.

Note

Staging laparotomy is no longer used for NHL.

PLATELET DISORDERS

Immune Thrombocytopenic Purpura (ITP)

Definition. Thrombocytopenia of unknown etiology.

Etiology. The idiopathic production of an antibody to the platelet, leading to removal of platelets from the peripheral circulation by phagocytosis by macrophages. The platelets are bound by the macrophage and brought to the spleen, leading to low platelet counts. ITP is often associated with lymphoma, CLL, HIV, and connective tissue diseases.

Clinical Presentation. Like all platelet disorders, the patient presents initially with signs of bleeding from superficial areas of the body such as the skin, nasal and oral mucosa, GI tract, urine, and vagina. The patient is generally young, more often female, and complains of epistaxis, bruising, hematuria, dysfunctional uterine bleeding, and sometimes GI bleeding. Petechiae, purpura, and ecchymoses are often found on exam. The patient is generally otherwise healthy. Splenomegaly should be absent.

Diagnosis. Thrombocytopenia is the major finding. A normal spleen on exam and on imaging studies such as an U/S is characteristic. Antiplatelet antibodies have a high sensitivity but poor specificity. The bone marrow should be filled with megakaryocytes indicating that there is a problem with platelet destruction and not platelet production. The bone marrow will also exclude other causes of thrombocytopenia such as primary or metastatic cancer, infiltration by infections such as tuberculosis or fungi, or decreased production problems such as drug, radiation, or chemotherapy effect on the bone marrow. The peripheral smear and creatinine should be normal, excluding other platelet destruction problems such as hemolytic uremic syndrome, thrombotic thrombocytopenic purpura, and disseminated intravascular coagulation.

Treatment. Prednisone is the initial therapy in almost all patients. Splenectomy is used in patients in whom very low platelet counts <10,000–20,000/mm^3 continue to recur despite repeated courses of steroids. IVIG or RhoGAM™ may be used in patients with profoundly low platelet counts (<10,000 μL) or in patients at risk for life-threatening bleeding. Note that RhoGAM may only be used in Rh-positive patients. In those who recur after splenectomy, we use thrombopoietin agents romiplostim or eltrombopag. Rituximab has also been used.

Von Willebrand Disease (vWD)

> A 22-year-old woman comes to the emergency department with epistaxis and heavy periods. She has a PT of 11 seconds (normal), a PTT of 40 seconds (prolonged), and 217,000/mm^3 platelets.

Definition. An increased predisposition to platelet-type bleeding from decreased amounts of von Willebrand factor.

Etiology. An autosomal dominant disorder resulting in a decreased amount of von Willebrand factor. This is the most common congenital disorder of hemostasis. vWD results in a decreased ability of platelets to **adhere** to the endothelial lining of blood vessels. This is different from platelets aggregating with each other, which is mediated by fibrinogen. In vWD, aggregation is normal, whereas adherence is abnormal. It is not necessary to know the difference between the different subtypes of vWD for the Step 2 exam.

Clinical Presentation. Patients with vWD manifest platelet-type bleeding such as that described above for ITP. This is mucosal and skin bleeding such as epistaxis, petechiae, bruising, and menstrual abnormalities. Both platelet problems as well as clotting factor abnormalities can result in GI and urinary tract bleeding. There is often a marked increase in bleeding after the use of aspirin.

Diagnosis. The platelet count and appearance are normal. The bleeding time is increased particularly after the use of aspirin. The level of von Willebrand factor, also known as factor VIII antigen, is low. The ristocetin platelet aggregation test, which examines the ability of platelets to bind to an artificial endothelial surface (ristocetin), is abnormal. The PTT may be elevated in some patients because of a concomitant decrease in levels of factor VIII coagulant portion.

Treatment. Desmopressin acetate (DDAVP) is used for mild bleeding or when the patient must undergo minor surgical procedures. It releases subendothelial stores of von Willebrand factor. Factor VIII replacement is used if desmopressin is not effective and the bleeding continues. Factor VIII replacement contains von Willebrand factor. This replaces the use of cryoprecipitate, which is now seldom necessary. Patients should not use aspirin. FFP is not useful.

COAGULOPATHY

Hemophilia A and B

Definition. The deficiency of factor VIII in hemophilia A and factor IX in hemophilia B resulting in an increased risk of bleeding.

Etiology. Both hemophilia A and B are X-linked recessive disorders resulting in disease in males. Females are carriers of the disease. Females do not express the disease because they would have to be homozygous, which is a condition resulting in intrauterine death of the fetus. Hemophilia A is far more common than B.

Clinical Presentation. Mild deficiencies (25% or greater activity) result in either the absence of symptoms or with symptoms only during surgical procedures or with trauma. More severe deficiency (<5–10% activity) can result in spontaneous bleeding. Factor-type bleeding is generally deeper than that produced with platelet disorders. Examples of the type of bleeding found with factor deficiencies are hemarthrosis, hematoma, GI bleeding, or urinary bleeding. Bruising and central nervous system bleeding can also occur. Severe hemophilia is obvious in most patients by the age of two. The disorder becomes apparent often at the time of circumcision.

Diagnosis. A prolonged PTT with a normal PT is expected. A factor deficiency is strongly suspected when a 50:50 mixture of the patient's blood is created with a normal control and the PTT drops to normal. This is known as a "mixing study." If the PTT does not correct with mixing, then an antibody inhibitor of the factor is suspected. The mixing study will only tell you that a deficiency is present; it will not tell you which specific factor is deficient. Specific factor VIII or IX levels are necessary to determine a precise diagnosis. This is true of both hemophilia A and B.

Treatment. Mild hemophilia can be treated with desmopressin (DDAVP). Desmopressin can also be used prior to surgical procedures in mild hemophiliacs. Desmopressin works by releasing subendothelial stores of factor VIII. More severe deficiencies are treated with replacement of the specific factor. Desmopressin does not work for hemophilia B.

Table 6-1. Causes of Prolonged PT or PTT

	Prolonged PT	Prolonged PTT	Prolonged PT and PTT
Inherited causes	Factor VII deficiency	vWF and factors VIII, IX, XI, or XII deficiencies	Prothrombin, fibrinogen, factor V, factor X, or combined factor deficiencies
Acquired causes	• Vitamin K deficiency • Liver disease • Warfarin use • Factor VII inhibitor	• Heparin • Antiphospholipid antibody	• Vitamin K deficiency • Liver disease • Disseminated intravascular coagulation • Supratherapeutic heparin or warfarin • Combined heparin and warfarin use • Direct thrombin inhibitors • Inhibitor of prothrombin, fibrinogen, or factor V or X

PT, prothrombin time; PTT, partial thromboplastin time; vWF, von Willebrand factor.

Vitamin K Deficiency

Definition. The deficiency of vitamin K resulting in decreased production of factors II, VII, IX, and X.

Etiology. Vitamin K deficiency can be produced by dietary deficiency, malabsorption, and the use of antibiotics that kill the bacteria in the colon that produce vitamin K.

Clinical Presentation. Bleeding may mimic that of hemophilia and may occur at any site. Look for oozing at venapuncture sites.

Diagnosis. Both the PT and PTT are elevated. The PT usually elevates first and more severely. A correction of the PT and PTT in response to giving vitamin K is the most common method of confirming the diagnosis.

Treatment. Severe bleeding is treated with infusions of fresh frozen plasma. Vitamin K is given at the same time to correct the underlying production defect.

Liver Disease

Definition. Coagulopathy from the decreased production of clotting factors by the liver.

Etiology. Any severe liver disease or cirrhosis leads to a decreased production of the majority of clotting factors that are generally all made in the liver, except for factor 8 and von Willebrand factor. Factor VII is first factor to be depleted.

Clinical Presentation. Bleeding may occur at any site, but the GI tract is the most common site.

Diagnosis. Patients have an elevation of both the PT and PTT, but the PT elevates first and is often more severely affected. The disorder is clinically indistinguishable from vitamin K deficiency except that there is no improvement when vitamin K is given. A clear history of liver disease is often present, suggesting the diagnosis. Low platelet counts are often present from the hypersplenism that accompanies the liver disease.

Treatment. Fresh frozen plasma is used acutely to correct severe bleeding such as melena. Long-term management is based on the nature of the liver disease.

Disseminated Intravascular Coagulation (DIC)

Definition. Consumptive coagulopathy from major underlying illness resulting in consumption of both platelet and clotting factor type and occasionally thrombosis. The bleeding is associated with a marked production of fibrin degradation products such as d-dimers.

Etiology. Although essentially an idiopathic disorder, there is almost always a major underlying disease in the case history. Look for evidence of sepsis most commonly. Almost any disorder that results is cellular destruction and the release of tissue factor can initiate the cascade of consumption of platelets as well as clotting factors. These problems include rhabdomyolysis, adenocarcinomas, heatstroke, hemolysis from transfusion reactions, burns, head trauma, obstetrical disasters such as abruptio placenta and amniotic fluid embolism, as well as trauma, pancreatitis, and snakebites. Promyelocytic leukemia (M3) is a classic association.

Gram-negative sepsis causes DIC by the releasing endotoxin. In acute promyelocytic leukemia (M3), the destruction of leukemic granulocyte precursors results in the release of large amounts of proteolytic enzymes from their storage granules, causing microvascular damage. Other malignancies may also cause DIC by augmenting the expression of various oncogenes that result in the release of tissue factor. DIC exists in acute and chronic forms.

- **Acute DIC** develops when sudden exposure of blood to procoagulants (tissue factor, tissue thromboplastin) generates intravascular coagulation. The compensatory hemostatic mechanisms are quickly overwhelmed, and, as a consequence, a severe consumptive coagulopathy leading to hemorrhage develops.

- In contrast, **chronic DIC** reflects a compensated state that develops when blood is continuously or intermittently exposed to small amounts of tissue factor. Compensatory mechanisms are not overwhelmed. Chronic DIC is more frequently observed in patients with solid tumors and in those with large aortic aneurysms.

Clinical Presentation. Bleeding from any site in the body is possible because of a decrease in both the platelet as well as clotting factor levels. Thrombosis is less common. Hemolysis is often present and may lead to acute renal failure, jaundice, and confusion.

Diagnosis. DIC is suspected when a patient has a serious underlying disorder as described above with bleeding and there is elevation in both the PT and PTT with a decrease in the platelet count. The fibrinogen level is often low because it has been consumed. D-dimers and fibrin-split products are present in increased amounts, suggesting the consumption of all available elements of the coagulation system. The peripheral blood smear often shows the schistocytes as fragmented cells consistent with intravascular hemolysis.

Treatment. Because most patients present with severe bleeding, fresh frozen plasma (FFP) and sometimes platelet transfusions are necessary to correct the bleeding. Heparin is controversial and is rarely used except in those patients presenting predominantly with thrombosis. Don't forget to correct the underlying disorder.

Heparin-Induced Thrombocytopenia (HIT)

HIT can occur with any form of heparin, though it is more common with IV unfractionated heparin than with low molecular weight (LMW) heparin. The amount of heparin administration, no matter how small, is irrelevant. That is because HIT is an immune-mediated process. If HIT is diagnosed, stop the heparin. When an acute form of anticoagulation is essential, use a direct-acting thrombin inhibitor such as argatroban or lepirudin.

Warfarin (coumadin) is the most widely prescribed anticoagulant used for the prevention and treatment of thromboembolic disease. It was initially introduced as a pesticide against rodents, and long-acting forms of warfarin are still used for this purpose.

Warfarin anticoagulates by inhibiting an enzyme that recycles oxidized vitamin K to its reduced form. Warfarin does not antagonize the action of vitamin K, but rather antagonizes vitamin K recycling. Once vitamin K is reduced, eventually the vitamin K dependent factors (factors 2,7,9,10) are also reduced (typically about 3-5 days after initiation of treatment).

Despite its efficacy, treatment with warfarin has several limitations. Many commonly used medications interact with warfarin, as do some foods—particularly green vegetables, since they typically contain large amounts of vitamin K. Its activity has to be monitored by the PT and international normalized ratio (INR) to ensure an adequate yet safe dose is taken (typically **INR 2-3** is considered adequate and safe anticoagulation). The pharmacologic action of warfarin may always be reversed by fresh vitamin K.

Table 6-2. Recommended Management of a Supratherapeutic INR

INR	Bleeding Present	Recommended Action
<Ther to 5.0	No	• Lower warfarin dose, **or** • Omit a dose and resume warfarin at a lower dose when INR is in therapeutic range, **or** • No dose reduction needed if INR is minimally prolonged
>5.0 to 9.0	No	• Omit the next 1–2 doses of warfarin, monitor INR more frequently, and resume treatment at a lower dose when INR is in therapeutic range, **or** • Omit a dose and administer 1–2.5 mg oral vitamin K*
>9.0	No	• Hold warfarin and administer 5–10 oral vitamin K. Monitor INR more frequently and administer more vitamin K as needed. Resume warfarin at a lower dose when INR is in therapeutic range.
>20	—	• Hold warfarin and administer 10 mg vitamin K by slow IV infusion; supplement with fresh frozen plasma, or recombinant human factor VIIa, depending on clinical urgency. Monitor and repeat as needed.
Any	Life-threatening	As per "INR >20" above

INR: International Normalized Ratio; Ther: therapeutic INR range for the patient in question.

*Preferred in patients at increased risk for bleeding (e.g., history of bleeding, stroke, anemia).

INTRODUCTION TO ANTIBIOTICS

Antibiotics can be grouped either by the type of organism they are effective against or by the chemical class of the medication. The organisms that cause specific diseases do not change very much over time. For example, *Staphylococcus aureus* is still the most common cause of osteomyelitis, and *Escherichia coli* is still the most common cause of pyelonephritis. What does change over time is the antibiotic that is effective against each organism and the sensitivity pattern of each organism.

Gram-Positive Cocci

Semisynthetic penicillinase-resistant penicillins (oxacillin, cloxacillin, dicloxacillin, nafcillin)

Staphylococcal and streptococcal organisms are effectively treated by medications such as the semisynthetic penicillins, including oxacillin, nafcillin, dicloxacillin, and cloxacillin. These agents are exclusively effective against Gram-positive cocci, in particular staphylococci.

Methicillin belongs to this group of antibiotics as well, and was one of the original drugs developed in the class. Methicillin is not used clinically, however, because it may cause interstitial nephritis. Hence the term "methicillin-sensitive" or "methicillin-resistant *Staphylococcus aureus*" (MRSA) is somewhat of a misnomer because we don't actually use methicillin. When this term is used, think of the drugs oxacillin, cloxacillin, dicloxacillin, and nafcillin. When *Staphylococcus* is sensitive to the semisynthetic penicillins and if concurrent Gram-negative infection is not suspected, these are the ideal agents. They are more efficacious than vancomycin is when the organism is sensitive. These drugs are also sometimes referred to as "beta-lactamase–resistant penicillins" or "antistaphylococcal penicillins." The latter term is somewhat misleading because they are also effective against a number of streptococci such as *S. pneumoniae*, the Viridans Strep group, and groups A, B, C, and G Strep.

MRSA is treated primarily with vancomycin. Linezolid, telavancin, daptomycin, ceftaroline, and tigecycline are alternatives for MRSA.

Penicillin G, penicillin VK, ampicillin, and amoxicillin

These agents are effective against streptococci, such as *S. pyogenes*, viridans group streptococci, and *S. pneumonia*, but *not* against staphylococci. Ampicillin and amoxicillin are only effective against staph when ampicillin is combined with the beta-lactamase inhibitor sulbactam or when amoxicillin is combined with clavulanate. Ampicillin also has some activity against *E. coli*. Both are effective against enterococci and *Listeria*. All of the agents can be useful against Gram-negative bacteria, such as *Neissera*.

Note

Do not use vancomycin if the organism is oxacillin-sensitive.

Cephalosporins (first-generation agents: cefazolin, cefadroxil, cephalexin; second-generation agents: cefoxitin, cefotetan, cefuroxime, cefprozil, loracarbef)

The first- and second-generation cephalosporins will all cover the same range of organisms that the semisynthetic penicillins will cover. In addition to staphylococci and streptococci, first- and second-generation cephalosporins will also cover some Gram-negative organisms. First-generation agents will only reliably cover *Moraxella* and *E. coli*. Second-generation agents will cover everything a first-generation cephalosporin covers, as well as a few more Gram-negative bacilli such as *Providencia*, *Haemophilus*, *Klebsiella*, *Citrobacter*, *Morganella*, and *Proteus*. In general, your answer should correspond most specifically to the organism you are treating. For example, if you are treating a sensitive *Staph aureus* or *Strep*, you should answer with a specific Gram-positive drug. Your answer should not be an extremely broad-spectrum agent such as imipenem or meropenem, even though these drugs will treat the organism. Don't give an answer that gives more coverage than you need unless there is definite evidence to support the presence of other organisms. In the case of Gram-positive infection, you should generally answer the use of a first-generation agent.

Third-generation agents, particularly ceftazidime, are not reliable in their staphylococcal coverage. Although the fourth-generation cephalosporin cefepime will cover staph and strep, you should never answer this agent when you have an exclusively Gram-positive infection.

Allergic Cross-Reactivity with Penicillins. For persons with a genuine allergy to penicillin, there is only a <1% risk of cross-reaction with cephalosporins. When this reaction occurs it is seldom an anaphylactic reaction. When the allergic reaction is described as a rash, you can safely use a cephalosporin. When the reaction is more severe, such as anaphylaxis, you should not answer a cephalosporin. For minor infections, use a macrolide (clarithromycin or azithromycin) or one of the new fluoroquinolones (levofloxacin, gemifloxacin, or moxifloxacin). For serious infections in those with a life-threatening penicillin allergy, you should use vancomycin, linezolid, or daptomycin.

Macrolides (erythromycin, clarithromycin, azithromycin), fluoroquinolones (levofloxacin, gemifloxacin, moxifloxacin), and clindamycin

These agents are alternatives to penicillins and cephalosporins for Gram-positive infection. Macrolides should not be used for serious staph infections. The new quinolones are very good for streptococcal infections, particularly *Strep pneumoniae* in the absence of outright penicillin resistance. They are also sufficient against staph. Ciprofloxacin is a quinolone as well but it does not cover *Strep pneumoniae*.

Vancomycin, linezolid, tigecycline, ceftaroline, telavancin

These agents are alternatives for Gram-positive infections. They are your answer when there is either a life threatening penicillin allergy or there is MRSA. Linezolid is the only oral medication available against MRSA. Linezolid, daptomycin, and quinupristin/dalfopristin are also effective against vancomycin-resistant enterococci. Ceftaroline is used like a third-generation such as ceftriaxone combined with an MRSA agent such as vancomycin. Ceftaroline is the only cephalosporin to cover MRSA. These medications should not be used if the organism is sensitive to methicillin.

Gram-Negative Bacilli

Penicillins (piperacillin, ticarcillin, mezlocillin)

These agents are fully active against the full range of Gram-negative bacilli, such as the Enterobacteriaceae as well as *Pseudomonas*. Enterobacteriaceae include *E. coli*, *Proteus*,

Note

Daptomycin, ceftaroline, and tigecycline are drugs also effective against MRSA.

Enterobacter, Citrobacter, Morganella, Serratia, and *Klebsiella*. They are only active against staph when they are combined with a beta-lactamase inhibitor such as piperacillin/tazobactam or ticarcillin/clavulanate. Ampicillin/Sulbactam and amoxicillin/clavulanate will also cover staph and Gram-negative bacilli, but not *Pseudomonas*. All penicillins will cover sensitive streptococci, but if the patient described has only a sensitive strep you should answer with a narrower agent, such as penicillin G or penicillin VK.

Cephalosporins (third-generation agents: ceftazidime, cefotaxime, ceftriaxone, cefotaxime; fourth-generation agent: cefepime)

Third- and fourth-generation agents are fully active against the full range of Gram-negative bacilli such as the Enterobacteriaceae. Only ceftazidime and cefepime will cover *Pseudomonas*. Cefepime also covers staph. Second-generation agents cover some of the Enterobacteriaceae, but not *Pseudomonas*. Although predominantly for use against Gram-negative organisms, ceftriaxone and cefotaxime are the best answers for penicillin-insensitive pneumococci-causing meningitis or pneumonia.

Quinolones (ciprofloxacin, levofloxacin, gemifloxacin, moxifloxacin, ofloxacin)

These agents all cover most of the Enterobacteriaceae, such as *E. coli, Proteus, Enterobacter, Haemophilius, Moraxella, Citrobacter, Morganella, Serratia,* and *Klebsiella*. Only ciprofloxacin will reliably cover *Pseudomonas*. The new fluoroquinolones (moxifloxacin, levofloxacin, and gemifloxacin) are also active against Gram-positive cocci, in particular *Strep pneumoniae*. They are amongst the first-line therapies for empiric treatment of pneumonia because they will also cover *Mycoplasma, Chlamydia,* and *Legionella*.

Aminoglycosides (gentamicin, tobramycin, amikacin) and monobactams (aztreonam)

These agents have essentially the same Gram-negative coverage as listed above for the other agents. Although aminoglycosides can be synergistic with a penicillin in the treatment of staph, they are essentially exclusively Gram-negative agents. Aztreonam is exclusively a Gram-negative agent, with no strep or staph coverage at all.

Carbapenems (imipenem, meropenem, ertapenem, doripenem)

Fully active against Enterobacteriaceae and *Pseudomonas*, they are similar in Gram-negative coverage to the aminoglycosides and third-generation cephalosporins. In addition, they have excellent staph and anaerobic coverage. Although effective in polymicrobial infections, they are best used in Gram-negative infections. Ertapenem will not cover *Pseudomonas*. All carbapenems are equally effective against anaerobes, as compared to metronidazole.

Anaerobes

The agent most active against anaerobes is metronidazole. Clindamycin is less active against intraabdominal anaerobes. Metronidazole has some advantages against the anaerobic Gram-negative bacteria in the bowel, such as *Bacteroides fragilis*. Metronidazole is also the first-line agent against *Clostridium difficile*. Clindamycin may have some advantages against the anaerobic streptococci found in the mouth. The other agents with excellent anaerobic coverage virtually equal to metronidazole are the carbapenems and the beta-lactam/beta-lactamase combination medications such as piperacillin/tazobactam, ticarcillin/clavulanate, ampicillin/sulbactam, or amoxicillin/clavulanate. The second-generation cephalosporins cefoxitin and cefotetan have fair activity against anaerobes, but they are not as good as the agents described above.

Note

Cephalosporins are safe in penicillin allergy if it is only a rash.

Clinical Pearl

Ceftriaxone does not have adequate pseudomonal coverage.

Note

Sensitive *Staph* should not be treated with TMP/SMZ, doxycycline, or clindamycin.

Skin MRSA

TMP/SMZ, clindamycin, doxycycline, and linezolid are oral agents useful for MRSA. Oral therapies such as these should only be used for minor MRSA infections. TMP/SMZ, clindamycin, and doxycycline cannot be used for MRSA bacteremia.

CENTRAL NERVOUS SYSTEM INFECTIONS

Meningitis

A 45-year-old man is brought to the emergency department with 1–2 days of fever, headache, nausea, and vomiting. On physical examination he is found to have neck stiffness and photophobia.

Definition. An infection or inflammation of the meninges, which is the connective tissue covering the central nervous system (CNS).

Etiology. Most cases of meningitis arise sporadically, and the precise method of spread of the microorganism into the central nervous stem is not determined. Overall, most cases of meningitis are due to viruses. *Streptococcus pneumoniae* is the most common cause of bacterial meningitis for all patients beyond the neonatal period. In the past, *Haemophilus influenzae* was the most common cause in children, but this has been markedly decreased by the use of the *Haemophilus* type B vaccine in children. *Neisseria meningitidis* is spread by respiratory droplets and is the most common cause of meningitis in adolescents. *Listeria monocytogenes* is more common in those with immune system defects, particularly of the cellular (T-cell) immune system and sometimes neutrophil defects. These defects include HIV, steroid use, leukemia, lymphoma, and various chemotherapeutic agents. Neonates and the elderly have decreased T-cell immune function; therefore, *Listeria* is more common in the very young and the very old.

Even with immune deficits, *Streptococcus pneumoniae* is still the *most* common etiology—it is just that *Listeria* is *more* common in these patients, as compared to fully immunocompetent patients. *Staphylococcus aureus* is more common in those who have had any form of neurosurgery because instrumentation and damage to the skin introduce the organism into the CNS. *Cryptococcus* is more common in those who are HIV positive and who have profound decreases in T-cell counts to levels <100 cells.

Rocky mountain spotted fever (RMSF) is common in those who have been exposed to ticks in the appropriate geographic area. The areas with the highest RMSF infection are in the mid-Atlantic areas, such as the Carolinas, Kentucky, Tennessee, etc. Lyme disease can also cause meningitis and is more common in the Northeast, such as Massachusetts, Connecticut, New York, and New Jersey. Tuberculosis and syphilis are also associated with meningitis. Viruses are the most common cause of aseptic meningitis, a syndrome in which patients present in a manner similar to bacterial meningitis, but CSF analysis mostly reveals a lymphocytic pleocytosis and bacterial cultures are negative. Viruses causing aseptic meningitis include entero viruses, arboviruses (St. Louis encephalitis virus, West Nile virus), HIV, herpes simplex, and lymphocytic choriomeningitis virus. In the past, most of these were not diagnosed, but with the availability of PCR-based testing, more cases of aseptic meningitis are being accurately classified. Group B *Streptococcus* (*Streptococcus agalactiae*) is the most common cause of meningitis in the neonatal period.

The spread of the organism into the CNS can be by sporadic (unknown) mechanisms or by means of contiguous local infection or by hematogenous spread. Local infections that can lead to meningitis include otitis media, sinusitis, mastoiditis, and dental infections. Hematogenous spread could possibly occur from any infection but is more common with endocarditis and pneumonia.

Clinical Presentation. Regardless of microbiologic etiology, all forms of meningitis present with fever, photophobia, headache, nuchal rigidity (neck stiffness, positive Kernig and Brudzinski signs), as well as nausea and vomiting. Altered mental status is possible as well and can make a patient seem like they have encephalitis. Any form of CNS infection can present with seizures. Focal neurologic deficits can also occur, the most common being visual field and cranial nerve deficits. The most common long-term neurologic deficit from bacterial meningitis is damage to the 8th cranial nerve.

Rash is associated with several different types of meningitis. A petechial rash is suggestive of *Neisseria*. A rash on the wrists and ankles with centripetal spread toward the body is suggestive of RMSF. Facial nerve palsy is suggestive of Lyme disease. The targetlike erythema migrans rash of Lyme disease is seldom present by the time the meningitis develops. Pulmonary symptoms or an abnormal chest x-ray suggest tuberculosis (TB).

Diagnosis. Lumbar puncture is essential for establishing the diagnosis. CT scan of the head is the best initial diagnostic test if the patient has papilledema, focal motor deficits, new onset seizures, or severe abnormalities in mental status, or is immunocompromised (HIV infection, immunosuppressive medications, post-transplantation, etc.). If none of the above is present, a lumbar puncture can be safely done without doing a CT scan of the head first, which can significantly delay the diagnosis. If the lumbar puncture is delayed >20–30 minutes for any reason, then the best initial step is to give an empiric dose of antibiotics.

The most accurate test for bacterial meningitis on the lumbar puncture is the culture of the CSF. The results are always delayed for several days, however, and are rarely, if ever, available at the time that the initial therapy must be instituted. Protein levels are elevated most commonly with bacterial meningitis, but they can be elevated in any type of meningitis. An elevated protein level and/or a decreased glucose level by themselves are relatively nonspecific findings. The opening pressure can be elevated with any cause of meningitis.

The Gram stain has a limited sensitivity and is positive in 50–70% of patients at most. When positive, however, the Gram stain has a high degree of specificity.

Initially, the most useful test is the cell count. Although elevated cell count by itself is nonspecific, the differential of the cells is useful. Only bacterial meningitis gives thousands of cells that are all neutrophils. A mild-to-moderate elevation in lymphocytes, with several dozen to several hundred cells, can occur with viral infection, *Rickettsia*, Lyme disease, tuberculosis, syphilis, or fungal (cryptococcal) etiology. A normal CSF cell count is <5 cells/mm^3, which should be predominantly lymphocytes.

Specific diagnosis of nonbacterial meningitis is based on the nature of the organism. Lyme disease and RMSF are best detected with a specific immunologic response and serology. *Cryptococcus neoformans* is detected initially with an India ink test and then later with an elevation in the serum and CSF cryptococcal antigen titer. Syphilis is confirmed by the presence of a positive VDRL or FTA on CSF. TB is rarely detected by AFB smear. Culture for TB has a much higher yield, particularly on several repeated LPs. PCR can also aid in the diagnosis of TB.

Treatment. Empiric therapy of bacterial meningitis in adults is best achieved with vancomycin (because of the increasing prevalence worldwide of pneumococci with decreasing sensitivity to penicillins) plus a third-generation cephalosporin, such as ceftriaxone. Ampicillin is added to those with immune defects to cover *Listeria* and for patients age >50 years or ≤ 1 month old.

Clinical Pearl

In patients presenting with symptoms and signs of meningitis, treat empirically for bacterial meningitis while awaiting test results from the lumbar puncture.

You will have to recognize the risks such as HIV, steroid use, pregnancy, or hematologic malignancies in the case description. *Listeria* is resistant to all forms of cephalosporins. Vancomycin is used if you know you have definite or suspected pneumococcal resistance to penicillin or if there is a chance of staphylococcal infection after neurosurgery. Lyme disease is best treated with ceftriaxone. *Cryptococcus* is treated initially with amphotericin. This is followed by fluconazole therapy in HIV-positive patients for life or until the patient is on HAART (highly active antiretroviral therapy) and is asymptomatic with a CD4 count >100/μL for at least 3–6 months. Neurosyphilis is treated with high-dose IV penicillin. TB meningitis is treated in the same fashion as you would use for pulmonary TB (though a longer duration of 9–12 months of therapy is given). Steroid use in adult meningitis is appropriate for TB meningitis and bacterial meningitis. There is no treatment currently proven useful for viral (or aseptic) meningitis.

Dexamethasone (corticosteroid) therapy for patients with bacterial meningitis decreases mortality and rates of deafness. The rationale for this is the inflammatory response elicited in the subarachnoid space due to bacterial cell wall lysis after antibiotics are administered; this inflammatory reaction can worsen morbidity and mortality due to bacterial meningitis. Accordingly, dexamethasone given 15–20 minutes before or concurrently with the administration of antibiotics resulted in improved outcomes (morbidity and mortality); the benefit is greatest for patients with pneumococcal meningitis. Dexamethasone should be continued for 4 days if bacterial meningitis is confirmed (a positive Gram stain of CSF fluid or >1000 WBCs within the CSF can be taken as confirmation of bacterial meningitis) and discontinued if the etiology is nonbacterial (viral, fungal, etc.).

Encephalitis

A young man is brought to the emergency department by his friends because of 1–2 days of confusion and strange behavior. He had been originally complaining of a headache and fever. On the day of admission, he became markedly worse and is now delirious. He is generally healthy. On physical examination, you find a lethargic, confused man with an elevated temperature. You are unable to determine if he has focal neurologic findings or to obtain an accurate neurologic exam because his confusion makes him unable to follow commands.

Definition. An infection of the brain. This includes both the meninges, as well as the brain parenchyma.

Clinical Pearl

Encephalitis usually presents with altered mental status, erratic behavior, etc (brain parenchyma involved).

Etiology. Although any bacterial, protozoal, or rickettsial infection can cause encephalitis, the majority is caused by viruses. Although virtually any virus can cause encephalitis, the most common cause is herpes simplex, usually type I (HSV-1). Varicella-zoster virus, CMV, enteroviruses, Eastern and Western equine encephalitis, St. Louis encephalitis, and West Nile encephalitis can also occur but are much less common than HSV.

Clinical Presentation. Fever and a headache occur but these findings are relatively nonspecific. Altered mental status with fever and headache is the primary clue to the diagnosis. Any level of neurologic deficit may occur, ranging from slight confusion to lethargy or coma. Focal deficits of any kind can occur. Neck stiffness similar to that found in meningitis can occur, making it difficult to distinguish encephalitis from meningitis. Seizures may also occur.

Diagnosis. Although CT or MRI scan of the head should be performed, it cannot give a specific diagnosis. HSV has a predilection for involvement of the temporal lobes, which can sometimes be seen on CT. A lumbar puncture is the key to the diagnosis. Formerly, a brain biopsy was necessary, but PCR (polymerase chain reaction) amplification techniques have virtually eliminated that need. PCR for HSV has a 98% sensitivity and >95% specificity, making it at least equal to the biopsy.

Treatment. HSV encephalitis is best treated with IV acyclovir. Although famciclovir and valacyclovir have activity against HSV, they are not available intravenously. Ganciclovir or foscarnet are active against CMV. Acyclovir-resistant herpes is treated with foscarnet.

Brain Abscess

An HIV-negative man is brought to the hospital because of a seizure. When he becomes more alert, you find that he has aphasia and weakness of the right hand and leg. A CT scan of the head with contrast shows enhancement of the lesion with a "ring" around the lesion.

Definition. A collection of infected material within the brain parenchyma.

Etiology. Bacteria can spread into the brain from contiguous infections such as otitis media, sinusitis, mastoiditis, or dental infections. Organisms may also spread through the bloodstream from endocarditis or pneumonia and seed the brain. Toxoplasmosis can reactivate in those with severe HIV disease when their CD4 counts are very low (<50–100/μL). Brain abscesses most commonly have *Streptococcus* in 60–70%, *Bacteroides* in 20–40%, Enterobacteriaceae in 25–35% and *Staphylococcus* in 10%, and are often polymicrobial. Because of the diversity of the organisms potentially involved, it is difficult to have a single standard therapy.

Clinical Presentation. Headache is the most common symptom. Fever can be present. Focal neurologic deficits are the initial complaint in about 60% of patients. Seizures may occur, as with any form of anatomic abnormality of the CNS. All CNS infections can cause seizures.

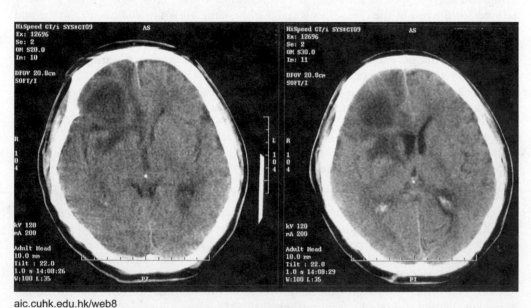

aic.cuhk.edu.hk/web8

Figure 7-1. CT Scan Demonstrating Large Cerebral Abscess

Diagnosis. The initial test is the CT scan. Contrast is used to help identify the lesion, although CNS malignancy enhances with contrast as well. MRI is even more accurate than is the CT scan. No radiologic test alone can give the precise etiology, however. In the case of bacterial brain abscess, examination of the abscess fluid (obtained by stereotactic aspiration or surgical excision of the abscess) for Gram stain and culture is essential. In HIV-positive patients, 90% of brain lesions will be either toxoplasmosis or lymphoma. This is the only circumstance where empiric therapy is sufficient to establish a specific diagnosis. If the lesion responds to 10–14 days of therapy with pyrimethamine and sulfadiazine, then the patient should simply continue to receive this therapy, as it accurately predicts cerebral toxoplasmosis.

Treatment. Almost always, successful treatment requires a combination of surgical and medical management. Stereotactic aspiration (preferred) and surgical excision of the abscess are the two methods used; the latter is rarely used nowadays because of significant complications.

With the exception of HIV-positive patients, who are best treated with pyrimethamine and sulfadiazine, therapy must be based on the specific etiology found. One example of a combination of therapy (but certainly not the only one) would be penicillin, metronidazole, and a third-generation cephalosporin, such as ceftazidime. Penicillin would cover the streptococci, metronidazole the anaerobes, and ceftazidime the Gram-negative bacilli.

HEAD AND NECK INFECTIONS

Otitis Media

Definition. An infection of the middle ear between the eustachian tube and the tympanic membrane.

Etiology. Viral upper respiratory infection can cause edema of the eustachian tube, which often leads to middle ear infection. The most common organisms are *Strep pneumoniae* (35–40%), *H. influenzae* (nontypeable; 25–30%), and *Moraxella catarrhalis* (15–20%). Viruses probably account for the rest of the cases. This is roughly the same breakdown of organism type and frequency that occurs in bronchitis and sinusitis.

Clinical Presentation. Patients complain of ear pain, fever, and decreased hearing. On physical examination you'll find a red, bulging tympanic membrane with loss of the light reflex. The most sensitive clinical finding is immobility of the membrane on insufflation of the ear with air. Perforation of the tympanic membrane with otorrhea occurs rarely.

Diagnosis. Physical examination of the ear is the chief means of establishing the diagnosis. Radiologic tests are not useful. A specific bacteriologic diagnosis can be obtained with tympanocentesis for culture, but this is rarely performed.

Treatment. Oral therapy with amoxicillin is still the best initial therapy. Amoxicillin-clavulanate is used if there has been recent amoxicillin use or if the patient does not respond to amoxicillin. Other alternatives to amoxicillin-clavulanate are second-generation cephalosporins, such as cefuroxime, loracarbef, or cefprozil, or third-generation agents, such as cefdinir or cefixime. Patients with severe penicillin allergies should receive macrolides such as azithromycin or clarithromycin. New fluoroquinolones such as levofloxacin, moxifloxacin, or gatifloxacin are certainly microbiologically acceptable but are broader coverage than necessary and should not be used in children (concern for arthropathy). TMP/SMZ is sometimes used but is poorly active against *Streptococcus pneumoniae*.

Sinusitis

A young woman comes to the office with several days of facial pain, a headache, cough, fever, and discolored nasal drainage. On physical examination, you find tenderness over the maxillary sinuses and decreased transillumination of the maxillary sinuses.

Definition. An infection of the sinuses. The most common site is the maxillary sinus, followed by ethmoid, frontal, and sphenoid sinuses.

Etiology. Viruses are responsible for most of the cases. Bacterial organisms that cause sinusitis are the same ones causing otitis media.

Clinical Presentation. Patients complain of facial pain, headache, postnasal drainage, and purulent nasal drainage. Headache is common and is worse when the patient leans forward. Fever occurs in about half of the cases. Tooth pain also occurs because of the proximity of the sinuses to the teeth.

Diagnosis. Obvious cases such as that described above do not always need radiologic confirmation prior to treatment. Sinus x-rays are of little value, and routine imaging as a rule is not recommended. However, if imaging is required because of concern of complications or the diagnosis is uncertain, or if there is no response to treatment, a CT scan of the sinuses is the test of choice. CT scans provide greater detail. Occasionally, a sinus puncture is necessary to confirm a specific bacteriologic etiology, particularly when the patient does not respond to therapy or if there are frequent recurrences.

Treatment. Mild or acute uncomplicated sinusitis can be managed with decongestants, such as oral pseudoephedrine or oxymetazoline sprays. More severe pain with discolored nasal discharge is treated with antibiotics. The drugs used are in the same order and type as those listed above for otitis media because the microbiology is almost identical.

Most cases of viral rhinosinusitis resolve in 7–10 days with symptomatic management (antihistamines, NSAIDS, and decongestants). If symptoms persist beyond that point or get worse, antibiotics should be considered.

Pharyngitis

Etiology. Although the majority of pharyngeal infections are from viruses, the most important cause is from group A beta-hemolytic streptococci (*S. pyogenes*). This is because of the possibility of the organism progressing on to rheumatic fever or glomerulonephritis. *S. pyogenes* only accounts for 15–20% of cases of pharyngitis.

Clinical Presentation. Sore throat with cervical adenopathy and inflammation of the pharynx with an exudative covering is highly suggestive of *S. pyogenes*. Most viruses do not give an exudate, although the Epstein-Barr virus can. Mild *S. pyogenes* infections may not give an exudate, and this is one of the reasons diagnostic testing is useful. Hoarseness and cough are not suggestive of pharyngitis.

Diagnosis. The rapid streptococcal antigen test is 80% sensitive but >95% specific. A positive test can be considered the equivalent of a positive culture, whereas a negative test should be confirmed with a culture.

Treatment. Penicillin remains the mainstay of therapy. Macrolides and oral, second-generation cephalosporins are alternatives in the penicillin-allergic patient.

Influenza

Definition/Etiology. A systemic viral illness from influenza A or B, usually occurring in an epidemic pattern and transmitted by droplet nuclei. Influenza can lead to damage to the respiratory epithelium, leading to sinusitis, otitis media, bronchitis, and pneumonia.

Clinical Presentation. Patients have a systemic illness characterized by fever, myalgias, headache, and fatigue. Upper respiratory symptoms tend to predominate. These include runny nose (coryza), nonproductive cough, sore throat, and conjunctival injection.

Diagnosis. Confirmation is best achieved initially with rapid antigen detection methods of swabs or washings of nasopharyngeal secretions. Viral culture is the most accurate test but is usually not available rapidly enough to make it useful in acute patient management.

Treatment. Symptomatic therapy with acetaminophen and antitussives is useful. Specific antiviral medications for both influenza A and B are the neuraminidase inhibitors oseltamivir and zanamivir. They should be used within 48 hours of the onset of symptoms to limit the duration of symptoms. Amantadine and rimantadine should not be used in the empiric therapy of influenza. Influenza vaccine is recommended annually in the general public.

The most important candidates for vaccination are those with chronic lung and cardiac disease, pregnant women in any trimester, residents of chronic care facilities, health-care workers, immunosuppressed patients, and those with diabetes and renal dysfunction. Influenza vaccine is contraindicated in those who are highly allergic to eggs and which would result in anaphylaxis.

Note

Flu vaccine is indicated annually for everyone age >6 months.

LUNG INFECTIONS

Bronchitis

> A 63-year-old man comes to the office with a cough productive of yellowish sputum for the last several days. He has smoked 1 pack of cigarettes a day for the last 30 years. On physical examination, he has clear lungs and a temperature of 101°F. His chest x-ray is normal.

Definition/Etiology. Bronchitis is an infection of the lung, which is limited to the bronchial tree with limited involvement of the lung parenchyma. Acute exacerbations of chronic bronchitis (COPD) are often difficult to distinguish from a pneumonia until after a chest x-ray is performed.

Acute bronchitis is an acute inflammation of the tracheobronchial tube. The vast majority of cases are caused by viruses. *S. pneumoniae* and *H. influenzae* have not been implicated. A small percentage of nonviral cases are due to *M. pneumoniae*, *C. pneumoniae*, and *B. pertussis*. The most common organisms responsible for *chronic bronchitis* are similar to those causing sinusitis and otitis media, which are *Streptococcus pneumoniae*, nontypeable *Haemophilus influenzae*, and *Moraxella*. Viruses account for a significant percentage but are often not confirmed. Cigarette smoking is the most common causative factor. Even a single cigarette a day is enough to paralyze the cilia, which clear the bronchial tree of mucus and inhaled impurities, for 24 hours.

Clinical Presentation. Patients present with a cough often accompanied by sputum production. A bacterial etiology is suggested by discolored sputum, but it is impossible to determine the specific bacterial etiology by sputum characteristics alone. Although the lung examination may reveal rales, patients most commonly have clear lungs. Signs of consolidation, such as increased fremitus, are absent. Low-grade fever may be present, but patients are most commonly afebrile.

Diagnosis. Signs of respiratory infection, such as cough and sputum, with a normal chest x-ray confirm the diagnosis.

Treatment. Mild acute cases often do not require therapy because they are often caused by viruses that resolve spontaneously. Acute exacerbations of chronic bronchitis can be treated with amoxicillin, doxycycline, or TMP/SMZ, if there has not been recent antibiotic use. Repeated infection or patients not responding to amoxicillin should be treated with any of the following: amoxicillin/clavulanate, clarithromycin, azithromycin, oral second- or third-generation cephalosporins, or the new fluoroquinolones, gemifloxacin, levofloxacin, or moxifloxacin.

Lung Abscess

A 58-year-old alcoholic man was admitted last night for several weeks of cough, sputum, and fever. He has lost 15 pounds and is feeling weak. On initial examination he is febrile and appears thin. He has very poor dentition. The lung examination is normal. The patient also exhibits a foul odor on the oral examination.

Definition. Necrosis of the pulmonary parenchyma caused by microbial infection.

Etiology

Microbiology

- 90% have at least some anaerobes involved
- The most commonly implicated anaerobes are *Peptostreptococcus*, *Prevotella*, and *Fusobacterium* species, which are oral anaerobes found in the gingival crevices
- 45% only anaerobic, 45% mixed with aerobes, 10% aerobes only
- Aerobic bacteria, most frequently involved are *S. aureus, E. coli, Klebsiella,* and *Pseudomonas*

Pathogenesis

- 85–90% have a clear association with periodontal disease or some predisposition to aspiration (e.g., altered sensorium, seizures, dysphagia).
- Pulmonary infarction, cancer, and vasculitis (like Wegener granulomatosis) are 3 examples of noninfectious causes of lung cavities.

Presentation. Besides the usual symptoms of pulmonary infection, such as fever, cough, sputum production, and chest pain, the features associated with lung abscesses are putrid, foul-smelling sputum in 60–70%, and a more chronic course. Several weeks of symptoms with weight loss, anemia, and fatigue have usually been present prior to diagnosis. This is probably due to the delay of 1–2 weeks between the aspiration of oral contents and the development of necrosis and cavitation.

Diagnosis. Sputum for Gram stain and culture will *not* be able to show the causative anaerobic organism in a lung abscess. The chest x-ray in an abscess will often show a thick-walled cavitary lesion. A chest CT scan is useful to help define the exact extent of the cavity. The lower lobes are the most common sites of aspiration in the upright position, and the posterior segment of the right upper lobe is the most common site in the supine position. Aspiration of the abscess fluid is necessary for a specific bacteriologic diagnosis.

Treatment. In the absence of specific microbiologic diagnosis, clindamycin is good empiric coverage for the "above the diaphragm" anaerobes most often found. Penicillin is also acceptable.

In contrast to most abscesses where drainage is the rule, lung abscesses rarely require drainage in the antibiotic era. Most respond to antimicrobial therapy and drain spontaneously by communicating with larger bronchi. Therefore, the answer to the question, *what is the best initial therapy for a lung abscess*, is antibiotics such as clindamycin, not drainage.

Pneumonia

Definition. An infection of the lung parenchyma.

Etiology. It is not necessary to have a particular predisposing condition to have pneumonia. Pneumonia is the only cause of death from an infectious disease in the top ten causes of death in the United States. It is the sixth leading cause of death. Some conditions do predispose to having pneumonia more commonly. These include cigarette smoking, diabetes, alcoholism, malnutrition, obstruction of the bronchi from tumors, and immunosuppression in general. Neutropenia and steroid use predispose to *Aspergillus* infection.

The most common cause of community-acquired pneumonia in all groups is *S. pneumoniae* when an actual cause is identified (however, viruses are the most common cause in children <5 years of age). The subsequent causes may vary, but *Strep pneumoniae* is always number one. Hospital-acquired or ventilator-associated pneumonia shows a predominance of Gram-negative bacilli such as *E. coli*, the other Enterobacteriaceae, or *Pseudomonas*, as well as MRSA.

Table 7-1. Frequency of Infectious Agents Causing Pneumonia

"Typical"	40–60%
Strep pneumoniae	15–35%
Haemophilus	2–10%
Moraxella	<5%
"Atypical"	10–30%
Legionella	0–15%
Mycoplasma	10%
Chlamydia	5–10%
Viral	2–20%
Unknown	30–60%

Specific predispositions are as follows:

- *Haemophilus influenzae*—smokers, COPD
- *Mycoplasma*—young, otherwise healthy patients
- *Legionella*—epidemic infection in older smokers, particularly when located near infected water sources, such as air-conditioning systems
- *Pneumocystis jiroveci* (formerly *carinii*) pneumonia—HIV-positive persons with <200 CD4 cells not on prophylaxis
- *Coxiella burnetti* (Q-fever)—exposure to animals, particularly at the time they are giving birth
- *Klebsiella*—alcoholics
- *Staphylococcus aureus*—following viral syndromes or viral bronchitis, especially influenza
- *Coccidioidomycosis*—exposure to the deserts of the American Southwest, particularly Arizona
- *Chlamydia psittaci*—birds
- *Histoplasma capsulatum*—exposure to bat or bird droppings, spelunking (recreational cave exploration)
- *Bordetella pertussis*—cough with whoop and post-tussive vomiting
- *Francisella tularensis*—hunters, or exposure to rabbits
- *SARS, Avian influenza*—travel to Southeast Asia
- *Bacillus anthracis, Yersinia pestis,* and *Francisella tularensis*—bioterrorism

Clinical Presentation. Patients with pneumonia present with cough, fever, and often sputum production. Severe pneumonia of any cause may present with dyspnea. The quality and degree of sputum produced might provide useful clues to the microbiologic etiology of pneumonia at the initial presentation. Bacterial infections such as *Streptococcus pneumoniae, Haemophilus,* and *Klebsiella* have significant purulent sputum production because they are infections of the alveolar air space. The sputum in patients with *S. pneumoniae* has been classically described as rusty. This "rust" is simply hemoptysis. As the blood oxidizes, it becomes brownish-red; hence, the comparison to rust. Any form of persistent cough may be associated with hemoptysis, however, and hemoptysis by itself is nonspecific. *Klebsiella pneumoniae* has been associated with sputum described as being like currant jelly. This is simply hemoptysis with mucoid characteristics from a combination of the necrotizing nature of *Klebsiella* with the organism's thick mucopolysaccharide coating. Interstitial infections such as those caused by *Pneumocystis* pneumonia (PCP), viruses, *Mycoplasma,* and sometimes *Legionella* often give a nonproductive or "dry" cough.

Any cause of pneumonia may be associated with pleuritic chest pain. This is pain worsened by inspiration. Commonly, pleuritic pain is associated with lobar pneumonia, such as that caused by *Pneumococcus.* This is because of localized inflammation of the pleura by the infection. Lobar pneumonia is the type most commonly associated with signs of consolidation on examination.

On physical examination pneumonia presents with rales, rhonchi, or signs of lung consolidation, including dullness to percussion, bronchial breath sounds, increased vocal fremitus, and egophony (E to A changes).

The respiratory rate is essential in determining the severity of a pneumonia. The respiratory rate is often a close correlate of the level of oxygenation. Severe pneumonia leads to hypoxia, which leads to hyperventilation.

Organism-specific presentations are as follows:

- *Mycoplasma*—Dry cough and chest soreness. Dyspnea is rare. Bullous myringitis and anemia from hemolysis from cold agglutinin disease is occasionally present. Patients with *Mycoplasma pneumoniae* rarely need to be admitted to the hospital; therefore, any patient presented to you as an inpatient is less likely to have *Mycoplasma*.

- *Legionella*—CNS manifestations such as confusion, headache, and lethargy. GI manifestations include diarrhea and abdominal pain.

- PCP—Marked dyspnea, particularly on exertion, with chest soreness with cough in an HIV-positive person. Patients invariably have AIDS with a CD4 count of <200/μL.

Diagnosis. The most important initial test for any type of pneumonia is the chest x-ray. Besides being able to simply show the presence of disease, the chest x-ray gives the initial clue to determining the diagnosis. The most important initial clue to the diagnosis is whether the infiltrates are localized to a single lobe of the lung or whether they are bilateral and interstitial. *S. pneumoniae* (and other causes of "typical" pneumonia) usually appear as a lobar pneumonia with parapneumonic pleural effusion. Interstitial infiltrates are associated with PCP, viral, *Mycoplasma, Chlamydia, Coxiella*, and sometimes *Legionella* pneumoniae. Sputum should be obtained for both Gram stain as well as culture. Sputum culture is the most specific diagnostic test for lobar pneumonia, such as with *S. pneumoniae, Staphylococcus, Klebsiella*, and *Haemophilus*. The other organisms (viral, *Mycoplasma, Chlamydia, Coxiella*, etc.), the so-called "atypical" organisms, will not show up on a Gram stain or regular bacterial culture for various reasons. Occasionally, more invasive tests are necessary to confirm the diagnosis such as bronchoscopy, thoracentesis, pleural biopsy, or culture of pleural fluid. Ultimately, the most specific diagnostic test for pneumonia is with an open lung biopsy.

Organism-specific diagnostic methods are as follows:

- *Mycoplasma*—Specific serologic antibody titers. Cold agglutinins have both limited specificity and sensitivity.

- *Legionella*—Specialized culture media with charcoal yeast extract, urine antigen tests, direct fluorescent antibodies, and antibody titers.

- PCP—Bronchoalveolar lavage, increased LDH

- *Chlamydia pneumoniae, Coxiella, Coccidioidomycoses*, and *Chlamydia psittaci*—All of these are diagnosed with specific antibody titers.

Note

CURB-65 indicates need for hospitalization in pneumonia:

Confusion

Uremia

Respiratory distress

Blood pressure low

Age >65

Treatment. Treatment depends on whether the patient has a mild disease that can be treated as an outpatient or a more severe illness that must be treated with IV antibiotics as a hospitalized inpatient. The major determinants of severity are the degree of hypoxia, such as a Po_2 <60 mm Hg, oxygen saturation <94% on room air, or a respiratory rate >30/min; confusion or disorientation; uremia; and hypotension (systolic BP <90 mm Hg and diastolic BP <60 mm Hg). Other markers of severity are high fever, hypothermia, leukopenia (WBC <4,000/mm^3), rapid pulse (>125/min), hyponatremia, or dehydration as determined by an elevated BUN. Patients with serious underlying diseases such as cancer, liver disease, renal disease, or chronic lung disease often do better in hospital with IV medications.

The specific organism causing pneumonia is rarely, if ever, known at the time that the initial therapeutic decision must be made. Empiric therapy for pneumonia managed as an outpatient is with a macrolide, such as azithromycin or clarithromycin. This is because of the high frequency of *Mycoplasma* and *Chlamydia pneumoniae* as the cause of less severe community-acquired pneumonia (CAP). New fluoroquinolones (levofloxacin, moxifloxacin, or gemifloxacin) are alternatives. Although oral second- and third-generation cephalosporins and amoxicillin/clavulanate are often used, they do not cover the atypical pathogens well.

Hospitalized patients with CAP should receive either levofloxacin, moxifloxacin, or gatifloxacin *or* a second- or third-generation cephalosporin such as cefotaxime or ceftriaxone combined with a macrolide antibiotic such as azithromycin or clarithromycin (or doxycycline).

Table 7-2. Empiric Therapy of Community-Acquired Pneumonia

Outpatient (Nonhospitalized)	Inpatient (Hospitalized)
First choice: macrolides: Azithromycin, clarithromycin *Alternatives: new fluoroquinolones:* Levofloxacin, moxifloxacin, gemifloxacin	New fluoroquinolones (levofloxacin, moxifloxacin, or gemifloxacin) *or* Second- or third-generation cephalosporins (cefuroxime or ceftriaxone) combined with a macrolide or doxycycline *or* Beta-lactam/beta-lactamase combination drug (ampicillin/sulbactam; ticarcillin/clavulanate; piperacillin/tazobactam) combined with doxycycline or a macrolide

Treatment of Hospital-Acquired Pneumonia. Those patients who develop pneumonia after 5–7 days in the hospital are at increased risk of infection from drug-resistant, Gram-negative bacilli (*Pseudomonas*, *Klebsiella*, *E. coli*, etc.) or gram-positive bacilli such as methicillin-resistant *Staphylococcus aureus* (MRSA). Empiric therapy of hospital-acquired pneumonia is with third-generation cephalosporins with antipseudomonal activity (such as ceftazidime) or carbapenems (such as imipenem) or with beta-lactam/beta-lactamase inhibitor combinations (such as piperacillin/tazobactam) and coverage for MRSA with vancomycin or linezolid. Aminoglycosides (gentamicin, tobramycin, amikacin) are often added to empiric gram-negative coverage for synergy and to ensure that the patient might be getting at least one drug if the bacteria is multidrug resistant. Antibiotic therapy can then be adjusted when results of cultures (sputum, blood, bronchoalveolar lavage, and/or pleural) become available.

Treatment of specific organisms is as follows:

- *Haemophilus influenzae*—Second- or third-generation cephalosporins
- *Mycoplasma*—Macrolides, doxycycline, or a quinolone
- *Legionella*—Macrolides, doxycycline, or a quinolone
- *Pneumocystis* pneumonia—Trimethoprim/Sulfamethoxazole (TMP/SMZ). Steroids should be used if the infection is severe. Severe is defined as an arterial P_{O_2} <70 mm Hg or an A-a gradient of >35 mm Hg. If the patient is allergic to TMP/SMZ, IV pentamidine or atovaquone should be used. Dapsone or atovoquone can be used prophylactically.
- *Coxiella brunetti* (Q-fever)—Doxycycline (or erythromycin as an alternative)
- *Klebsiella*—Third-generation cephalosporins and the other drugs for Gram-negative bacilli
- *Staphylococcus aureus*—Semisynthetic penicillins (oxacillin, nafcillin, etc.) if methicillin sensitive. In the nosocomial setting, isolates are invariably methicillin-resistant, and vancomycin or linezolid is administered.
- *Coccidioidomycosis*—Primary pulmonary disease does not need to be treated. Treatment is only used for disseminated disease or in those with pulmonary disease who are immunosuppressed. Life-threatening disease is treated with amphotericin. Mild disease is treated with fluconazole or itraconazole.

Pneumococcal vaccine

Those patients at increased risk for pneumonia should receive pneumococcal vaccine. Those who should receive the vaccine include all patients age >65, as well as those with any serious underlying lung, cardiac, liver, or renal disease. Immunocompromised patients, such as those on steroids, HIV-positive persons, splenectomized patients, diabetics, and those with leukemia or lymphoma, should be vaccinated at the earliest possible opportunity. The vaccine is 60–70% effective. Re-dosing in 5 years is only necessary for those with severe immunocompromise or in those who were originally vaccinated before the age of 65. In generally healthy persons vaccinated age >65, a single dose of vaccine is enough to confer lifelong immunity.

Tuberculosis

A 37-year-old resident of a maximum-security correctional facility has been having a cough, voluminous sputum production, and fever for the last few weeks. He has had a 10-pound weight loss and feels very weak.

Definition/Etiology. Tuberculosis is an infection with *Mycobacterium tuberculosis* (TB). Worldwide, TB is one of the top 3 causes of all deaths. Nearly a quarter of the entire world's population has been exposed and would be reactive to PPD testing. Up until the middle of this century, TB was the most common cause of death in the United States, but at present TB is at an all-time low in the United States with an incidence of <15,000 cases per year. More than half of all cases are in recent immigrants. TB is spread exclusively by person-to-person transmission by means of respiratory droplet infection. There is no animal reservoir of the disease. Bacillus Calmette-Guérin (BCG) vaccination is used in many parts of the world outside of the United States to try to prevent infection. It is, at best, 50% effective and is never indicated for routine use in the United States. Besides immigrants, TB predominantly occurs in persons with specific risks for exposure such as alcoholics, healthcare workers, prisoners, residents of homeless shelters and nursing homes, and in chronically debilitated patients whose weakened immune systems allow for more frequent re-activation of latent infection. Impairment of T-cell–mediated cellular immunity is the most significant defect associated with re-activation. This is why steroid use, organ transplantation, leukemia, lymphoma, and HIV are such important risk factors.

Clinical Presentation. Patients present with cough, sputum, fever, and an abnormal lung examination. They may be impossible to distinguish clinically from those with pneumonia. Weight loss is common because of the chronicity of the infection. Even when untreated, tuberculosis usually takes up to 5 years to become fatal. Night sweats may occur. TB occurs outside of the lungs in 15–20% of cases. The presentation is dependent on the site involved. Any part of the body may be involved, although the lymph node, meningeal, GI, and genitourinary are the most frequent sites involved in extrapulmonary TB. Lymph node involvement (adenitis) is the most frequently involved extrapulmonary site.

Diagnosis. Chest x-ray is the best initial test, as it is with all forms of pulmonary infections. Apical involvement with infiltrates and sometimes cavitation is the most common finding. Adenopathy, effusion, and calcified nodules (Ghon complex) are associated findings. Sputum examination with specific staining for acid-fast bacilli (AFB) allows specific diagnosis. AFB stain has limited sensitivity, and you need 3 negative smears to reach >90% sensitivity. AFB-positive sputum staining is usually the trigger to start therapy for TB. Culture is the most specific test, but because it routinely takes 4–6 weeks to grow, the culture is often not available to guide initial therapy. The culture is also necessary in order to do sensitivity testing. Other diagnostic modalities sometimes necessary if the sputum AFB stain is unrevealing are thoracentesis (to examine the pleural fluid), gastric aspirate in children, biopsy or needle aspiration of the specific extrapulmonary organ involved, and lumbar puncture with meningitis. Pleural biopsy is the single most sensitive diagnostic test. A single pleural biopsy can have up to 75% sensitivity. TB will give caseating necrosis on biopsy of any tissue.

Do not use PPD testing to diagnose acute cases of TB. PPD is relatively insensitive and nonspecific particularly with acute illness.

Treatment. Initial therapy of TB before the results of sensitivity testing are known consists of 4-drug therapy with isoniazid (INH), rifampin (Rif), pyrazinamide (PZA), and ethambutol (ETB). All 4 drugs are continued for the first 2 months or until sensitivity testing is known. PZA and ETB are then discontinued, and therapy continues with INH and rifampin for another 4 months. This makes routine therapy last for a total of 6 months. The fourth drug, ETB, is given if the sensitivity is not known. The only forms of TB that definitely must be treated for longer than 6 months are TB meningitis (12 months), TB in pregnancy (9 months), and osteomyelitis. HIV-positive persons may be treated for 6–9 months, but there is no clear evidence that 9 months is necessary, i.e., even in HIV-positive persons, 6 months of therapy is effective. INH use should generally be combined with vitamin B_6 (pyridoxine) to prevent peripheral neuropathy that can be a side effect of INH.

Pregnant patients should not receive PZA or streptomycin. Steroid use with TB medications is only your answer for TB meningitis and TB pericarditis.

All of the TB medications can cause liver toxicity, except streptomycin. INH also causes peripheral neuropathy because of pyridoxine deficiency. Rifampin is associated with causing a benign change in the color of all bodily fluids to orange/red. This color is dangerous only because it could stain contact lenses and white underwear. Ethambutol is associated with optic neuritis, which can cause color blindness and other visual disturbances. PZA can cause a benign hyperuricemia. Don't treat the hyperuricemia unless there are symptoms of gout associated with it, which rarely occurs.

Diagnosis and treatment of latent TB infection. The PPD test and interferon gamma release assay (IGRA) are used to screen asymptomatic populations at risk of TB to see if they have been exposed and are at increased risk of re-activating the disease. The AFB stain and culture of the affected tissues should be performed. PPD is considered positive based on the amount of induration of the skin 48–72 h after the intradermal (not subcutaneous) injection of the PPD. Erythema is irrelevant. A positive PPD or IGRA roughly indicates a 10% lifetime risk of developing TB in HIV-negative persons. Most of the active cases will develop within the first 2 years after converting to a positive test. HIV-positive persons have a roughly 7–10% risk per year of developing active disease. Previous BCG vaccination does not alter these recommendations. The cutoffs are as follows:

≥5 mm:

- Close contacts of active TB cases
- HIV-positive persons
- Abnormal chest x-ray consistent with old, healed TB
- Steroid use or organ transplantation recipients

≥10 mm: High-risk groups, such as healthcare workers, prisoners, and nursing home residents; recent immigrants (within 5 years) from areas with a high prevalence; homeless patients; persons with immunocompromise other than those described above, such as those with leukemia, lymphoma, diabetics, dialysis patients, and injection drug users who are HIV-negative or whose HIV status is unknown; and children <4 years of age, or infants, children, and adolescents exposed to adults at high risk of TB.

≥15 mm: Low-risk populations, i.e., *not* the people described above, i.e., people who should never have been tested in the first place.

Clinical Pearl

Newer tests may provide TB sensitivity testing in a few weeks, thus the period of using 4 drugs is significantly shortened.

Two-stage testing: Those in whom there has not been a recent PPD test and now show some reactivity that is <10 mm should have a second test within 2 weeks. This is to make sure the first test was not a false negative. A reaction of >10 mm on the second test is simply a positive test, not a recent converter. You cannot make a PPD-negative person become positive with repeated testings.

All patients who test positive on the PPD test or IGRA should have a chest x-ray to see if they have early asymptomatic evidence of TB on their film. Those with abnormal chest x-rays should have 3 sputum AFB stains done to see if they have active disease. Positive AFB smears indicate the need for the start of 4 TB drugs as described above.

Patients with positive PPD tests or IGRA and no evidence of active disease should receive therapy with 9 months of INH and vitamin B_6. A normal chest x-ray or an abnormal x-ray and 3 negative AFB stains of sputum are sufficient to exclude active disease. Although 6 months of INH/B6 is an acceptable alternative, the recommendation is that *all* patients, including those who are HIV positive, should receive the same 9-month course of therapy. Previously, this was referred to as "prophylaxis." The proper designation is now "treatment of latent TB."

The IGRA is not altered at all with previous BCG vaccine. The IGRA has the same meaning and treatment as a positive PPD skin test. Previous BCG vaccination does not alter these recommendations in any way. Previous BCG will not make the IGRA positive.

GASTROINTESTINAL INFECTIONS

Infectious Diarrhea/Food Poisoning

A 27-year-old medical student leaves the Step 2 class at 12:30 to go to lunch. At 3 P.M. she starts having repeated episodes of diarrhea. The diarrhea contains blood and mucus. She is also febrile and has abdominal pain.

Definition. Most infectious diarrhea is caused by contaminated food and water, so the overlap between food poisoning and infectious diarrhea is considerable. There are several types of food poisoning, such as *Bacillus cereus* and *Staphylococcus aureus*, that present predominantly with vomiting, so the two terms are not entirely synonymous.

Etiology. A wide variety of agents can cause food poisoning.
- The most common agent causing food poisoning is *Campylobacter*.
- The most commonly associated agent with contaminated poultry and eggs is *Salmonella*.
- *E. coli* is still the most common cause of travelers' diarrhea; it produces a wide spectrum of disease depending on whether it makes toxin or is invasive.
  - *E. coli 0157:H7* is associated with undercooked hamburger meat.
  - *Bacillus cereus* is associated with fried rice; the rice becomes contaminated with bacillus spores, and as it is prepared for serving it is warmed only at a moderate temperature not hot enough to kill the spore.
  - *Giardia lamblia* and cryptosporidiosis are acquired from contaminated water sources that have not been appropriately filtered, such as fresh water found on a camping trip.
    ° Cryptosporidiosis is also associated with HIV, particularly when there is profound immunosuppression and CD4 count drops <50 cells.

- There are several types of Vibrio causing human disease.
  - *V. cholera* is very rare in the United States.
  - *V. parahaemolyticus* is associated with ingestion of contaminated shellfish such as clams, oysters, and mussels.
  - *V. vulnificus* is associated with ingestion of raw shellfish; it causes severe disease in those with underlying liver disease; it is also associated with iron overload and the development of bullous skin lesions.
- Viral infections such as rotavirus or Norwalk agents are most commonly associated with outbreaks in children.
- Clostridia associations are as follows:
  - *C. difficile* with previous antibiotic use
  - *C. botulinum* with ingestion of infected canned foods
  - *C. perfringens* with ingestion of meat contaminated with spores due to unrefrigeration

Although it is important to be familiar with these associations, remember that virtually any food can be contaminated by almost any organism. In reality, the most important thing is not what food you eat but whose dirty hands touched your food and what were they contaminated with.

Clinical Presentation. The single most important feature of any person presenting with possible food poisoning is the presence or absence of blood in the stool. Blood is most commonly associated with invasive enteric pathogens, such as *Salmonella, Shigella, Yersinia*, invasive *E. coli*, and *Campylobacter*. The time between the development of the diarrhea from the ingestion of the food is not as important as the presence of blood. Incubation times are helpful only if you have a group outbreak and you can pinpoint a common source of contamination. In other words, the last thing you eat is not necessarily the thing that was contaminated. The invasive enteric pathogen may be causing infection in the absence of blood, however, and the absence of blood does not exclude them. *Campylobacter* is rarely associated with Guillain-Barré syndrome.

Ingestion of ciguatera toxin causes symptoms within 2–6 hours, which includes paresthesias, numbness, nausea, vomiting, and abdominal cramps. In severe cases symptoms can be neurologic (weakness, reversal of hot-cold sensations), and cardiovascular (hypotension) can develop. Neurologic symptoms can be severe, progressive, and debilitating. There is no specific therapy to reverse ciguatera poisoning. The most commonly implicated fish are barracuda, red snapper, and grouper.

E. coli 0157:H7 and *Shigella* are associated with hemolytic uremic syndrome (HUS).

Bacillus cereus and *Staphlococcus* predominantly present with vomiting within 1–6 hours of their ingestion because they contain a preformed toxin. They can give diarrhea later.

Giardia, Cryptosporidium, Cyclospora, and most other protozoans do not give bloody diarrhea. The major protozoan associated with blood in the stool is *Entamoeba histolytica*.

Viruses can give voluminous watery diarrhea but do not result in bloody diarrhea.

Scombroid is a type of poisoning that occurs after ingesting scombroid fish (tuna, mackerel, mahi mahi), which may contain a large amount of histamine. When ingested, scombroid can give symptoms within a few minutes: rash, diarrhea, vomiting, and wheezing, along with a burning sensation in the mouth, dizziness, and paresthesias.

Diagnosis. When there is no blood present in the stool, the best initial method of determining the etiology of the diarrhea is to test the stool for the presence of WBCs with methylene blue testing. WBCs will tell you that you have an invasive pathogen but will not distinguish the specific type. Culture is necessary to determine the specific type.

Giardia and *Cryptosporidia* are detected by direct examination of the stool for the parasites, as well as for their eggs. A special modified AFB stain is necessary to detect *Cryptosporidia*. Stool ELISA is also used for *Giardia*.

Treatment. Therapy is determined by the severity of disease. Mild infections with the invasive pathogens and viruses usually require only oral fluid and electrolyte replacement. More severe infections, such as those producing high fever, abdominal pain, tachycardia, and hypotension, require IV fluids and oral antibiotics. You rarely, if ever, have the luxury of a specific etiology identified when the initial therapeutic decision must be made. The best initial empiric antibiotic therapy of an invasive pathogen is with a fluoroquinolone such as ciprofloxacin.

Organism-specific therapy is as follows:

- *Campylobacter*—Erythromycin
- *Giardia*—Metronidazole
- *Cryptosporidium*—Control of underlying HIV disease with antiretrovirals, nitazoxanide
- Nitazoxanide is the first truly useful therapy for cryptosporidiosis.
- Scombroid—Antihistamines such as diphenhydramine

ACUTE VIRAL HEPATIC INFECTIONS

> An 18-year-old woman comes to the emergency department because of several days of nausea, vomiting, and fever. She uses no medications. She reports unprotected sex. Her stool is light in color. On physical examination she is jaundiced.

Definition. Viral hepatitis is an infection of the liver caused by hepatitis A, B, C, D, or E.

Etiology.

- **Hepatitis A and E** are transmitted by contaminated food and water. They are orally ingested and have an asymptomatic incubation period of several weeks, with an average of 2–6 weeks. They cause symptomatic disease for several days to weeks, have no chronic form, and do not lead to either cirrhosis or hepatocellular carcinoma.
- **Hepatitis B, C, and D** are transmitted by the parenteral route. They can be acquired perinatally or through sexual contact, blood transfusion, needlestick, and needle sharing.
- **Hepatitis G** has been identified in a small number of patients through screening of the blood supply but has not yet been associated with clinical disease.
- **Hepatitis B and C** can lead to a chronic form, which can cause cirrhosis and hepatocellular carcinoma. Four million people in the United States are infected with Hepatitis C. Hepatitis C is the most common disease leading to the need for liver transplantation in the United States.

All forms of hepatitis can occasionally present with fulminant hepatic necrosis and acute liver failure.

Clinical Presentation. The most common presentation of acute hepatitis of any cause is jaundice, dark urine, light-colored stool, fatigue, malaise, weight loss, and a tender liver. On physical examination the liver may be enlarged. You cannot distinguish the precise viral etiology of the hepatitis by initial presentation alone. In fact, drug-induced hepatitis, such as that from isoniazid or massive alcohol use, may present with the same symptoms. Hepatitis B and C can also give symptoms similar to serum sickness, such as joint pain, rash, vasculitis, and glomerulonephritis. They also lead to cryoglobulinemia. Hepatitis B has been associated with the development of polyarteritis nodosa (PAN). Hepatitis E has been associated with a more severe presentation in pregnant women.

Table 7-3. Comparative Features: Hepatitis A, B, C, E, and Delta

Feature	Hepatitis A	Hepatitis B	Hepatitis C	Delta	Hepatitis E
Incubation period (wk)	2–6 (avg. 4)	4–26 (avg. 13)	2–20	4–8	—
Transmission	Fecal-oral	Sexual > parenteral	Parenteral > sexual	Parenteral, sexual	Fecal-oral
Severity	Mild	Occasionally severe	Usually subclinical	Co-infection with B	Mild, except in pregnant women
Fulminant hepatitis	Rare	Very rare (1% of icteric patients	Extremely rare	Co-infection occasional	Rare
Symptoms	Fever, malaise, headache, anorexia, vomiting, dark urine, jaundice	As with A, but 10–20% with serum sickness-like (joint pain, rash)	Only 20% acutely symptomatic	As with A	As with A
Carrier state	None	Yes	Yes	Yes	None
Chronicity (%)	0	5–10	80	5	0
Associated with blood transfusion (%)	Very rare	5–10	Almost negligible 2% to routine screening	Occurs, but frequency unknown	Rare
Serology	Anti-HAV IgM fraction IgG fraction	HBsAg, HBsAb HBeAg Anti-HBs Anti-HBc Anti-HBe	Antibody to hepatitis C PCR-RNA	Anti-delta IgM fraction IgG fraction	Anti-Hep E IgM IgG
Postexposure prophylaxis	Immunoglobin Hep A vaccine	HBIg/Hep B vaccine	None effective	None	Unknown
Association with cirrhosis	No	Yes	Yes	Yes	No
Association with primary hepatocellular carcinoma	No	Yes	Yes	Yes	No

Diagnosis. All forms of viral and drug-induced hepatitis will produce elevated total and direct bilirubin levels.

- Viral hepatitis will produce both elevated ALT and AST, but ALT is usually greater than the AST.
- With drug- and alcohol-induced hepatitis, AST is usually more elevated than the ALT.
- Alkaline phosphatase and GGTP are less often elevated because these enzymes usually indicate damage to the bile canalicular system or obstruction of the biliary system.
- If there is very severe damage to the liver, prothrombin time and albumin levels will be abnormal.

Hepatitis A, C, D, and E are diagnosed as **acute** by the presence of the IgM antibody to each of these specific viruses. IgG antibody to hepatitis A, C, D, and E indicates old, resolved disease.

- Hepatitis C activity can be followed with PCR-RNA viral load level. However, do not use PCR to establish the initial diagnosis.
- Hepatitis B is diagnosed as acute with the presence of the hepatitis B surface antigen, which is the first viral marker to elevate. The hepatitis B e antigen and IgM core antibody also help establish acute infection.
    - The e antigen indicates high levels of viral replication and is a marker for greatly increased infectivity.
    - Resolution of the infection is definitively indicated by the loss of surface antigen activity and the development of hepatitis B surface antibody.
    - Hepatitis B core antibody of the IgG type and hepatitis e antibody also indicate that the acute infection is about to resolve and may be the only marker present in the period of 2-6 weeks between the loss of surface antigen activity and development of the surface antibody.

Treatment. There is no effective therapy for acute hepatitis B. Chronic hepatitis B can be treated with either interferon, entecavir, adefovir, or lamivudine.

With the approval of the newest hepatitis C drugs, the goal of HCV treatment is to cure the virus, which can be done with a combination of drugs. The specific medications used and the duration of treatment depend on a number of factors:

- HCV genotype
- Viral load
- Past treatment experience
- Degree of liver damage
- Ability to tolerate the prescribed treatment
- Whether patient is waiting for a liver transplant or is transplant recipient

There are a number of approved therapies to treat HCV, such as sofosbuvir/ledipasvir (Harvoni), simeprevir (Olysio), sofosbuvir (Sovaldi) and Viekira Pak (ombitasvir, paritaprevir and ritonavir tablets co-packaged with dasabuvir tablets that may be prescribed with or without ribavirin). Sofosbuvir and simeprivir may be prescribed together with or without ribavirin, or each may be separately combined with ribavirin and in some cases peginterferon as well.

Sofosbuvir/ledipasvir, the current preferred HCV treatment, is 2 drugs formulated in to one daily pill. For genotype 1 success rates of sofosbuvir/ledipasvir are around 94–99%, while treatment duration is 8–12 weeks. Both are direct-acting antivirals (DAAs) which means they directly

Note

Entecavir, adefovir, tenofovir, and telbivudine, can also be used in place of lamivudine for the treatment of hepatitis B.

interfere with hepatitis C virus replication. Sofosbuvir is a polymerase inhibitor while ledipasvir, an NS5A inhibitor. Patients who have never been treated for HCV—whether they have cirrhosis or not—take sofosbuvir/ledipasvir for 12 weeks. Treatment-naïve patients without cirrhosis whose pre-treatment viral load (HCV RNA) is <6 million IU/mL may be considered for **8 weeks of treatment.**

When hepatitis C treatment is working, the virus will become undetectable within 4-12 weeks and will remain that way throughout treatment. Patients are considered cured when they have achieved what is known as a sustained virologic response (SVR), or continuation of this undetectable status, 12-24 weeks after completing therapy.

After a needlestick from a hepatitis B surface-antigen–positive patient, the person stuck should receive hepatitis B immunoglobulin (HBIg) and hepatitis B vaccine. If the person stuck already has protective levels of surface antibody to hepatitis B present in the blood, then no further therapy is indicated. There is no effective postexposure prophylaxis to hepatitis C, and there is no vaccine. All healthcare workers, IV drug users, and others at risk should be vaccinated for hepatitis B. All newborn children are vaccinated against hepatitis B and A. Hepatitis A vaccine should be given to those traveling to countries that may have contaminated food and water, those with chronic liver disease, and those with high risk sexual behavior.

GENITAL AND SEXUALLY TRANSMITTED INFECTIONS

Urethritis

A 31-year-old man is in your clinic today with several days of urinary frequency, urgency, and burning.

Definition. Inflammation of the urethra.

Etiology

- Gonococcal urethritis caused by *Neisseria gonorrhoeae*
- Nongonococcal urethritis caused by either *Chlamydia trachomatis* (50%), *Ureaplasma urealyticum* (20%), *Mycoplasma hominis* (5%), *Trichomonas* (1%), herpes simplex

Clinical Findings. Purulent urethral discharge; dysuria, urgency, and frequency in urination.

Diagnosis. Smear can show the Gram-negative, coffee bean–shaped diplococci intracellularly. Serology (fluorescent antibodies) for chlamydia by swabbing the urethra, or by ligase chain reaction test of voided urine. Culture for gonorrhea is the most specific test for gonorrhea.

Treatment. Single-dose ceftriaxone intramusculary and single-dose azithromycin orally is now the treatment of choice. An alternative regimen with doxycycline for 7 days can also be used. Gonorrhea can also be treated with single-dose cefixime. This is the same treatment as that for cervicitis. Ciprofloxacin should not be used as first-line therapy for gonorrhea.

Pelvic Inflammatory Disease

Definition. Infections involving the fallopian tubes, uterus, ovaries, or ligaments of the uterus.

Etiology. *N. gonorrhoeae*, *Chlamydia*, *Mycoplasma*, anaerobic bacteria, or Gram-negative bacteria. Intrauterine devices predispose to PID.

Clinical Findings. Lower abdominal and pelvic pain on palpation of the cervix, uterus, or adnexa; fever, leukocytosis, and discharge are common. Cervical motion tenderness is key. Discharge from the cervix may be present.

Diagnosis. Culture on Thayer-Martin for gonococcus and Gram stain of discharge, increased ESR. Laparoscopy is the only definitive test. If there is fluid in the retrouterine cul-de-sac, a culdocentesis will rarely be performed. A pregnancy test should be done. Ultrasonography of the pelvis may also be helpful to exclude other pathology, such as an ovarian cyst or tubo-ovarian abscess. Clinical presentation is the main method (CMT/adnexal tenderness).

Treatment. Doxycycline and cefoxitin (or cefotetan) for inpatient therapy. Outpatient therapy is with single-dose ceftriaxone intramuscularly and doxycycline orally for two weeks. The main reason to treat in hospital is a high WBC or high fever. Outpatient therapy can also be with 2 weeks of oral ofloxacin and metronidazole as a second-line agent.

Complications. Infertility and ectopic pregnancy.

Syphilis

> A 43-year-old man comes to the clinic with several days of an ulcerated genital lesion. He also has some surrounding adenopathy.

Definition. A systemic contagious disease caused by a spirochete; characterized by periods of active manifestations and by periods of symptomless latency.

Etiology. *Treponema pallidum.*

Clinical Findings. Syphilis can be classified as being congenital or acquired.

Congenital

- **Early:** symptomatic; seen in infants up to age 2
- **Late:** symptomatic, Hutchinson teeth, scars of interstitial keratitis, bony abnormalities (saber shins)

Acquired

- Early infectious syphilis
  - **Primary stage:** Chancre that appears within the third week and disappears within 10–90 days; also, regional lymphadenopathy is painless, rubbery, discrete, and nontender to palpation. Primary chancres are usually found on the penis, anus, rectum in men, and vulva, cervix, and perineum in women (may be found in other places such as lips, tongue, etc.).
  - **Secondary stage:** Cutaneous rashes appear 6–12 weeks after infection, usually found symmetrically and more marked on the flexor and volar surfaces of the

body (pinkish or pale red in white persons; pigmented spots, copper-colored macules in blacks). Lymphadenopathy, papules that develop at mucocutaneous junctions and moist areas, are termed condylomata lata (extremely infectious), and alopecia can be seen.

- Latent stage: Asymptomatic; may persist for life, and one-third of patients develop late or tertiary syphilis.
- Late or tertiary syphilis: Most commonly neurologic

These patients are symptomatic but not contagious. Benign tertiary develops 3–20 years after the initial infection, and the typical lesion is the gumma (a chronic granulomatous reaction), found in any tissue or organ. It will heal spontaneously and leave a scar. Cardiovascular syphilis and neurosyphilis are the other manifestations of tertiary syphilis. The Argyll Robertson pupil (usually only with neurosyphilis) is a small irregular pupil that reacts normally to accommodation but not to light. Tabes dorsalis (locomotor ataxia) results in pain, ataxia, sensory changes, and loss of tendon reflexes. Neurosyphilis is rare and is essentially the only significant manifestation of tertiary syphilis likely to be seen. The FTA on CSF is far more sensitive for neurosyphilis than a VDRL.

Note

Use the FTA to exclude neurosyphilis in CSF.

Diagnosis

- Screening tests are the VDRL and RPR; specific tests are the FTA-ABS, MHA-TP, and Darkfield exam of chancre.
- False–positives VDRL with EBV, collagen vascular disease, TB, subacute bacterial endocarditis

Treatment. Penicillin is the drug of choice for all stages of syphilis. A reaction called Jarisch-Herxheimer can occur in >50% of patients (general malaise, fever, headache, sweating rigors, and temporary exacerbations of the syphilitic lesions 6–12 hours after initial treatment).

- Primary, secondary, and latent syphilis are treated with 2.4 million units of intramuscular benzathine penicillin given once a week. Primary and secondary syphilis receive one week of therapy. Late latent syphilis is treated with 3 weeks of therapy and diagnosed when the VDRL or RPR titers are elevated >1:8 without symptoms.
- Tertiary syphilis is treated with penicillin 10–20 million units/day IV for 10 days.
- Penicillin-allergic patients receive doxycycline for primary and secondary syphilis, but must be desensitized in tertiary syphilis. Pregnant patients must also undergo desenitization.

Chancroid

Definition. An acute, localized, contagious disease characterized by painful genital ulcers and suppuration of the inguinal lymph nodes.

Etiology. *Haemophilus ducreyi* (Gram-negative bacillus).

Clinical Findings. Small, soft, painful papules that become shallow ulcers with ragged edges. They vary in size and coalesce. Inguinal lymph nodes become very tender and enlarged.

Diagnosis. Made on clinical findings; usually Gram stain initially with culture to confirm; PCR testing is useful.

Treatment. Azithromycin single dose or ceftriaxone intramuscularly (single dose). Erythromycin for 7 days or cipro for 3 days are alternatives.

Lymphogranuloma Venereum

Definition. A contagious, sexually transmitted disease having a transitory primary lesion followed by suppurative lymphangitis.

Etiology. *Chlamydia trachomatis.*

Clinical Findings. A small, transient, nonindurated lesion that ulcerates and heals quickly; unilateral enlargement of inguinal lymph nodes (tender); multiple draining sinuses buboes develop (purulent or bloodstained); scar formation occurs, sinuses persist or recur; fever, malaise, joint pains, and headaches are common.

Diagnosis is made by clinical examination, history, and a high or rising titer of complement fixing antibodies. Isolate chlamydia from pus in buboes.

Treatment. Doxycycline (or erythromycin as an alternative).

Granuloma Inguinale

Definition. A chronic granulomatous condition, probably spread by sexual contact.

Etiology. Donovania granulomatis, *Calymmatobacterium granulomatis.*

Clinical Findings. A painless, red nodule that develops into an elevated granulomatous mass. In males, usually found on the penis, scrotum, groin, and thighs; in females on the vulva, vagina, and perineum. In homosexual males, the anus and buttocks are common areas. Healing is slow, and there is scar formation. Looks like condyloma lata or carcinoma.

Diagnosis

- Clinically and by performing a Giemsa or Wright stain (Donovan bodies) or smear of lesion
- Punch biopsy

Treatment. Doxycycline ceftriaxone or TMP/SMZ. Erythromycin as an alternative.

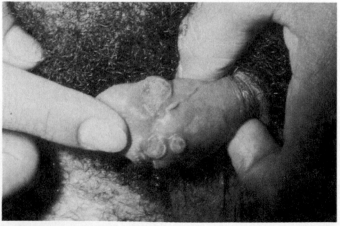

phil.cdc.gov

Figure 7-2. Lesions of Granuloma Inguinale Due to *Calymmatobacterium Granulomatis* Infection

Genital Herpes

Etiology. Herpes virus, Type II, although Type I can be seen in genital herpes.

Clinical Findings. Vesicles develop on the skin or mucous membranes; they become eroded and painful and present with circular ulcers with a red areola. Itching and soreness usually precede them. The ulcers are scarring; there can be inguinal lymphadenopathy. Lesions are commonly seen in the penis in males and on the labia, clitoris, perineum, vagina, and cervix in females.

Diagnosis. Tzanck test and culture.

Treatment. Oral acyclovir, famciclovir, or valacyclovir. Must explain to the patient the relapsing nature of the disease. Those with frequent recurrence should be given **chronic suppressive therapy**.

Genital Warts

Definition. Also known as condylomata acuminata or venereal warts.

Etiology. Papilloma virus.

Clinical Findings. Genital warts commonly found on warm, moist surfaces in the genital areas. They appear as soft, moist, minute, pink, or red swellings that grow rapidly and become pedunculated. Their cauliflower appearance makes them unique in appearance.

Diagnosis. Clinical appearance. Differentiation must be made between flat warts and condylomata lata of secondary syphilis.

Treatment

- Destruction (curettage, sclerotherapy, trichloroacetic acid)
- Cryotherapy
- Podophyllin
- Imiquimod (an immune stimulant)
- Laser removal

URINARY TRACT INFECTIONS

Cystitis

A 32-year-old woman is in your office because of dysuria. For the last several days, she has burning on urination with increased frequency and urgency to urinate.

Definition. Infection of the urinary bladder.

Epidemiology

- Very common; 6 million office visits per year in the United States
- Majority in women

> **Clinical Pearl**
>
> Transmission of genital herpes commonly occurs during an asymptomatic phase, when a person who is shedding the virus inoculates virus onto a mucosal surface of the sexual partner.

> **Note**
>
> Refer to the discussion of mulluscom contagiosum in Dermatology chapter.

Etiology

- Roughly the same as for pyelonephritis
- Any cause of urinary stasis or any foreign body predisposes
- Tumors/stones/strictures/prostatic hypertrophy/neurogenic bladder
- Sexual intercourse in women ("honeymoon cystitis")
- Catheters are a major cause, and the risk is directly related to the length of catheterization (3–5% per day).
- Microbiology: *E. coli* in >80%; second are other coliforms (Gram-negative bacilli) such as *Proteus, Klebsiella, Enterobacter*, etc.; enterococci occasionally, and *Staph. saprophyticus* in young women.

Presentation

- Dysuria, frequency, urgency, and suprapubic pain are common.
- Hematuria, low-grade fever; foul-smelling and cloudy urine are less common.
- On exam, suprapubic tenderness but no flank tenderness.

Diagnosis

- Best initial test is the urinalysis looking for WBCs, RBCs, protein, and bacteria; WBCs is the most important.
- Nitrites are indicative of Gram-negative infection.
- A count of <5 WBCs is normal.
- Urine culture with >100,000 colonies of bacteria per mL of urine confirmatory but not always necessary with characteristic symptoms and a positive urinalysis.

Treatment

- For uncomplicated cystitis, 3 days of trimethoprim/sulfamethoxazole, nitrofurantoin, or any quinolone is adequate.
- Seven days of therapy for cystitis in diabetes
- Quinolones should not be used in pregnancy.
- Fosfomycin is a single-dose oral therapy for cystitis only

Acute Bacterial Pyelonephritis

Definition. An acute patchy, most often unilateral, pyogenic infection of the kidney.

Etiology

- Infection usually occurs by ascension after entering the urethral meatus.
- Predisposing factors: obstruction due to strictures, tumors, calculi, prostatic hypertrophy, or neurogenic bladder, vesicoureteral reflux
- More common in women, in childhood, during pregnancy, or after urethral catheterization or instrumentation
- *E. coli* is the most common pathogen; others include: *Klebsiella, Proteus*, and *Enterococcus*. Patients who are immunosuppressed and subjected to indwelling catheters are more prone to *Candida*.

Pathology. Polymorphonuclear neutrophils, leukocytes (in interstitial tissue and lumina of tubules).

Clinical Findings. Chills, fever, flank pain, nausea, vomiting, costovertebral angle tenderness, increased frequency in urination, and dysuria.

Diagnosis. Dysuria, flank pain and confirmation with:

- Clean-catch urine for urinalysis, culture, and sensitivity
- >100,000 bacteria/mL of urine in the majority of cases.

Routine imaging is not required. However, if the patient does not improve in 48–72 hours or complications are suspected (obstruction, renal, or perinephric abscess), U/S or CT scan can be done.

Treatment. Antibiotics for 10–14 days (fluoroquinolone), or ampicillin and gentamicin, or a third-generation cephalosporin are all acceptable. Essentially, any of the antibiotics for Gram-negative bacilli are effective.

Most patients can be treated as outpatients, though pregnant women who appear very ill and those unable to tolerate oral medication due to nausea or vomiting should initially be hospitalized. Because of increasing resistance to TMP/SMZ, which has approached almost 20% in some parts of the United States, this agent is no longer recommended for empiric therapy until culture results and antibiotic sensitivity results are available.

Perinephric Abscess

Definition. A collection of infected material surrounding the kidney and generally contained within the surrounding Gerota fascia. Very uncommon.

Etiology. Although any factor predisposing to pyelonephritis is contributory, stones are the most important and are present in 20–60%. Other structural abnormalities, recent surgery, trauma, and diabetes are also important.

Pathophysiology

- Arises from contiguous pyelonephritis that has formed a renal abscess
- Rupture occurs through the cortex into the perinephric space
- Microbiology: *1)* The same coliforms as in cystitis and pyelonephritis; *2)* *E. coli* most common, then *Klebsiella*, *Proteus*; *3)* *Staph. aureus* sometimes accounts for hematogenous cases

Signs and Symptoms

- Often insidious; 2–3 weeks of symptoms prior to first physician visit
- Fever is the most common symptom
- Flank pain/palpable abdominal mass/abdominal pain
- Persistence of pyelonephritis-like symptoms despite treatment for pyelonephritis

Diagnosis. Urinalysis (normal 30%) and urine culture (normal 40%) are the best initial tests. Fever and pyuria with a negative urine culture or a polymicrobial urine culture are suggestive.

- Imaging is essential; U/S is the best initial scan but CT or MRI scan offers better imaging.
- Aspiration of the abscess is necessary for definitive bacteriologic diagnosis.

Treatment

- Antibiotics for Gram-negative rods
- Third-generation cephalosporins, antipseudomonal penicillin, or ticarcillin/clavulanate, often in combination with an aminoglycoside, for example
- Antibiotics alone are unlikely to be successful. Drainage (usually percutaneous) is necessary.

BONE AND JOINT INFECTIONS

Osteomyelitis

A 59-year-old man was admitted last night because of a painful leg for 2 weeks. Over the last 4 days, he developed an ulcer over the proximal portion of his tibia just below the knee. He has a history of peripheral vascular disease and diabetes. He is afebrile. He has a sinus tract in the center of the red, inflamed ulcer that is draining purulent material.

Definition. Infection of any portion of the bone including marrow, cortex, and periosteum.

Etiology. There are 3 types:

- **Acute hematogenous:** Occurs mostly in children in the long bones of the lower extremities and is secondary to a single organism 95% of the time. The most common organism is *Staphylococcus aureus*. The most commonly involved bones are the tibia and femur, and the location is usually metaphyseal due to the anatomy of the blood vessels and endothelial lining at the metaphysis. In adults, hematogenous osteomyelitis accounts for about 20% of all cases and the most common site is the vertebral bodies (lumbar vertebrae are most frequently involved). The infection can extend posteriorly to form an epidural abscess. A patient with this diagnosis would present with fever and back tenderness.
- **Secondary to contiguous infection:** Can occur in anyone with recent trauma to an area or placement of a prosthetic joint. Although this is secondary to a single organism most of the time, a higher percentage is polymicrobial in origin. *S. aureus* is the most common organism.
- **Vascular insufficiency:** Majority are age >50, with diabetes or peripheral vascular disease, resulting in repeated minor trauma, which is not noticed because of neuropathy and decreased sensation. It is most common in small bones of the lower extremities. The majority is polymicrobial, but the single most common organism is still *S. aureus*.

Presentation. Pain, erythema, swelling, and tenderness over the infected bone. With vascular insufficiency, there is often an obvious overlying or nearby ulceration or wound. Occasionally, a draining sinus tract is present.

Diagnosis. The earliest tests to detect osteomyelitis are the technetium bone scan and the MRI. Both have equal sensitivity for early pick-up, but the MRI can allow better differentiation between the overlying soft-tissue infection and bone. The MRI can be less readily available, however.

Note

Injection drug use is a significant risk factor for vertebral osteomyelitis in adults.

- *Plain x-ray:* Usually the initial test because it is more easily obtained, easily read, and inexpensive. Periosteal elevation is the first abnormality visible. The disadvantage is that 50–75% of bone calcification must be lost before the bone itself appears abnormal, which usually takes at least two weeks to develop.

- *Erythrocyte sedimentation rate (ESR):* Nonspecific. It is useful to follow during treatment. A normal value strongly points away from osteomyelitis.

- *Bone biopsy and culture:* This is the best diagnostic test but also the most invasive.

- *CT scan, indium, and gallium:* All 3 can be abnormal in osteomyelitis, but none are as specific or sensitive as the tests listed above.

Treatment. Acute hematogenous osteomyelitis in children can usually be treated with antibiotics alone; however, osteomyelitis in adults requires a combination of surgical (wound drainage and debridement, removal of infected hardware) and antibiotic therapy. Antibiotic therapy depends on the specific isolate obtained, which must be as precise as possible because empiric treatment for 6–12 weeks would be undesirable. A semisynthetic penicillin (oxacillin, nafcillin) or vancomycin (if MRSA is suspected) plus an aminoglycoside or a third-generation cephalosporin would be adequate until a specific diagnosis is obtained. Chronic osteomyelitis must be treated for as long as 12 weeks of antibiotic therapy, and in some cases, even longer periods of antibiotics may be required. The other MRSA drugs are daptomycin, linezolid, ceftaroline, and tigecycline.

Septic Arthritis

A 73-year-old woman was admitted to your service today with a swollen right knee for the last several days. The knee has an obvious effusion and decreased mobility. There is also redness and tenderness of the knee.

Definition. Infection of a joint due to virtually any agent. The most common etiology is bacterial; specifically, *Neisseria gonorrhoeae*, staphylococci or streptococci, but *Rickettsia*, viruses, spirochetes, etc., may also cause it. Generally, bacterial arthritis is divided into gonococcal and nongonococcal types.

Etiology

Pathogenesis. Sexual activity is the only significant risk factor for gonococcal septic arthritis. A total of 1–5% of people with gonorrhea will develop disseminated disease, and 25% will have a history of recent symptomatic gonorrhea. Nongonococcal bacterial arthritis is usually spread by the hematogenous route. Additional routes may include bites (animal or human), direct inoculation of bacteria into the joint through surgery or trauma, or spread of infection from surrounding structures such as bone. Even though both normal or damaged joints can get infected, any previous damage to a joint, such as from rheumatoid arthritis or osteoarthritis, previous surgery, prothesis placement, gout, sickle cell disease, or the presence of certain risk factors such as IV drug abuse, diabetes mellitus, or HIV infection can predispose a joint to infection. Any cause of bacteremia can seed the joint because the synovium does not have a basement membrane.

Microbiology. Nongonococcal:

- Gram-positive (>85); (*S. aureus* [60%], *Streptococcus* [15%], *Pneumococcus* [5%])
- Gram-negative (10–15%)
- Polymicrobial (5%)

Presentation

Nongonococcal. Monoarticular in >85%, with a swollen, tender, erythematous joint with a decreased range of motion. Knee is the most common. Skin manifestations are rare.

Gonococcal. Polyarticular in 50%; a tenosynovitis is much more common. Effusions are less common. Migratory polyarthralgia are common. Skin manifestations with petechiae or purpura are common.

Diagnosis

Nongonococcal. Culture of joint aspirate fluid is positive in 90–95% and Gram stain is positive in 40–70%. The cell count of the synovial fluid is high (>50,000) and is predominantly PMNs with a low glucose. Blood culture is positive in 50%.

Gonococcal. Much harder to culture. Only 50% of joint aspirates have positive synovial fluid culture; <10% of blood cultures are positive. Other sites such as cervix, pharynx, rectum, and urethra may also be positive. In the aggregate, culture of the other sites has a greater yield than culturing the joint itself.

Treatment. Bacterial arthritis is usually treated by a combination of joint aspiration and antimicrobial therapy.

Nongonococcal. In the absence of a specific organism seen on a stain or obtained from culture, good empiric coverage is nafcillin or oxacillin (or vancomycin) combined with an aminoglycoside or a third-generation cephalosporin. Combine an antistaphylococcal/antistreptococcal drug with a Gram-negative drug.

Gonococcal. Ceftriaxone is the drug of choice.

Gas Gangrene (Clostridial Myonecrosis)

Definition. The necrotizing destruction of muscle by gas-producing organisms, associated with signs of sepsis.

Epidemiology. Gas gangrene is uncommon; a large referral center may admit 10 cases per year; there are 1,000–3,000 cases per year in the United States, though incidence markedly increases during times of war.

Etiology. Gas gangrene is largely due (80%) to the spread of infection from wounds contaminated by *Clostridium perfringens* (the toxins produced by clostridia play a significant role in tissue damage). It is strongly associated with traumatic injury (50%), shrapnel in war, and motor vehicles in peacetime. The trauma may be as minor as an intramuscular injection; however, the wound must be deep, necrotic, and without exit to the surface. Postoperative (30%), nontraumatic (20%). Uterine gangrene was formerly a major complication of improper abortion.

Signs and symptoms. Symptoms usually begin <1–4 days of incubation after the wound and include pain, swelling, and edema at the site of the wound. Later hypotension, tachycardia, and fever can occur. Crepitation over the site and renal failure are late developments, usually prior to death.

Diagnosis. A Gram stain of the wound shows Gram-positive rods, but no white cells. A culture may be positive for *C. perfringens* as early as 1 day; however, this is not necessarily diagnostic because up to 30% of wounds can be colonized by *Clostridia*. Gas bubbles on x-ray are suggestive but may be caused by streptococci as well. Direct visualization (usually at surgery) of pale, dead muscle with a brownish, sweet-smelling discharge is ultimately diagnostic.

Treatment. High-dose penicillin (24 million/day) or clindamycin (if penicillin allergic) is necessary, but surgical debridement or amputation is the absolute center of treatment. Hyperbaric oxygen is of possible benefit, but this is still controversial.

CARDITIS

Infective Endocarditis

A 40-year-old man is brought to the hospital because of fever. He has a history of IV drug use. On physical examination, there is a systolic murmur at the lower left sternal border.

Definition. Colonization of heart valves with microbial organisms causing friable infected vegetations and valve injury. Bacterial endocarditis produces large vegetations and may affect any value in the heart, although left-sided lesions of the aortic and mitral valves are more common.

Epidemiology and etiology. There are several important invasive and other predisposing factors to bacterial endocarditis:

- Dental procedures that cause bleeding
- Oral and upper respiratory tract surgery
- Genitourinary surgery
- Prosthetic heart valves
- Catheters in the right heart
- Pressure-monitoring catheters
- IV drug use

Table 7-4. Relative Risk of Various Predisposing Conditions for Infective Endocarditis

High Risk	Intermediate Risk	Low/Negligible Risk
Prosthetic valves*	Mitral valve prolapse with regurgitation	Mitral prolapse without regurgitation
Aortic valve disease	Mitral stenosis	Atrial septal defect
Mitral regurgitation	Tricuspid valve disease	Luetic aortitis
Patent ductus arteriosus	Hypertrophic obstructive cardiomyopathy	Transvenous pacemakers
Arteriovenous fistula	Calcific aortic sclerosis Tetralogy of Fallot	Surgically corrected congenital lesions (no prosthesis) >6 mo after surgery
Coarctation of the aorta Indwelling right heart catheters (hyperalimentation)	Indwelling right heart and pulmonary artery catheters	Aortocoronary bypass surgery Cardiac pacemakers
Previous infective endocarditis	Nonvalvular intracardiac prosthesis	—
Marfan syndrome	—	—

*Indication for endocarditis prophylaxis.

Table 7-5. Microorganisms Responsible for Infective Endocarditis

Organism	Incidence, %
Native valves *Streptococcus viridans*	50–60
Enterococci	5–15

Other streptococci:
  Staphylococcus aureus
  Staphylococcus epidermidis
	15–20
	20–30
	1–3

Gram-negative bacilli	<5
Fungi (*Candida, Aspergillus, Histoplasma*)	<3
Culture negative	<5

In narcotic addicts
  Staphylococcus aureus
  Staphylococcus epidermidis
	
	60–95
	5–10

Streptococci	10–20
Enterococci	8–10
Gram-negative bacilli	4–8
Fungi	4–5
Diphtheroids	1–2

Prosthetic valves
  Staphylococcus epidermidis
  Streptococcus viridans
  Staphylococcus aureus
	Acutely: first 2 months after surgery
	
	40–50 acutely; 10–20 later
	5–20 acutely; 40–60 later
	15–20 acutely; 20–30 later

Enterococci	5–10
Other streptococci	1–5
Culture negative	<5

Pathogenesis. Acute infective endocarditis is caused by bacteremia.

- *S. aureus* is the most common cause of *acute* endocarditis
- Seed previously *normal* valves, producing necrotizing, ulcerative, invasive infection
- Produces large, bulky vegetations (2 mm to 2 cm) on the atrial side
- IV drug use a major risk factor
- Rapid onset with fever and sometimes sepsis
- Splenomegaly
- Associated with invasion of myocardium (abscess cavities) and rapid valve destruction
- Embolic complications, particularly to the lungs with right-sided lesions

With subacute infective endocarditis, viridans group streptococci is the most common organism and is associated with low virulence.

- Seed previously *abnormal* valves
- Produce smaller vegetations composed of fibrin, platelets, debris, and bacteria
- *Risk factors:* 1) Ventricular septal defect with shunt, 2) stenosis of any valve, 3) prosthetic valves, 4) indwelling catheters, 5) bicuspid aortic valve, 6) mitral valve prolapse, and 7) Marfan syndrome
- *Clinical course:* 1) Slow onset with vague symptoms; 2) malaise, low-grade fever, weight loss, flulike symptoms; 3) destruction of valves is also present; and 4) less fatal than acute, with 5-year survival 80–90% with treatment

Clinical manifestations

Table 7-6. Incidence of Clinical Findings in Infective Endocarditis

Symptoms, %	Signs, %
Chills, 41	Heart murmur or changing murmur, 80–90
Weakness, 38	Fever, 90
Dyspnea, 36	Embolic events, 50
Sweats, 24	Skin manifestations, 50
Anorexia, weight loss, 24	Splenomegaly, 28
Malaise, 24	Septic complications, 19
Cough, 24	Mycotic aneurysms, 18
Skin lesions, 21	Glomerulonephritis, 10
Stroke, 18	Digital clubbing, 12
Nausea, vomiting, 17	Retinal lesions, 5
Chest pain, 16	

Table 7-7. Peripheral Manifestations of Infective Endocarditis

Physical Findings (Frequency)	Pathogenesis	Most Common Organisms
Petechiae (20–30%): red, nonblanching lesions in crops on conjunctivae, buccal mucosa, palate, extremities	Vasculitis or emboli	*Streptococcus, Staphylococcus*
Splinter hemorrhages (15%): linear, red-brown streaks most suggestive of IE when proximal in nailbeds	Vasculitis or emboli	*Staphylococcus, Streptococcus*
Osler's nodes (5–10%): 2–5 mm painful nodules on pads of fingers or toes	Vasculitis	*Streptococcus*
Janeway lesions (10–15%): macular, red, or hemorrhagic, painless patches on palms or soles	Emboli	*Staphylococcus*
Roth's spots (<5%): oval, pale, retinal lesions surrounded by hemorrhage	Vasculitis	*Streptococcus*

Complications of infective endocarditis are as follows:

- CHF (most common cause of death)
- Septic embolization (related to infarctions and metastatic infections): brain ("mycotic" aneurysm); spleen (greater with subacute); kidneys; coronary arteries
- Glomerulonephritis with nephrotic syndrome or renal failure (immune complex)

Diagnosis. The major criteria for the diagnosis of endocarditis are a combination of positive blood cultures and an abnormal echocardiogram. The sensitivity of transthoracic echo is <60%, but its specificity is excellent. Transesophageal echo is >90% sensitive and >95% specific.

If 1 of the major criteria is absent, a combination of 1 major and 3 minor criteria will constitute a diagnosis. The minor criteria are:

- Fever
- Predisposing cardiac lesion
- IV drug use
- Vascular phenomena (arterial embolic, septic pulmonary infarcts, Janeway lesions), immunologic phenomena (such as Osler nodes, Roth spots, glomerulonephritis, or a positive rheumatoid factor)
- Microbiologic evidence (positive blood cultures not meeting major criteria or evidence of active infection with an organism consistent with infective endocarditis)

Treatment. Treatment decisions for infective endocarditis should be based on the identification of the specific organism found in blood culture and its specific antimicrobial sensitivities. Prior to the results of blood cultures, therapy can be started if the patient is very ill or there is very clear evidence of endocarditis such as fever, a clearly new or changing murmur, and embolic phenomena. Acceptable empiric therapy would be a combination of an antistaphylococcal drug such as nafcillin (or oxacillin), a streptococcal drug such as penicillin (or ampicillin), and gentamicin. You *must* alter therapy as soon as a specific microbiologic agent is known. Vancomycin and gentamicin are the standard empiric treatment of infective endocarditis.

Table 7-8. Therapy of Specific Microorganisms Causing Endocarditis

Organism	Medication	Duration
Strep. viridans	Penicillin	4 weeks
	Penicillin-allergic: ceftriaxone *or* vancomycin	4 weeks
	Penicillin or ceftriaxone + 2 weeks of gentamicin	2 weeks
Staph. aureus, **native valve** (Methicillin-sensitive)	Nafcillin (+ 5 days of gentamicin)	4–6 weeks
	Penicillin-allergic: cefazolin *or* vancomycin + gentamicin for first 5 days	4–6 weeks
(Methicillin-resistant)	Vancomycin	4–6 weeks
Enterococcal	Penicillin (or ampicillin) *and* gentamicin (vancomycin if penicillin-allergic)	4–6 weeks
	Penicillin-allergic or resistant: vancomycin *and* gentamicin	4–6 weeks

Criteria for Surgery in Infective Endocarditis

Major criteria

- CHF, progressive or unresponsive to "simple" measures
- Recurrent systemic emboli
- Persistent bacteremia despite adequate antibiotic therapy
- Fungal etiology
- Extravalvular infection (atrioventricular block, purulent pericarditis)
- Prosthetic valve dehiscence or obstruction
- Recurrence of infection despite adequate therapy

Minor criteria

- CHF, resolved with medical therapy
- Single systemic embolic event
- Large aortic or mitral vegetations on echocardiography
- Premature mitral valve closure in acute aortic insufficiency
- Prosthetic valve infection due to organisms other than highly penicillin-sensitive streptococci
- Tricuspid endocarditis due to Gram-negative bacilli
- Persistent fever without other identifiable cause
- New regurgitation in an aortic prosthesis

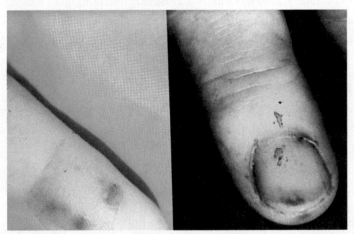

Gold Standard Multimedia Inc., 2007

Figure 7-3. Embolic Features of Acute Endocarditis

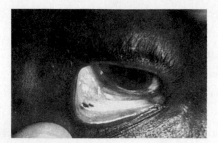

phil.cdc.gov

Figure 7-4. Petechial Hemorrhage, an Embolic
Phenomenon Due to Septicemia/Endocarditis

Prevention of bacterial endocarditis

The number of cardiac lesions which are an indication for endocarditis prophylaxis has markedly diminished over the years. AS, MS, AR, and MR **no longer** need prophylaxis, even for dental procedures. Prophylactics are indicated when there is both a serious underlying cardiac defect and a procedure causing bacteremia.

- **Dental procedures:** amoxicillin; for penicillin-allergic patients, use clindamycin, azithromycin, clarithromycin, or cephalexin

- **Urinary or GI procedures:** no longer require prophylaxis

Cardiac Conditions Which <u>Do Require</u> Prophylactic Therapy

- Prosthetic cardiac valves, including bioprosthetic and homograft valves
- Previous bacterial endocarditis, even in the absence of heart disease
- Most congenital cardiac malformations, especially cyanotic lesions (negligible risk with isolated ASD) if <u>**not**</u> repaired

Conditions Which <u>Do Not Require</u> Prophylactic Therapy

- Surgically corrected systemic pulmonary shunts and conduits
- Rheumatic and other acquired valvular dysfunction, even after valvular surgery
- Hypertrophic cardiomyopathy
- Mitral valve prolapse with valvular regurgitation
- Surgically repaired intracardiac defects

Dental or Surgical Procedures Which Predispose to Endocarditis

- Dental procedures known to induce gingival or mucosal bleeding, including professional cleaning
- Tonsillectomy and/or adenoidectomy

Procedures in Which Indication for Prophylaxis Is Unclear

- Surgical operations that involve intestinal or respiratory mucosa

Anatomic Defects or Conditions Which Require Prophylaxis

- Prosthetic valves
- Unrepaired cyanotic heart disease
- Previous endocarditis
- Transplant status

LYME DISEASE

A couple comes to your office after a recent camping trip. The woman has sustained a tick bite but did not develop any symptoms. The man has developed a red skin lesion that resolved and was followed by the onset of facial palsy. He does not recall having sustained a tick bite.

Definition/Etiology. Lyme disease is spread by the bite of the *Ixodes scapularis* (dammini) tick. On the basis of animal studies we know that the tick needs at least 24 hours of attachment to transmit the *Borrelia burgdorferi* organism. The tick is small, and the bite is often not remembered.

Clinical presentation. Symptoms begin 3–30 days after the bite of the tick. Eighty percent of patients develop the erythema migrans rash at the site of the bite. (An erythematous patch, which may enlarge in the first few days, may have partial central clearing, giving it a "bull's-eye" appearance, although this is not commonly seen.) Even without treatment, the rash resolves in several weeks. A flulike illness with fever, chills, and myalgias occurs in half of patients.

Neurologic symptoms develop several weeks later in 10–20% of patients. This is most commonly paralysis of the seventh cranial nerve (facial paralysis) and may be bilateral. Meningitis, encephalitis, headache, and memory disturbance may develop as well. Cardiac symptoms develop in <10% of patients and is most commonly AV heart block. Myocarditis, pericarditis, and various forms of arrhythmias may develop as well. Joint involvement may develop months to years later in up to 60% of patients, most commonly as a migratory polyarthritis, although a small percentage can have chronic monoarticular arthritis, most commonly affecting the knee.

Diagnosis. Definite diagnostic criteria for Lyme are the development of the erythema migrans rash combined with the presence of at least one late manifestation, as well as laboratory confirmation of the presence of the organism. Most patients are treated on the basis of the presence of the rash alone. Serologic testing is the most commonly used test. An ELISA test combined with a western blot is the standard method of establishing the diagnosis. The problem with the serologic test is that it often does not distinguish between current and previous infection. Also, in early disease when patients have the rash, testing is often negative because patients have not had sufficient time to mount an immune response. In such circumstances, treatment should be given based on strong clinical suspicion, and serologic testing should not be done. Serology will almost always be positive later in the course of the disease.

Treatment. Minor symptoms are treated with doxycycline or amoxicillin. The rash, facial palsy, and joint pain can be treated with oral doxycycline. More serious manifestations such as heart block, meningitis, myocarditis, or encephalitis are treated with IV ceftriaxone. In other words, all cardiac and serious neurologic manifestations should be treated with IV ceftriaxone.

ROCKY MOUNTAIN SPOTTED FEVER

Etiology. *R. rickettsi* is transmitted by the wood tick. Mid-Atlantic coast, upper South, and Midwest are the most common areas.

Clinical Findings

- More common in spring and summer
- Triad: abrupt onset of fever, headache, and rash (erythematous maculopapules). This disease starts at wrist and ankles and spreads centripetally (can involve palms and soles).
- Differential diagnosis with syphilis

Signs and Symptoms. Confusion, lethargy, dizziness, irritability, stiff neck, and GI symptoms. Rash starts before day 6.

Diagnosis. Specific serology: Biopsy of skin lesion

Treatment. Doxycycline

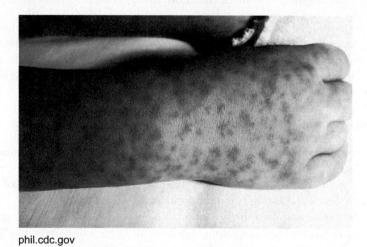

phil.cdc.gov

Figure 7-5. Rash of Rocky Mountain Spotted Fever on an Infant

ACQUIRED IMMUNE DEFICIENCY SYNDROME (AIDS)

Etiology. AIDS is caused by the human immunodeficiency virus (HIV). The primary mechanism of HIV is infection of a particular subset of T lymphocytes called CD4 cells, often just referred to as T cells. Over time, HIV decreases the number of CD4 cells. As a person's CD4 count drops, he becomes at increasing risk of developing opportunistic infections and certain malignancies.

The mode of HIV acquisition is different in different parts of the world. In the United States, the earlier part of the epidemic was fueled by men who had sex with men (MSM) and injection drug use. Nowadays, the most common risk factors are MSM and heterosexual intercourse. In women, the most common mode is heterosexual transmission. In most developing countries, including Africa, Asia, and Latin America, heterosexual transmission is the primary mode.

There is often a 10-year lag between contracting HIV infection and developing the first symptoms. This is because CD4 cells drop at a rate of 50–100/μL/year without therapy. It would take 5–10 years to drop from a normal level of around 700/mm^3 to a CD4 count of 200/mm^3.

Opportunistic Infections in AIDS

Pneumocystis jirovecii (formerly carinii) (CD4 count <200/μL)

Principle Manifestations. Pneumonia; dyspnea on exertion; dry cough; fever; chest pain; usually subacute onset and progression.

Principle Diagnostic Test. Bronchoscopy with bronchoalveolar lavage for direct identification of the organism. Chest x-ray reveals bilateral, interstitial infiltrates. Pneumothorax may be present and it is possible to have PCP pneumonia with a normal chest x-ray. Serum LDH is usually moderately elevated.

Treatment and Side Effects

- Trimethoprim-sulfamethoxazole (TMP-SMZ) is the first-line therapy for mild-severe disease and may cause a rash. Alternative therapy for mild-moderate disease is a combination of dapsone and trimethoprim or primaquine and clindamycin or atovaquone or trimetrexate (with leucovorin).
- Pentamidine—pancreatitis, hyperglycemia, hypoglycemia
- Steroids are used as adjunctive therapy for any patient with severe pneumonia. Severe is defined with a PaO_2 of <70 mm Hg or an A-a gradient of >35 mm Hg.

Prophylaxis (in Order of Preference)

- TMP/SMZ orally—this is most effective.
- Dapsone
- Atovaquone
- Aerosolized pentamidine—fails the most
- Prophylaxis of PCP may be discontinued if antiretrovirals raise CD4 count >200/μL for >6 months.

Cytomegalovirus (CD4 <50/μL)

Principle Manifestations

- *Retinitis:* blurry vision, double vision, or *any* visual disturbance in a patient with a very low CD4 count
- *Colitis:* diarrhea (<20% of patients)
- *Esophagitis:* odynophagia, fever, retrosternal chest pain (endoscopy reveals multiple *shallow ulcers in the distal esophagus*)
- *Encephalitis:* altered mental status, cranial nerve deficits

Principle Diagnostic Tests

- Funduscopy for retinitis
- Colonoscopy with biopsy for diarrhea or upper GI endoscopy with biopsy of ulcers

Treatment and Side Effects

- Valganciclovir—an oral prodrug of ganciclovir, achieves levels in the serum comparable to IV ganciclovir. This drug can be used to treat CMV retinitis (along with intravitreal ganciclovir) and GI manifestations of CMV disease. IV ganciclovir is reserved for serious CNS infections and for patients that cannot tolerate oral medications. Foscarnet and cidofovir are used when ganciclovir resistance or failure occurs.

- Ganciclovir—neutropenia *or* foscarnet-renal toxicity

- Cidofovir—renal toxicity

Prophylaxis. Valganciclovir is used for maintenance therapy. Primary prophylaxis is not indicated.

Mycobacterium avium complex (CD4 <50/mL)

Principle Manifestations. A ubiquitous atypical mycobacteria found in the environment; mode of infection is inhalation or ingestion. Fevers, night sweats, bacteremia, wasting, anemia, diarrhea.

Principle Diagnostic Tests

- Blood culture

- Culture of bone marrow, liver, or other body tissue or fluid

Treatment. Clarithromycin *and* ethambutol ± rifabutin.

Prophylaxis

- Azithromycin orally once a week *or* clarithromycin twice a day

- Prophylaxis may be discontinued if antiretrovirals raise the CD4 count >100/μL for several months.

Toxoplasmosis (CD4 <100/μL)

Principle Manifestation. Brain mass lesion: headache, confusion, seizures, and focal neurologic deficits

Principle Diagnostic Tests

- CT or MRI scan of the head showing a "ring" (contrast) enhancing lesion with edema and mass effect. A trial of specific therapy is given for 2 weeks, and the scan is repeated. Shrinkage of the lesions is considered diagnostic.

- Brain biopsy is occasionally necessary if there is no shrinkage of the lesions with treatment for toxoplasmosis.

Treatment. Pyrimethamine and sulfadiazine. Clindamycin can be substituted for sulfadiazine in the sulfa-allergic patient. Leucovorin is given to prevent bone marrow suppression.

Prophylaxis

- TMP/SMZ

- Dapsone

Cryptococcosis (CD4 <100/µL)

Principle Manifestation. Meningitis; patients mostly present with fever, headache, and malaise.

Principle Diagnostic Tests

- Lumbar puncture with initial evaluation by India ink and then specific cryptococcal antigen testing. A lower CSF cell count implies worse disease.
- Serum cryptococcal antigen testing. A high antigen titer, high opening pressure, and low CSF cell count all imply a worse prognosis.

Treatment. Amphotericin intravenously for 10–14 days at least (with flucytosine), followed by fluconazole orally for maintenance and surpressive therapy.

Prophylaxis. Oral fluconazole is not recommended for general use as a prophylaxis. This is because the incidence of cryptococcal meningitis is too low to demonstrate a mortality benefit with its use.

Vaccinations

All HIV-positive persons should receive vaccinations for pneumococcus, influenza, and hepatitis B. If the CD4 level is >200, even varicella vaccine can be given.

Monitoring the Immune System

CD4 count monitoring and viral load testing can be compared to the staging of cancer in terms of assessing prognosis for the patient. They are indispensable for determining appropriate treatment.

CD4 cell count

The CD4 count is the most accurate method for determining what infections or other diseases the patient is at risk for. At the present time the CD4 count provides an assessment of the extent of immunologic damage at the time of diagnosis and is usually the most important factor when deciding the timing of therapy. It is also the strongest predictor of disease progression and survival. Without treatment, CD4 count drops 50–100 cells per year.

The following is an approximate breakdown of when the risk of certain diseases begins to increase.

CD4 Count	
700–1,500/µL:	Normal
200–500/µL:	Oral thrush, Kaposi sarcoma, tuberculosis, Zoster
100–200/µL:	*Pneumocystis carinii* pneumonia, disseminated histoplasmosis and coccidiomycosis
<100/µL:	Toxoplasmosis, *Cryptococcus*, cryptosporidiosis, disseminated herpes simplex
<50/µL:	Cytomegalovirus, *Mycobacterium avium* complex. Progressive, multifocal leukoencephalopathy (PML), CNS lymphoma

In addition to determining the risk of opportunistic infections, the other uses of the CD4 count are to determine:

- When to start prophylactic medications
- When to initiate antiretroviral medications (<500)
- Adequacy of response to antiretroviral medications (though the best test to monitor response to therapy is the HIV-RNA viral load)

Viral load monitoring

Tests now exist to give a numerical value to the quantity of HIV in the blood. Viral load can be compared to glucose level for patients with diabetes. Monitoring of viral load is the best method to monitor adequate response to therapy when the patient is on antiretroviral medications and the goal is undetectable viremia. High viral loads indicate a greater risk of complications of the disease and a worse prognosis. **A high viral load generally indicates that the level of CD4 cells is going to drop more rapidly.**

Other uses of viral load testing are to determine:

- When to initiate antiretroviral medications
- The adequacy of response to antiretroviral medications; usually with current assays, the goal is complete suppression of viremia with <50 to 70 copies of HIV-RNA/mL

Viral sensitivity/resistance monitoring

Viral sensitivity testing is done to determine which antiviral medications will be effective in an individual patient. Sensitivity testing should always be done if a patient is failing a combination of medications and a change in therapy is necessary. It should also be done in any pregnant woman who has not been fully suppressed on the initial combination of medications.

Antiretroviral Therapy

Currently available agents and their major adverse effects

Nucleoside Reverse Transcriptase Inhibitors

- Zidovudine (ZDV or AZT)—Leukopenia, anemia, GI
- Didanosine (DDI)—Pancreatitis, peripheral neuropathy
- Stavudine (D4T)—Peripheral neuropathy
- Lamivudine (3TC)—Nothing additional to placebo
- Emtricitabine—Structurally related to lamivudine; few side effects as for lamivudine
- Tenofovir is a nucleo*tide* analog as compared to the others that are nucleo*side* analogs.
- Abacavir—Most important side effect is a hypersensitivity reaction that usually occurs in the first 6 weeks of therapy. Patients may have a rash, fever, nausea/vomiting, muscle and joint aches, and shortness of breath. In these cases, the drug should be immediately stopped and never restarted because recurrence of hyperactivity symptoms can be rapid and life-threatening.
- Zalcitabine (DDC)—Pancreatitis, peripheral neuropathy, lactic acidosis

Protease Inhibitors. Hyperlipidemia, hyperglycemia, and elevated liver enzymes for all in the group; abnormal fat loss (lipoatrophy) from the face and extremities with redistribution of fat in the back of the neck and abdominal viscera can be seen.

- Nelfinavir—Gastrointestinal
- Indinavir—Nephrolithiasis (4%), hyperbilirubinemia (10%)
- Ritonavir—Severe GI disturbance
- Saquinavir—Gastrointestinal
- Amprenavir
- Lopinavir/Ritonavir combination—Diarrhea
- Atazanavir—Diarrhea, asymptomatic hyperbilirubinemia

Non-Nucleoside Reverse Transcriptase Inhibitors. These drugs are noncompetitive inhibitors of reverse transcriptase.

- Efavirenz—Neurologic; somnolence, confusion
- Nevirapine—Rash, hepatotoxicity
- Delavirdine—Rash
- Rilpivirine

Guidelines for starting therapy

Guidelines for starting therapy are:

- CD4 <500/μL *or*
- Viral load (by PCR-RNA) >55,000–100,000 by RNA

Regarding what to start:

- Use 2 nucleosides combined with a protease inhibitor *or*
- Use 2 nucleosides combined with efavirenz
- Emtricitabine, tenofovir, and efavirenz are available as a single pill once a day.

A combination therapy (highly active antiretroviral therapy, HAART) should be used with medications having synergistic activity by acting at different sites of the virus replicative process; hence current guidelines recommend two NRTIs (usually tenofovir/emtricitabine or zidovudine/lamivudine) combined with either a NNRTI (efavirenz preferred) *or* a PI (atazanavir/ritonavir, fosamprenavir/ritonavir, or lopinavir/ritonavir).

Giving **"boosted protease inhibitors"** is the practice of giving most protease inhibitors in combination with a low dose of ritonavir (also a PI). Ritonavir given alone as a PI has modest efficacy and significant drug interactions, but when given in a low dose with other PIs, it decreases their metabolism and enables higher drugs levels of the "boosted" PI over a prolonged period of time. This increases chances of success and also decreases pill burden.

Any regimen that increases the CD4 count and drops the viral load to undetectable amounts or close to undetectable amounts is considered **adequate therapy**. When starting medication, a drop of at least 50% of viral load in the first month is expected to indicate adequate therapy.

Pregnant Patients

Without treatment, approximately 25–30% of children born to HIV-positive mothers will truly be HIV positive. All children at birth will carry the maternal antibody to the virus and will be positive by ELISA testing, but only 25–30% will remain truly infected.

- Pregnant women with serious disease (i.e., low CD4 or high viral load) should be treated fully for their HIV infection. That is, they should get triple antiretroviral therapy as you would in a nonpregnant person.
- C-section is only used routinely in those whose CD4 count and viral load are not controlled with medications (when viral load is >1000 copies/mL of HIV-RNA at the time of delivery).
- Treatment is indicated in *all* pregnant women. Zidovudine (AZT) should be used in combination with 2 other antiretroviral medications. Even when the CD4 is high and viral load is <1000, you should start therapy as soon as you know the patient is pregnant.
- The only known teratogen is efavirenz in animal studies.

Breast Feeding

Breast feeding is associated with transmission of virus to the infant. If a pregnant woman is already on antiretrovirals, she should continue on them. She should start immediately regardless of gestational age. If the woman has high CD4 cells and does not need treatment for herself, combination therapy can end after delivery. The majority of women can deliver with a normal vaginal delivery. Avoid efavirenz in pregnancy.

Postexposure Prophylaxis (e.g., Needlestick Injury)

All persons with serious exposure to blood containing body fluids of HIV-positive patients should receive AZT, lamivudine, and nelfinavir or raltegravir or any other fully suppressive 3-drug combination for 4 weeks. Modify the regimen as needed to ensure compliance. The point is to use any fully suppressive combination for at least 4 weeks; we know zidovudine alone will decrease the risk of transmission by 80%. We don't know how much the combination will decrease transmission.

Tetanus

Etiology. A severe infectious complication of wounds caused by the toxin of *Clostridium tetani* (neurotoxin); takes 1–7 days to develop; spore forming, Gram-positive rod.

Clinical Findings. Tonic spasms of voluntary muscles; respiratory arrest; difficulty in swallowing (dysphagia); restlessness; irritability; stiff neck, arms, and legs; headache; lockjaw; flexion of the arms and extension of the lower extremities; and high mortality rate.

Diagnosis. Clinical.

Treatment. Prophylactic.

- Tetanus toxoid (Tdap) boosters every 10 years
- Immediate surgical care, débride wound
- Antitoxin, tetanus immunoglobulin
- Penicillin 10–14 days

Wound Management		
Patient	**Not Tetanus Prone**	**Tetanus Prone**
	Linear, 1 cm deep cut, without devitalized tissue, without major contaminants, <6 hours old	Blunt/missile, burn, frostbite, 1 cm deep; devitalized tissue present + contaminants (e.g., dirt, saliva); any wound 6 hours old
Not completed primary or vaccination history unknown	Vaccine	Vaccine and TIG*
Completed primary series	Vaccine if >10 years since last booster	Vaccine if >5 years since last booster

*TIG = tetanus immunoglobulin (human)

Aspergillosis

Definition. A fungus that is widespread in the environment; primarily causes pulmonary disease in the immunocompromised.

Etiology
- 90% species known, with *A. fumigatus* the most common
- Ubiquitous in natural decaying organic matter, ceiling tile, and ventilation systems
- Spores can be isolated from air anywhere on earth

Signs and Symptoms
- Various degrees of respiratory tract invasion
- Rarely it can disseminate to any organ but starts in the lung
- Allergic bronchopulmonary-like asthma with cough/fever/wheezing
- Mycetoma—literally a "fungal ball": *1*) Sets up residence in a pre-existing cavity, with hemoptysis as chief complaint; and *2*) it is *not* invasive.
- Invasive pulmonary
- 90% have 2 of these 3 risks: *1*) neutropenia <500, *2*) steroid use, and *3*) cytotoxic drugs (e.g., azathioprine, cyclophosphamide).

Diagnosis. Depends on the type of disease being caused; however, all can have an abnormal chest x-ray and aspergillus in sputum.
- Allergic bronchopulmonary elevation of markers of allergy/asthma, such as eosinophil/IgE levels
- Positive skin testing
- Mycetoma: abnormal sputum culture/serum precipitins/x-ray
- Invasive: Sputum culture not sufficient; biopsy to show invasion necessary. CT scan (or sometimes chest x-ray) will show a "halo" sign, a zone of low attenuation around a nodular lesion; this is often an early finding in invasive pulmonary aspergillosis.

Note

Voriconazole and caspofungin are used to treat aspergillosis and some other fungal infections.

Treatment. Depends on syndrome (really, they are separate diseases).

- Allergic: steroid taper and asthma medications, not antifungals
- Mycetoma: surgical removal
- Invasive: Voriconazole is superior to amphotericin; there are fewer failures seen with it (and caspofungin) as compared with amphotericin. Itraconazole for very mild disease or after initial treatment with amphotericin. Caspofungin is active against *Aspergillus* and may be superior to amphotericin. Caspofungin is an echinocandin. The other echinocandins are micafungin and anidulafungin. Echinocandins have virtually no toxicity.

ACUTE RENAL FAILURE

Definition. Acute renal failure (ARF), or better referred to as acute kidney injury (AKI), is defined as a rapid rise in blood urea nitrogen (BUN) or creatinine over a period of several hours to days. There is no precise duration to define it as acute. ARF may, in fact, develop over a period as short as several hours, such as in the case of rhabdomyolysis or contrast-induced renal failure. It can also happen several weeks later, such as from aminoglycoside toxicity or from poststreptococcal glomerulonephritis.

There are several terms for renal failure, which all roughly mean a rise in creatinine and a decrease in renal function or decrease in glomerular filtration rate.

- **Renal insufficiency** means renal failure, but generally not to the point of needing dialysis. **Azotemia** can be used interchangeably with the term renal insufficiency; literally, azotemia means the buildup of azole groups or nitrogen in the blood.

- **Uremia** describes a syndrome of very severe renal failure in which there is the need for dialysis to save life. Uremia, which literally means "urea in the blood," is more severe than azotemia.

- In uremia there is severe acidosis, mental status changes, hyperkalemia, and fluid overload, as well as anemia, hypocalcemia, and possible pericarditis. Patients also develop bleeding diathesis.

- Uremia can be used interchangeably with the phrase **end-stage renal disease**. Both mean such severe renal dysfunction as to be life threatening and both require dialysis.

- Uremia does **not** necessarily mean the same thing as **chronic renal failure**. Although most patients develop uremia only after years of renal insufficiency such as from diabetes or hypertension, it is possible to become uremic in as little as 1–2 weeks with a severe illness such as tumor lysis syndrome or rhabdomyolysis.

- ARF or AKI is also classified as prerenal, postrenal, or intrarenal to determine the site of the defect.

  - **Prerenal azotemia** means decreased perfusion of the kidney.

  - **Postrenal azotemia** means decreased drainage from the kidney or decreased forward flow of urine. In both prerenal and postrenal azotemia, the kidney is not intrinsically defective. If the kidney in prerenal or postrenal azotemia were taken out and transplanted into another person, it would function normally.

  - **Intrarenal** means there is a tubular or glomerular problem, and the kidney itself is defective.

Diagnostic Tests. The BUN becomes abnormally elevated in all forms of renal failure. It can also be falsely elevated even when renal function is normal, in response to an increased protein load in the diet or from GI bleeding. This is also from increased catabolism. The BUN is derived from protein waste products; blood in the gut acts like a big protein meal. This is also from increased catabolism.

The BUN improves after a session of dialysis. The BUN can be falsely low when there is liver disease, malnutrition, or SIADH. The BUN level corresponds to the degree of renal failure; the higher the BUN, the worse the kidney function is.

Creatinine is our main measure of renal function. Creatinine clearance is our closest approximation of glomerular filtration rate (GFR) without the use of more cumbersome testing such as the clearance of inulin. Inulin does not naturally exist in the human body. Creatinine is a metabolic product of skeletal muscle. Creatinine clearance slightly overestimates GFR because there is some tubular secretion of creatinine. Creatinine can be falsely low just because of a decrease in muscle mass. That is why the creatinine clearance is always adjusted for weight. More muscles mean more creatinine. A bodybuilding weight lifter with 100 kg of muscle will naturally have a higher creatinine than a wimpy librarian who weighs 50 kg. The higher creatinine in the bodybuilder does not necessarily mean worse renal function.

Creatinine needs some time to rise. Even if the patient becomes anuric, the creatinine will only rise at a rate of 0.5 to 1.0 point per day. This rise will be faster if the body muscle mass is greater. Hence, if the patient has a renal injury and the creatinine goes from 1 to 3 over a 2-day period, this is consistent with fully dead or nonfunctioning kidneys.

Prerenal Azotemia

Prerenal azotemia is a form of renal insufficiency caused by diminished perfusion of the kidney on any basis. The kidney itself is normal. If the kidney could receive adequate perfusion, the BUN and creatinine would normalize. The causes of prerenal azotemia include: hypovolemia on any basis (dehydration, burns, poor oral intake, diuretic, vomiting, diarrhea, sweating, hemorrhage), hypotension on any basis (septic shock, cardiogenic shock, anaphylactic shock), and third spacing of fluids such as peritonitis, osmotic diuresis, or low aldosterone states such as Addison disease. Addison disease results in intravascular volume depletion. This leads to diminished tissue perfusion.

Decreased perfusion from a decrease in cardiac output also results in prerenal azotemia. Although there may be total body fluid overload with significant edema, all that matters in terms of renal function is how much fluid is still in the vascular space and how much can provide meaningful perfusion of the kidney. With severe CHF, constrictive pericarditis, or coarctation of the aorta, you may experience edema and fluid overload, but the kidney is receiving virtually no perfusion, hence the rising BUN and creatinine. This is the concept of effective arterial volume.

The first clue to the diagnosis of prerenal azotemia is a BUN:creatinine ratio of 20:1. There is also a low urine sodium and low fractional excretion of sodium (FeNa <1%). This is because the kidney perceives the body as being volume-depleted; hence, there will be a vigorous sodium and water reabsorption by the kidney. This results in a very high urine osmolality as well. This is because the kidney attempts to retain all the water it can in the kidney and therefore excretes very concentrated urine. Concentrated urine has a high specific gravity (>1.010) and a high urine osmolality (>500). These laboratory findings are irrespective of the etiology of the prerenal azotemia. In other words, the BUN:creatinine ratio rises to 20:1, urine sodium is low, and the urine osmolality is high no matter what the etiology of the decreased perfusion or hypotension.

Low albumin states also lead to decreased renal perfusion. Nephrotic syndrome and other malabsorptive states lead to a low albumin level. This leads to renal failure.

Renal artery stenosis

Renal artery stenosis results in a high BUN and creatinine with a high BUN:creatinine ratio. Although the systemic blood pressure may be markedly elevated, the result is still a form of pre-renal azotemia. There is markedly diminished renal perfusion because of the obstruction in the renal artery. The systemic blood pressure does not matter. All that matters is how much is getting to the kidney. Hence, to the kidney, renal artery stenosis functions like hypotension. This effect is greatly exaggerated with the use of ACE inhibitors, which markedly diminish renal perfusion. This is because of the extremely high aldosterone state in renal artery stenosis.

Hepatorenal syndrome

Hepatorenal syndrome is defined as renal failure based entirely on the presence of hepatic failure. The kidneys are normal. The etiology of the rise in BUN and creatinine is thought to be from an intense vasoconstriction of the afferent arteriole, resulting in decreased renal perfusion. Because the defect is at the afferent arteriole, the laboratory numbers are consistent with prerenal azotemia, i.e., a high BUN:creatinine ratio above 20:1. In addition, those with hepatorenal syndrome have a urine sodium that is low (<10) and a fractional excretion of sodium <1%. It is important to measure the urine sodium off of antibiotics. Intrinsic renal disease should be excluded to make a diagnosis. No improvement in renal failure after 1.5 L of colloid, like albumin, is diagnostic of hepatorenal syndrome.

The treatment of hepatorenal syndrome is to correct the underlying liver disease. Midodrine, an alpha agonist, and octreotide may be beneficial in hepatorenal syndrome. However, the best treatment is liver transplantation.

ACE inhibitor effect on the kidney

ACE inhibitor–induced renal failure is from vasodilation of the efferent arteriole. Angiotensin has a significant vasoconstrictive effect on the efferent arteriole; ACE inhibitors block this. This results in a decrease in GFR that is usually transient. However, in patients who are elderly, diabetic, hypertensive, or who have baseline renal disease such as from myeloma, an ACE inhibitor can result in quite a marked decrease in renal function. Hence, there can be a rise in BUN and creatinine after initiating ACE inhibitors if there is underlying renal insufficiency. Severe decline in renal function may be observed in patients with bilateral renal artery stenosis after initiation of ACE inhibitors.

Despite the ability of ACE inhibitors to potentially worsen renal function, the overall effect on the kidney is diminishing the rate of progression to uremia and renal failure. This beneficial effect is most likely secondary to the decrease in intraglomerular hypertension. ACE inhibitors and angiotensin receptor blockers decrease hypertension inside the glomerulus. ACE inhibitors decrease proteinuria by 35–45%. ACE inhibitors give a brief decrease in GFR in the short term with a long-term beneficial effect on decreasing proteinuria and the rate of progression of renal failure. This is particularly true in patients with diabetes.

Postrenal Azotemia

This is caused by any decrease in the outflow of urine. The precise etiology of the obstruction is not particularly relevant when it comes to the degree of renal failure. All that matters is that there is an obstruction bilaterally to the flow of urine out of the kidney. You cannot get renal failure by the obstruction of only a single kidney if a patient has both kidneys in place. In other words, a large stone in 1 ureter cannot cause renal failure because the creatinine does not rise if there is a loss of only 1 kidney. A small stone or clot in the bladder can obstruct both kidneys and this can cause postrenal azotemia. Other causes of postrenal azotemia are bladder cancer, prostate hypertrophy or cancer, bilateral ureteral disease such as retroperitoneal fibrosis, neurogenic bladder, or any other cause of bilateral obstructive disease. Strictures can cause this problem but only if they are bilateral in location. The complete obstruction of only 1 kidney does not cause renal failure because you only need one-third of 1 kidney in order to live. Creatinine will only begin to rise when you have lost at least 70–80% of renal function. Hence, you lose a greater percentage of renal function as you go from a creatinine of 1 to 2 than you do when going from a creatinine of 2 to 10. Patients usually have a preceding history of obstructive symptoms followed by sudden onset of oliguria or anuria. Neurologic causes such as multiple sclerosis, spinal cord lesions, and neuropathy may lead to poor function of the urinary bladder and obstruction.

Initially, the BUN and creatinine will elevate in a ratio of 20:1 as it does with prerenal azotemia. There will also be a low fractional excretion of sodium (FeNa) and low urine sodium. When the obstruction continues for such a long time that there is permanent damage to the kidney and the kidney tubule cells die, then the BUN:creatinine ratio will lower to closer to 10:1, such as that seen in acute tubular necrosis (ATN). Early diagnosis is, therefore, essential. Complete recovery is possible until 10 to 14 days of obstruction.

ATN is the most common cause of ARF (intrinsic) in hospitalized patients.

The diagnosis of postrenal azotemia is determined by finding a distended bladder on examination, bilateral hydronephrosis on renal sonogram or CT scan, or by finding large volumes of urine in the bladder after passing a Foley urinary catheter. After urinating (voiding), there should be no more than 50 mL of urine left in the bladder. If this post-void residual is markedly elevated, it implies an obstruction to the flow of urine out of the bladder.

The treatment of postrenal azotemia is based on relieving the cause of the obstruction.

Intrarenal: Tubulointerstitial Disease

Acute tubular necrosis

Acute tubular necrosis (ATN) is defined as acute renal failure on the basis of tubular damage as opposed to glomerular damage, or simply decreased perfusion of the kidney or drainage out of the kidney.

- About 85% of acute renal failure is secondary to intrinsic renal disease such as ATN.
- ATN is from either hypoperfusion of the kidney leading to such severe ischemia that there is cellular death or from a toxic injury to the kidney such as aminoglycoside toxicity or from amphotericin. This is from sepsis, or after cardiac or aortic surgeries.
- ATN often occurs from a combination of both toxic and ischemic injury. If tissue ischemia seems similar in concept to what was described above for prerenal azotemia, that is because there is overlap. It is like the difference between myocardial ischemia and a myocardial infarction.
  - If there is modest hypotension or hypovolemia, the BUN and creatinine will rise in a 20:1 ratio consistent with prerenal azotemia. Prerenal azotemia is essentially reversible.
  - If the ischemia becomes more severe, the tubular cells will necrose and slough off into the urine and become visible as granular, muddy brown, or pigmented casts.
- At the point of necrosis, the renal insufficiency can be permanent. In less severe disease and nonoliguric ATN, urinalysis may be relatively normal.

The hypotension causing tubular ischemia can be of any etiology. This can be either from surgery or medical problems. The degree and especially the duration of hypotension are extremely important. The longer the duration of hypotension/hypoperfusion, the greater the chance of ATN. The risk of ATN goes up even further when there is a toxic injury as well as hypotension. In other words, the likelihood of rhabdomyolysis causing renal failure is markedly increased when there is hypoperfusion of the kidney. The same can be said of cisplatin toxicity, tumor lysis syndrome, or injury from hemoglobin toxicity.

Three Phases (Not Seen in All Patients)

- **Prodromal**—This is the time between the acute injury and the onset of renal failure.

- **Oliguric** (<400 mL per 24 hours) or anuric (<100 mL per 24 hours)

- **Postoliguric**—This is a diuretic phase when all the water not previously excreted will now leave the body in a vigorous polyuria.

Diagnosis. The initial clue is a BUN:creatinine ratio close to 10:1. By itself, the BUN:creatinine ratio simply implies the damage is intrarenal, or inside the kidney itself, as opposed to abnormalities of perfusion (prerenal) or drainage (postrenal). Further clues to the diagnosis of ATN are a high urine sodium (>40), high fractional excretion of sodium (>1%), and low urine osmolality (<350). This is because tubular cells are responsible for forming either concentrated or dilute urine. If the tubular cells die from ischemia, then the kidney can neither concentrate nor dilute the urine. Dead cells don't work.

Table 8-1. Diagnosis: How to Confirm the Difference between Prerenal and ATN (Based on Lab Values)

	Prerenal	ATN
Urine osmolarity	>500	<350
Urine Na$^+$	<20	>40
FeNa$^+$	<1%	>1%
Urine sediment	Scant	Full (brownish pigmented granular casts, epithelial casts)

Note: In ATN, the urine cannot concentrate. In prerenal, you hold on to all free H_2O and Na$^+$.

Treatment of ATN. There is no specific therapy for ATN to reverse the renal failure. The underlying cause must be corrected. Hydration is often given to make sure there is no prerenal component. Diuretics such as furosemide or mannitol do not reverse the ATN. Hydration can prevent contrast-induced renal failure, but it does not reverse it once it occurs. Another form of ineffective therapy is dopamine at low dose to increase renal perfusion. This is a nice idea, but it does not work. ATN is a combined ischemic/toxic disease. It is like a sunburn for the kidney. Once it occurs, all you can do is support the patient and wait to see if the renal tubular cells can restore themselves. No medical therapy reverses ATN.

If the degree of renal failure is severe and life threatening, then dialysis is used.

Allergic interstitial nephritis

Allergic interstitial nephritis (AIN) accounts for 10–15% of intrinsic renal failure. It can be distinguished from other causes of renal failure by the presence of fever and rash on physical examination and many WBCs, occasionally eosinophils.

Note

Other Meds
- NSAIDS
- Allopurinol
- Proton pump inhibitor

The etiology of AIN is usually from an adverse effect to medications in 70% of cases. The medications most likely to be allergenic in general are the medications most likely to cause AIN. For example, skin rash from an allergic drug reaction can be from penicillins, cephalosporins, sulfa drugs, allopurinol, rifampin, and quinolones.

These are the same medications to cause AIN. In addition, many of these same drugs cause drug-induced hemolysis as well. In other words, 10% of the population is allergic to penicillins or sulfa drugs. This allergic reaction can take the form of a rash, Stevens-Johnson syndrome, hemolysis, or AIN. In the same way, calcium channel blockers rarely cause a rash. Calcium blockers also rarely cause nephritis or hemolysis. Most patients require several weeks of drug exposure before developing renal injury.

It is important to remember that any sulfa drug can cause allergic reactions. Besides antibiotics, other examples of sulfa drugs are diuretics such as thiazides, furosemide, or acetazolamide.

AIN is also caused by infections themselves, such as viruses, bacteria, and fungi. The most common infections to result in AIN are leptospirosis, legionella, CMV, rickettsia, and streptococci. The least common causes of AIN are several autoimmune disorders such as systemic lupus erythematosus (SLE), Sjögren syndrome, sarcoidosis, and cryoglobulins. Cryoglobulins can cause renal failure from membranous glomerulonephritis as well. Eight percent of cases are idiopathic.

Fever is present in 80% of those with AIN. It can be very difficult to determine if the fever is from the underlying illness or from the AIN. Rash is present in 25–50% of patients. Joint pain is common because AIN acts somewhat like serum sickness.

Laboratory abnormalities include eosinophilia, eosinophiluria, hematuria, proteinuria, and an increase in serum IgE levels. Although hematuria is present in 95% of patients, this finding is rather nonspecific. More people with AIN have eosinophils in the urine rather than in the blood. The level of proteinuria is mild and nearly always <2 grams per 24 hours. The best initial test for AIN is a urinalysis (UA) looking for white cells. Remember that the UA cannot distinguish eosinophils from other white cells. The most accurate test for urine eosinophils is a Hansel stain or Wright stain of the urine. Although the single most accurate test for AIN is a kidney biopsy, this is essentially not necessary if you have some of the other findings described above. NSAID-induced injury typically lacks fever, rash, and eosinophilia.

There is no specific therapy necessary for AIN in the majority of patients. AIN resolves spontaneously after stopping the offending agent. If renal failure persists or worsens after stopping the offending agent, you may use a short course of steroids.

Pigments (hemoglobin/myoglobin)

A 25-year-old man is undergoing a physical examination to become a firefighter. He must carry a 200-pound bag up a flight of stairs followed by push-ups and a walk across a balance beam. He becomes very weak afterward and is brought to the emergency department with painful muscles and dark urine. What is the most important test to do first?

Etiology. Rhabdomyolysis is caused by sudden, severe crush injury; seizures; severe exertion; and sometimes by hypokalemia, hypophosphatemia, or medications such as statins. Massive hemoglobinuria severe enough to cause renal failure is generally only caused by an ABO incompatibility. Both of these disorders result in enough pigment release in the bloodstream to cause nephrotoxicity. The toxicity is because the pigment is directly toxic to the tubular cells as well as from precipitation of the pigment in the tubules. The degree of toxicity is related to the duration of contact of the tubular cells with the hemoglobin or myoglobin. This toxicity is compounded by dehydration. Hence, a person who has run a marathon has both myoglobin release as well as poor kidney perfusion. This is cumulative in the risk of renal failure.

Laboratory Testing. The most important test when there has been a severe crush injury or seizure and the rhabdomyolysis is potentially life threatening is an EKG or potassium level. This implies that you know how a patient with rhabdomyolysis will die. Acidosis and hyperkalemia can lead to an arrhythmia. If there are peaked T-waves on the EKG, you will give calcium chloride or calcium gluconate. The best initial test that is specific for rhabdomyolysis is a UA in which you find a dipstick that is positive for blood but in which no red cells are seen. This is because myoglobin can react with the reagent on the dipstick and come out as if there were red cells present. Hemoglobin will do the same thing. The dipstick of the UA cannot distinguish among hemoglobin, myoglobin, and RBCs. This is because myoglobin has heme in it.

Rhabdomyolysis is confirmed with a markedly elevated serum CPK level. Elevated serum CPK is a biochemical marker of skeletal muscle neurosis. In order for nephrotoxicity to occur, the level must be enormously elevated into the 10,000 to 100,000 range with a normal value generally <500 or less. You will also find metabolic acidosis with a decreased serum bicarbonate, hyperphosphatemia secondary to muscle breakdown, and hypocalcemia secondary to the deposition of calcium in muscles that have been damaged. Severe hyperuricemia may develop because of release of purines from damaged muscles.

Rhabdomyolysis is associated with a very rapidly rising creatinine level. This is because of both the renal failure and massive release of muscle products. Thus, the BUN:creatinine ratio may be low, below 10:1.

Treatment. If there are EKG abnormalities from the hyperkalemia the best initial therapy is calcium chloride or gluconate. In general, therapy consists of hydration and mannitol as a diuretic to decrease the duration of contact between the nephrotoxic hemoglobin or myoglobin and the kidney tubule. Alkalinizing the urine with bicarbonate may help prevent the precipitation of the pigment in the tubule.

Proteins

Bence-Jones proteins, such as in myeloma, also cause tubular damage. Myeloma is most prominently a cause of nephritic syndrome, however, not tubular damage.

> A man with myeloma is being evaluated for an elevated creatinine. His UA shows trace positive for protein, but the 24-hour urine shows 5 grams of protein. What is the etiology of this discrepancy?

Crystals

Oxalate. The most common cause of hyperoxaluria resulting in acute renal failure is from ethylene glycol overdose in a suicidal person who ingests antifreeze. Look for an intoxicated person with a metabolic acidosis with an elevated anion gap who is found to have renal insufficiency. The diagnosis is confirmed by finding oxalate crystals on a UA. Oxalate crystals are shaped like envelopes.

Acute ethylene glycol overdose is treated with fomepizole infusion to prevent the formation of the toxic metabolite of ethylene glycol, which is oxalic acid. Fomepizole is preferred. It is the oxalic acid that causes the renal failure. Dialysis must also be used to then remove the ethylene glycol. Sodium bicarbonate can be given to correct acidosis.

Chronic hyperoxaluria and kidney stones can be caused by Crohn's disease because of fat and calcium malabsorption.

Urate. Acute renal failure from uric acid toxicity occurs in the setting of tumor lysis syndrome. This is why patients with leukemia or lymphoma receive vigorous hydration and allopurinol prior to being given chemotherapy. Allopurinol reduces the production of uric acid by inhibiting conversion of xanthine to hypoxanthine to uric acid. Uric acid stones precipitate in an acidic urine, unlike oxalate crystals, which precipitate in alkaline urine. Allopurinol treatment with alkalinization of urine markedly reduces the risk of uric acid nephropathy. Chronically, gout causes renal impairment through a slower and milder version of the same mechanism. The diagnosis is by finding uric acid crystals in the urine.

Hypercalcemia

Calcium precipitates in the kidney tubule, forming stones. In addition, hypercalcemia can lead to distal RTA and nephrogenic diabetes insipidus. The most common cause of hypercalcemia is primary hyperparathyroidism. If there is no renal damage or decrease in GFR and there are no symptoms, then mild hyperparathyroidism is not treated surgically. If the hyperparathyroidism is associated with evidence of renal impairment, then surgical resection of the glands is performed.

Toxins

The most common toxins to be associated with renal insufficiency and ATN are NSAIDs, aminoglycosides, cephalosporins, contrast agents, amphotericin, chemotherapy such as cisplatin, radiation effect, heavy metals such as lead, mercury, or gold, and cyclosporine. The difference between the basis of allergic interstitial nephritis and direct toxins is that allergic nephritis occurs with the first dose and is associated with fever, rash, joint pain, and eosinophils in both blood and urine.

Direct acting toxins can take several days to weeks to result in enough cumulative toxicity to lead to renal failure and are not associated with eosinophils, fever, joint pains, or rash. There is no specific test to confirm a specific toxin as the etiology of the renal failure. You must exclude the other causes of renal failure and find the toxin in the history. There is no specific therapy to reverse the renal insufficiency of any of the direct acting toxins.

Aminoglycosides. Tobramycin is the least nephrotoxic compared with gentamicin and amikacin. Aminoglycoside toxicity generally takes 5–10 days of administration to result in toxicity. The likelihood of toxicity is associated with trough levels. Renal failure due to aminoglycosides is frequently non-oliguric (K+ levels not elevated). Hypokalemia and hypomagnesemia predispose the patient to aminoglycoside toxicity. The ability of antibiotics to kill bacteria is associated with the peak level, but the likelihood of toxicity is associated with the trough level. This is most likely because a low trough allows time for the renal tubular cells and neural cells of the inner ear to regenerate themselves. Aminoglycosides also exert a bactericidal effect after their level has become low because they enter the bacteria and continue to kill. This ability to exert an effect despite low or absent levels is called *postantibiotic effect*. Hence, aminoglycosides should be given once a day. Once-a-day dosing allows high bactericidal levels with the same efficacy and very low trough levels. The low trough levels reduce toxicity. Aminoglycoside-related nephrotoxicity is estimated to be between 10–20% of all drug-induced nephrotoxicity and is usually reversible.

Amphotericin B. This medication is associated with renal insufficiency as well as distal renal tubular acidosis. It is expected that after several days or weeks of amphotericin use, the patient will develop a high creatinine as well as a decreased magnesium, bicarbonate, and potassium level. These often revert to normal after the medication is stopped. This form of toxicity is from cumulative dosing.

Atheroembolic Disease. Look for a patient who undergoes a vascular catheter procedure such as angioplasty who develops renal failure several days later. Atheroemboli are also associated with eosinophilia, low complement levels, bluish discoloration of the fingers and toes, and livedo reticularis. Although the most accurate test is a skin biopsy to see cholesterol crystals in the skin, this is rarely done. There is no therapy for atheroemboli. High doses of statins have been tried.

Contrast Agents. Radiocontrast material for CT scanning can result in renal failure in as little as 12–24 hours after the use of the agent. This is one of the main ways to distinguish this form of renal failure from aminoglycoside or amphotericin toxicity, which need several days to weeks of cumulative exposure. The rise in creatinine peaks at 3–5 days after the injury. The BUN and creatinine may be up in a 20:1 ratio, such as in prerenal azotemia, because the hypertonicity of the agent provokes an intense vasospasm of the afferent arteriole. The worse the underlying renal parenchyma, the more likely the patient is to have renal failure secondary to contrast material. If you are elderly, diabetic, and hypertensive with myeloma, you are far more likely to experience contrast-induced renal insufficiency.

Other Toxins. Pentamidine is associated with renal failure in addition to its toxicity on the pancreas. Vancomycin, cyclosporine, and lithium can all cause renal failure in a dose-dependent fashion. Indinavir is a protease inhibitor that results in renal failure usually from the drug precipitating out in the kidney tubules. Indinavir stones need contrast to be identified on a spiral CT scan.

Analgesic nephropathy

NSAIDs are a frequent cause of renal failure. NSAIDS cause renal failure by several mechanisms:

- Interstitial nephritis
- Direct toxic effect on the tubules
- Papillary necrosis
- Inhibition of vasodilatory prostaglandins in the afferent arteriole
- Membranous glomerulonephritis

A person without underlying renal insufficiency should not experience a rise in creatinine from the use of NSAIDs. This only occurs in those with significant impairment such as the elderly or those with hypertension or diabetes. NSAIDs can also cause toxicity by a combination of these. More than half the patients have pyuria, which if persistently associated with sterile urine can be an important clue to diagnosis. There is no specific test to confirm that NSAIDs caused the renal failure. You see a rise in BUN and creatinine and a history of the use of NSAIDs. There is no specific therapy.

Papillary necrosis

Acute papillary necrosis occurs in patients with a history of sickle cell disease, diabetes, urinary obstruction, or chronic pyelonephritis. It can be brought on acutely by the ingestion of NSAIDs. The presentation is with the sudden onset of flank pain, hematuria, pyuria, and fever. This can be very similar in presentation to acute pyelonephritis. In a patient with the risks described above, symptoms for papillary necrosis will come on very suddenly. The findings of white and red cells on UA will not distinguish them. However, papillary necrosis will not grow any organisms on culture. The most accurate diagnostic test for papillary necrosis is a CT scan. The CT scan will show "bumpy" contours in the renal pelvis where the papillae have sloughed off. There is no specific therapy for papillary necrosis.

Prevention of contrast-induced renal failure

In those patients with significant underlying renal disease who have an unavoidable radiologic procedure requiring contrast, you must hydrate with 1–2 liters of normal saline over 12 hours before the procedure. Hydration has been shown to decrease the likelihood of contrast-induced renal failure. Bicarbonate and N-acetyl cysteine have also been shown to decrease the risk of renal failure. Ineffective preventive measures are diuretics such as furosemide or mannitol. If the question asks, "Which of the following is most likely to prevent the development of renal failure with contrast?" you should answer hydration.

GLOMERULONEPHRITIS

Glomerulonephritis (GN) is an inflammation of the glomerulus, often on the basis of an autoimmune event, circulating antibodies, or vasculitis. Diabetes and hypertension cause glomerular disease and are certainly the most common causes of nephrotic syndrome and end stage renal disease. Diabetes and hypertension, however, do not have the acute inflammatory stage of glomerulonephritis characterized by hematuria.

All forms of GN can be characterized by edema, hematuria, red cell casts, and hypertension. The red cells develop an abnormal shape as they squeeze through the abnormal glomerulus and are termed "dysmorphic." The edema of GN is found first in areas of low tissue tension, such as the periorbital area or the scrotum. When more severe, edema can be found anywhere. With the salt and water retention leading to edema, you also develop hypertension. GN is also characterized by modest amounts of protein in the urine with the daily total being <2 grams per 24 hours, although by definition nephrotic syndrome does not begin until there are >3.5 grams per 24 hours. The most important distinction between GN and nephrotic syndrome is the degree of proteinuria.

Glomerulonephritis is also characterized by low urine sodium with a fractional excretion of sodium of <1%.

Many, but not all, forms of GN have a characteristic blood test such as ANCA, basement membrane antibodies, ANA, or antistreptolysin. However, the single most important test to diagnose GN is the renal biopsy. Unlike in tubular diseases, the renal biopsy is extremely important in GN because it guides therapy. There are few treatments to reverse a form of ATN based on the specific etiology. In GN, however, there are cytotoxic medications such as cyclophosphamide to use, or other treatments such as mycophenolate for SLE nephritis or plasmapheresis for Goodpasture syndrome. Hence, before we commit a patient to long-term therapy with potentially harmful medications (cyclophosphamide causes hemorrhagic cystitis), we should obtain a precise diagnosis.

Table 8-2. Causes of Glomerulonephritis Disease Spectrum

Vascular Disease	Glomerular Disease
Wegener granulomatosis	Goodpasture syndrome
Churg-Strauss syndrome	Postinfectious glomerulonephritis
Henoch-Schönlein purpura	IgA nephropathy (Berger disease)
Polyarteritis nodosa	SLE
Thrombotic thrombocytopenic purpura (TTP)	Idiopathic rapidly progressive glomerulonephritis
Hemolytic uremic syndrome (HUS)	Alport syndrome
Cryoglobulinemia	Diabetes and hypertension (most common causes)
	Amyloid

Wegener Granulomatosis

Wegener granulomatosis (WG) is characterized by systemic vasculitis that most often involves the kidney, lung, and upper respiratory tract such as the sinuses or middle ear. In a patient with chronic upper and lower respiratory illness, not responding to antibiotics should evoke WG as a possibility. If there is renal disease as well, then WG is the most likely diagnosis. In addition, WG can have involvement of the skin (50%), joints, eyes (50%), and GI tract, as well as neuropathy.

Laboratory abnormalities are elevated ESR, anemia, and leukocytosis. Rheumatoid factor is positive in 50%. These findings are rather nonspecific and could be found in almost any vasculitis or chronic infectious or inflammatory condition. The best initial test that is specific for WG is the anti-proteinase-3 antibody, which is also known as cytoplasmic antineutrophil cytoplasmic antibody, or C-ANCA. The perinuclear pattern, or P-ANCA, is found in a much smaller number. The other name for P-ANCA is antimyeloperoxidase antibody. Complement levels are normal in WG.

The most accurate test for WG is a biopsy of the kidney, nasal septum, or lung looking for granulomas. Sinus biopsy, specifically the nasal septum, is less sensitive and has more false negative results. Treatment is with cyclophosphamide and steroids.

Churg-Strauss Syndrome

Churg-Strauss syndrome (CS) is a vasculitis similar to Wegener granulomatosis and is also characterized by chronic lung involvement, neuropathy, skin lesions, GI, cardiac, and renal involvement. All forms of vasculitis are characterized by fever, weight loss, and a generalized malaise. CS is characterized by a history of asthma, eosinophilia, and other atopic diseases. The characteristic diagnostic tests are the elevated eosinophil count and positive P-ANCA or antimyeloperoxidase. The most accurate test is a lung biopsy showing the granulomas and eosinophils. Treatment is with glucocorticoids and cyclophosphamide.

Goodpasture Syndrome

Goodpasture syndrome (GP) is an idiopathic disorder of renal and lung disease characterized by a unique antibasement membrane antibody. Unlike Wegener or Churg-Strauss, GP does not affect multiple organs or sites in the body besides the lung and the kidney. Hence, the absence of skin or eye findings is a clue to the diagnosis. One-third of patients have no lung involvement and they only present with hematuria and proteinuria. Lung involvement is characterized by hemoptysis, cough, and shortness of breath. There will be hemosiderin-laden macrophages. The macrophages are cells that phagocytose free hemoglobin in the lung where it is metabolized to hemosiderin. The best initial test to confirm the diagnosis is the level of antibasement membrane antibodies to type IV collagen. The single most accurate test is a lung or kidney biopsy. The biopsy shows linear deposits on immunofluorescence. Therapy is with plasmapheresis and steroids. Cyclophosphamide may also help.

Polyarteritis Nodosa

Polyarteritis nodosa (PAN) is a systemic vasculitis of small- and medium-sized arteries that affects virtually every organ in the body with the exception of the lung. In PAN, renal involvement is common and manifests as hypertension, renal insufficiency, and hemorrhage due to microaneurysms. The most accurate diagnostic test is a biopsy, and treatment is with cyclophosphamide and steroids.

Like all vasculitides, PAN is associated with fever, weight loss, and malaise. Like WG and Churg-Strauss, there is involvement of the skin, eyes, muscles, GI tract, heart, kidneys, and neurologic system. Although the liver is involved, there is usually no clinically evident hepatic effect. Hepatitis B is associated with 10–30% of patients. This is especially true in injection drug users. Abdominal pain and joint pain may be prominent. The abdominal pain may mimic mesenteric ischemia, and the pain will occur with eating. In this case, an angiogram of the involved vessels in the GI tract may eliminate the need for a biopsy. The sural nerve is a frequent location for the biopsy. Anemia and an elevated sedimentation rate are present but are too nonspecific to be useful diagnostically. P-ANCA is only present in a minority of patients. Treatment of PAN is with steroids and cyclophosphamide.

IgA Nephropathy (Berger Disease)

Note

Most common glomerulopathy worldwide.

IgA nephropathy presents with mild hematuria that resolves spontaneously in 30% of patients. About 40–50% of patients progress to end stage renal disease. Like HSP, this is a disorder of the deposition of IgA, however, symptoms arise only from the kidney. Hypertension is frequent. This is most likely secondary to abnormally increased salt and water retention by the kidney. Look for an Asian patient under 35 years of age who has had a recent viral illness or pharyngitis who develops hematuria 1–2 days later. This is to distinguish it from poststreptococcal glomerulonephritis, in which the renal involvement occurs 1–2 weeks later or longer. Although this is an IgA deposition disease, blood IgA levels are elevated in only 50% of patients. Complement levels are normal. The diagnosis is based on finding IgA deposited in the kidney on biopsy.

The treatment of IgA nephropathy is difficult. There is no proven effective therapy. Anyone with proteinuria should receive ACE inhibitors or angiotensin receptor blockers (ARB). When the proteinuria is massive, steroids should be tried. The value of fish oil is marginal. You trade fishy breath for a minimal possibility of improvement that is not proven. The presence of proteinuria and hypertension imply a worse course.

Postinfectious Glomerulonephritis

In addition to group A beta hemolytic streptococci (*Streptococcus pyogenes*), numerous other infections can be associated with postinfectious glomerulonephritis. Virtually any infectious agent can cause it, including hepatitis B and C, CMV, and chronic staphylococcal infections such as endocarditis. In the pre-antibiotic era, glomerulonephritis was the most common cause of death in endocarditis. Poststreptococcal glomerulonephritis (PSGN) can occur with either throat or skin infection with *Streptococcus pyogenes*, although rheumatic fever only occurs with the strains that cause pharyngitis. PSGN occurs in about 10–15% of patients with pharyngitis infected with a nephritogenic strain.

The presentation is characterized by smoky, cola, or tea-colored urine. This abnormal urine color is from hematuria, red cell casts, and proteinuria. Periorbital edema and hypertension are common. The best initial test is the antistreptolysin (ASO) test and the antihyaluronic acid (AHT) test. Complement levels, particularly C3, are low. The most accurate test is the renal biopsy showing "humps" on electron microscopy. IgG and C3 will be deposited in the mesangium as subepithelial humps.

Treatment is largely supportive, with management of the fluid overload and hypertension with diuretics. The vast majority of cases resolve spontaneously. This is why a biopsy is rarely needed. Antibiotics should be given to eradicate the organism from the pharynx.

Thrombotic Thrombocytopenic Purpura/Hemolytic Uremic Syndrome

Thrombotic thrombocytopenic purpura (TTP) and hemolytic uremic syndrome (HUS) are two varieties of the same disease process with considerable overlap. There is no specific diagnostic test, so the diagnosis is based on the clinical triad (HUS) or pentad (TTP).

- Most cases of TTP are idiopathic and arise from inhibition of the enzyme ADAMTS13, which is responsible for cleaving large multimers of von Willebrand factor into smaller units. The increase in circulating multimers of vWF increase platelet adhesion to areas of endothelial injury, particularly the arteriole-capillary junctions.

- Some cases of TTP are associated with specific diseases (cancer, HIV) and drugs (ticlopidine, clopidogrel, cyclosporine, and interferon) and are referred to as secondary TTP. ADAMTS13 activity is generally not as depressed in secondary TTP.

HUS predominantly affects children. Most cases are caused by a shiga-like toxin produced by *E. coli* O157:H7 although Campylobacter, shigella and some viruses have also been implicated. It is one of the most common causes of acute renal failure in childhood and carries up to 10% mortality.

HUS consists of a triad of hemolytic anemia, uremia, and thrombocytopenia. TTP has the same 3 findings, and is also associated with fever and neurologic problems. You do not have to have all 5 findings simultaneously to be considered to have TTP. The anemia in both will be intravascular in nature and will have an abnormal blood smear showing schistocytes, helmet cells, and fragmented red cells. LDH and reticulocyte count will be elevated and haptoglobin decreased.

If TTP is very severe, the treatment is plasmapheresis. Plasmapheresis is used to treat severe cases of HUS but is not established in the treatment of mild disease. Mild disease resolves spontaneously. Dipyridamole may help treat TTP by preventing platelet aggregation.

Do not give antibiotics to those with possible HUS; if antibiotics are given, organism may release more toxins as it dies and may worsen the disease.

Do not transfuse platelets. Even if the platelet count is low, administering platelets can actually worsen the CNS and renal abnormalities by giving more platelets as a substrate to precipitate. Small platelet plugs are actually the cause of the problem.

Cryoglobulinemia

Renal disease from cryoglobulinemia is associated with chronic hepatitis C or less commonly B. Besides the renal disease, cryoglobulinemia is associated with joint pain, neuropathy, and purpuric skin lesions. This is similar to other types of vasculitis. There is no GI involvement as there is with Henoch-Schönlein purpura. Cryoglobulinemia is associated with an elevated ESR and low levels of complement and is confirmed with a test for the cryoglobulins. A positive rheumatoid factor is a marker for the disease as well. The main treatment is to manage the underlying chronic hepatitis with interferon and ribavirin. For severe disease, pulse doses of steroids and occasionally plasmapheresis are also used.

Diabetes

The incidence of glomerular involvement in diabetes is directly proportional to the duration of the diabetes. The standard dipstick becomes positive for albumin at a level 150–300 mg per 24 hours of excretion. Microalbuminuria is a level of protein excretion that is abnormal but is <300 mg. If albumin is not present on dipstick all patients with diabetes should be screened for microalbuminuria annually. Annual screening with a serum creatinine level should also be performed. Treatment for albuminuria is with an ACE inhibitor or ARB. The blood pressure goal is also lower in diabetes, and <130/80 is optimal. Although a renal biopsy is the most accurate test for renal involvement in diabetes, it is not routinely performed unless there is the possibility of another disease causing the renal failure.

SLE

SLE is associated with an enormously wide variation in the degree of renal involvement. There may be asymptomatic proteinuria or hematuria, or there may be severe renal disease requiring dialysis. Double-stranded DNA levels go up and complement levels go down as a marker of severity in flare-ups of the disease. The most accurate test is a biopsy. Biopsy is essential with lupus nephritis in order to guide therapy.

Sclerosis: No therapy needed. This is simply scarring of the kidney.

Proliferative disease: Use steroids combined with mycophenolate. Mycophenolate is superior to cyclophosphamide.

Alport Syndrome

Alport syndrome is the combination of glomerular disease with congenital eye and ear abnormalities. There is sensorineural hearing loss.

Idiopidly Rapidly Progressive Glomerulonephritis

RPGN may occur with any of the glomerular diseases described above, in which case it simply refers to a time course of the disease. In addition, there is an idiopathic form associated with crescent formation in the kidney and the presence of ANCA negative. Diagnosis is with renal biopsy, and the treatment is with steroids and cyclophosphamide.

Amyloidosis

There are two common types of amyloidosis:

1) AL: Plasma cell dyscrasia causing deposition of protein derived from immunoglobulin light chains. This may be associated with multiple myeloma.

2) AA: Amyloid is produced as a proteinaceous material in association with multiple chronic infectious or inflammatory conditions, such as rheumatoid arthritis, inflammatory bowel disease, or myeloma. The amyloid protein builds up in the kidney, causing glomerulonephritis, and in the GI tract, nerves, and muscles. In the heart, amyloid is associated with restrictive cardiomyopathy, rhythm disorders, and heart block. A large tongue (macroglossia) is also characteristic. Neural involvement produces carpal tunnel syndrome. Malabsorption may occur from GI involvement.

The diagnosis of amyloidosis is established by biopsy of an involved organ such as the kidney. Other unique methods of diagnosis are aspirating the abdominal fat pad or taking a sample of the rectum. Congo red testing shows green birefringence. Amyloidosis treatment is very difficult and consists of controlling the underlying disease. Melphalan and prednisone can control protein production.

Nephrotic Syndrome

Nephrotic syndrome is defined as the presence of renal disease sufficient to produce a level of proteinuria >3.5 grams per 24 hours, hyperlipidemia, edema, and a low serum albumin level. Nephrotic syndrome refers to the severity of glomerular disease and does not, by itself, imply one specific etiology. The edema is from increased salt and water retention by the kidney, as well as low oncotic pressure in the serum. Hyperlipidemia is of unclear etiology but is most likely from the loss of the lipoprotein markers or signals on the surface of chylomicrons and LDL that lead to the clearance of these lipids from the bloodstream.

One-third of nephrotic syndrome is associated with systemic diseases such as diabetes, hypertension, or amyloidosis. In addition, patients with any of the diseases associated with glomerulonephritis described above may develop nephrotic syndrome if the severity of disease is bad enough to cause massive proteinuria and low serum albumin levels. Nephrotic syndrome is a descriptor of severity, not a specific etiology. When the glomerular basement membrane loses its negative charges, protein is spilled into the urine.

Nephrotic syndrome is associated with hyperlipiduria, which gives a droplet found on urinalysis that may form the shape of Maltese crosses.

Hypercoagulable states or thrombophilia develops from the urinary loss of natural anticoagulant proteins such as antithrombin, protein C, and protein S. Patients can develop spontaneous arterial or venous thrombosis. There is also iron, copper, and zinc deficiency from the urinary loss of their transport proteins such as transferrin and ceruloplasmin.

Diagnosis. The diagnosis of nephrotic syndrome is based on the presence of a high protein level in the urine, a low protein level in the blood, edema, and hyperlipidemia. The 24-hour urine shows >3.5 grams of protein; however, this test is cumbersome to perform. An easier test with equal accuracy is a single spot urine for albumin and creatinine. When you correct the albumin level in a single spot urine, the ratio that is found is equivalent to the 24-hour urine. In other words, if you find a protein:creatinine ratio of >3.5 on a single urine, this is equal to 3.5 grams of protein on a 24-hour urine. Remember that Bence-Jones protein is not found on the routine urine dipstick, which only detects albumin. You must do a urine immune electrophoresis to detect Bence-Jones protein.

The most accurate test to determine the specific etiology of nephrotic syndrome is a renal biopsy.

Figure 8-1. Maltese cross

Treatment. Treatment of nephrotic syndrome is to control the underlying disease. In addition, steroids are used to treat all forms of idiopathic primary renal causes of nephrotic syndrome, such as membranous, nil lesion, membranoproliferative, mesangial, and focal-segmental disease. If steroids do not work, the next best step in therapy is to add cyclophosphamide or mycophenolate. Azathiaprine is sometimes useful. ACE inhibitors or ARBs are used for all patients with proteinuria, but they do not reverse the underlying disease.

All of the following syndromes are diagnosed as described above and treated with steroids and sometimes cyclophosphamide or mycophenolate.

Focal-Segmental Glomerulosclerosis (FSGS). Associated with the use of heroin as well as HIV. Limited response (only 20–40%) to steroids. May progress to end stage renal disease (ESRD) over 5–10 years. FSGS is the **most common cause of nephrotic syndrome** in adults.

Membranous. Associated with cancer such as lymphoma or breast cancer, and infections such as endocarditis or chronic hepatitis B or C. Other etiologies are lupus, penicillamine, gold salts, and NSAIDs.

Nil Lesion (Minimal Change Disease). Most common form in children, although it may account for 15% of adult disease. NSAIDs have also been associated with nil lesion disease. Light microscopy is normal and electron microscopy is needed to see fusion of foot processes. Nil lesion disease is treated with steroids. Hodgkin's lymphoma has an association with nil lesion disease.

Mesangial. Mostly idiopathic, steroid-resistant type of nephrotic syndrome. Immunofluorescent staining shows IgM deposits in an expanded mesangium.

Membranoproliferative. Associated with chronic hepatitis and low serum complement levels. Dipyridamole and aspirin are also useful therapeutically. Cryoglobulins are treated with interferon and ribavirin, which address the hepatitis.

DIAGNOSTIC TESTING IN RENAL DISEASE

Urinalysis

There is no recommendation for routine testing of the general population by urinalysis. Diabetics or those with systemic diseases such as hypertension are not the general population.

Proteinuria. The urine dipstick detects albumin but no other proteins, such as immunoglobulin light chains. This can be from either glomerular or tubular diseases, although glomerular diseases can give greater amounts. Microalbuminuria is defined as levels 30–300 mg per 24 hours. Mild amounts of proteinuria under 1 gram per day can be seen in up to 10% of the population and most often resolve spontaneously. Proteinuria can also occur from stressors such as fever, CHF, and severe exercise. Proteinuria is also caused by prolonged standing, which is known as orthostatic proteinuria. It is diagnosed by splitting the 24-hour urine sample. If you find no protein in the first 8 hours and then find it in the second part, it is orthostatic proteinuria, which is considered benign.

Hematuria. Red cells can be found in the urine from any cause of disease in the bladder or kidney. Etiologies are stones, cancer, bleeding disorders, trauma to urinary system, and treatment such as cyclophosphamide (which causes hemorrhagic cystitis or glomerular disease). Hematuria is also from infections such as cystitis or prostatitis. The red cells change shape in glomerular disease and can be dysmorphic.

Nitrites. Gram-negative bacteria reduce nitrate to nitrite, which is a marker of infection.

Bacteriuria. By itself, the isolated finding of bacteria in the urine is of very limited significance. The most important exception is in pregnant women, whom you should screen for bacteria and treat. About 30% of pregnant women with bacteriuria progress to pyelonephritis.

Table 8-3. Casts

Casts	Significance
Hyaline	Dehydration. These casts develop as an accumulation of the normal amount of tubular protein. They do not necessarily mean disease.
Red cell	Glomerulonephritis
Broad, waxy	Chronic renal failure
Granular	Also called "dirty" or "muddy." They are associated with acute tubular necrosis and represent accumulated epithelial cells.
White cell	Pyelonephritis, interstitial nephritis

END-STAGE RENAL DISEASE/DIALYSIS

The most common causes of end stage renal disease (ESRD) that require dialysis are diabetes and hypertension. Glomerulonephritis is the etiology of about 15%, with cystic disease and interstitial nephritis causing 4–5% each.

The indications for dialysis are life-threatening abnormalities that cannot be corrected another way, such as fluid overload refractory to diuretics, acidosis, pericarditis, encephalopathy, and other severe neuropathies including myoclonus, wrist or foot drop, and hyperkalemia. Another indication is persistent nausea, vomiting, and bleeding diathesis attributable to uremia.

Hemodialysis is used in 85% of patients and peritoneal dialysis in 15%. The most common complication of peritoneal dialysis is peritonitis.

Other complications of ESRD are as follows.

Anemia. This is from the loss of production of erythropoietin from the kidney. It is treated with replacement of erythropoietin. The anemia of ESRD is normochromic and normocytic.

Hypocalcemia/Hyperphosphatemia. This is from the loss of 1,25-dihydroxyvitamin D production. The hypocalcemia is treated with vitamin D replacement. Hyperphosphatemia is from the inability of the kidney to excrete phosphate. High phosphate levels contribute to low calcium levels by precipitating out in tissues in combination with the calcium. High phosphate levels are treated with phosphate binders, such as calcium carbonate or calcium acetate. Sevelamer and lanthanum are two phosphate binders that do not contain either aluminum or calcium. They are used when the calcium level is abnormally high because of vitamin D replacement. Cinacalcet is a substance that simulates the effect of calcium on the parathyroid. Cinacalcet is used in severe, refractory cases. Cinacalcet will tell the parathyroid to shut off parathyroid hormone production and helps decrease phosphate in this way.

Aluminum-containing phosphate binders should not be used. Aluminum is associated both with CNS accumulation and dementia as well as bone abnormalities.

Osteodystrophy. This is also known as osteitis fibrosa cystica. Bone abnormalities occur because dead kidneys don't make 1,25 vitamin D. This leads to a low calcium level. The low calcium leads to secondary hyperparathyroidism, which removes calcium from the bones. In addition, bones buffer acidosis by removing calcium from bone. When you want to demineralize a piece of bone in a lab, you soak it in acid; this is what is happening in the body. Renal osteodystrophy is controlled with improving calcium and phosphorous levels and treating the secondary hyperparathyroidism.

Hypermagnesemia. Magnesium accumulates because of decreased renal excretion. Treatment is by restricting magnesium intake.

Hypertension and Accelerated Atherosclerosis. Renal disease results in a rapidly progressive coronary artery disease. The reason for this is not precisely clear, however, this is the most common cause of death for those on dialysis. This is why the goal of blood pressure management is lower at <130/80 for those with renal impairment.

Infection. ESRD patients are at increased risk of infection because neutrophils and other white cells do not work normally in a uremic environment. This is the second most common cause of death in dialysis patients. The most common organism is *Staphylococcus* because of the constant need to penetrate the skin to place someone on dialysis for 4–6 hours 3–4 times a week.

Bleeding. Although nephrotic syndrome gives thrombophilia because of the urinary loss of protein C, protein S, and antithrombin, the most common coagulation problem with ESRD is bleeding. This is because of uremia-induced platelet dysfunction. It gives an increased bleeding time. Uremia-induced bleeding is treated with desmopressin, which releases subendothelial stores of von Willebrand factor and factor VIII, which increase platelet aggregation and adherence. Rarely, estrogen or cryoprecipitate are used.

Dietary Treatment. Patients with severe renal disease should be on a diet restricted in potassium, sodium, protein, magnesium, and phosphate.

Other abnormalities associated with ESRD are pruritus, hyperuricemia, decreased libido from low testosterone levels, weakness, fatigue, and glucose intolerance. Although not life threatening, they do have a significant impact on function. The only way to improve them is with dialysis, although, by themselves, they are not indications for dialysis (the indications for dialysis are hyperkalemia, acidosis, fluid overload, encephalopathy, and pericarditis).

RENAL TRANSPLANTATION

The duration of survival is by far superior with transplantation when compared with maintenance on dialysis.

Table 8-4. Duration of Survival

Live related donor	95% at 1 year, 72% at 5 years
Cadaver donor	88% at 1 year, 58% at 5 years
Dialysis alone	30–40% at 5 years
Diabetics on dialysis	20% at 5 years

The average wait to obtain a kidney for transplantation is 2–4 years and becoming longer because of an insufficient donor supply.

Post-transplantation renal graft rejection is prevented by using cyclosporine, tacrolimus, and mycophenolate. These are all medications that inhibit T-cell function.

FLUID AND ELECTROLYTE DISORDERS

Hyponatremia

Hyponatremia is defined as a low serum sodium concentration with a level <135 mEq. This generally occurs from either increased free water retention or urinary sodium loss. About 85–90% of sodium is extracellular. Serum osmolality is largely a function of the serum sodium level.

$$\text{Serum osmolality} = (2 \times \text{sodium}) + \text{BUN}/2.8 + \text{glucose}/18$$

When the glucose and BUN are normal, this roughly comes out to be $2 \times$ sodium + 10.

Presentation. The symptoms of hyponatremia are predominantly neurologic. They range from mild confusion and forgetfulness to disorientation and obtundation to seizure or coma, depending on the severity of the hyponatremia. The symptoms do not correspond to a specific level of sodium because the symptoms largely depend on how fast the level dropped. An acute 15–20 point drop in sodium level can result in a seizure or coma. If the level drops gradually, the patient can sustain an extremely low sodium level with no symptoms at all. Generally, there should be no symptoms at all unless the level drops below 125.

Treatment. Mild hyponatremia should resolve with fluid restriction. "Mild" refers to the absence of symptoms, not a specific level.

Moderate hyponatremia can be managed with normal saline administration combined with a loop diuretic such as furosemide. The saline gives sodium, and the loop diuretic causes a net free water loss.

Severe and chronic hyponatremia such as that resulting in seizure or coma should be managed with 3% hypertonic saline or the V2 receptor-antagonists conivaptan and tolvaptan. It would be unusual to see severe symptoms with a sodium level >120.

The rate of rise of the sodium level should be monitored so as not to cause central pontine myelinolysis. This is what occurs if the sodium level is corrected too rapidly. Generally, the rate of rise should not exceed 0.5–1 mEq per hour. This means no more than a 12-point rise in a 12–24-hour period. Hyponatremia can be corrected as rapidly as 2 mEq per hour if the patient is seizing and it is extremely urgent. Fludrocortisone is used for cerebral salt wasting disease.

Specific etiologies

Pseudohyponatremia. These are conditions in which the total body sodium level is truly normal and the sodium blood level is artificially low. Treatment is directed at etiology of the lab artifact, not specifically the sodium level.

- Hyperglycemia: The sodium level is decreased by 1.6 mEq/L for every 100 mg/dL increase in glucose above normal. The high glucose load causes a transcellular shift of water out of the cell into the vascular space unaccompanied by sodium. This drops the serum sodium level. Mannitol and sorbitol can do the same.
- Hyperlipidemia: In this case, there is a normal sodium level and this is simply a lab artifact.

Hypervolemic States (Increased ECF). These are all conditions in which there is a decrease in intravascular volume resulting in an increase in ADH secretion from the posterior pituitary. This is a form of appropriate increased ADH syndrome.

- CHF
- Nephrotic syndrome and low albumin states
- Cirrhosis
- Renal insufficiency: When renal failure becomes advanced, the impaired free water excretion will drop the sodium level.

Hypovolemic States (Decreased ECF). For most of these, the hyponatremia develops because of the loss of sodium through body fluids and replacement with free water. For example, sweating is a cause of hypernatremia because sweat is mostly free water and only has a little sodium. However, when you sweat and replace only with free water, the sodium level drops over time.

- GI loss: vomiting, diarrhea, gastric suction
- Skin loss: burns, sweating, cystic fibrosis
- Diuretics: you urinate out a little salt but replace with only free water
- Renal sodium loss: The kidney can lose the ability to reabsorb sodium in the proximal convoluted tubule as the kidney is damaged. Damaged tubules cannot reabsorb sodium.
- Adrenal insufficiency (Addison disease): Aldosterone reabsorbs sodium from the kidney. Without aldosterone, you lose sodium.
- ACE inhibitors: unclear etiology

Table 8-5. Causes of Hypovolemic Hyponatremia

Urine Na <20	Urine Na >20
Dehydration	Diuretics
Vomiting	ACE inhibitors
Diarrhea	Renal salt wasting
Sweating	Addison disease
	Cerebral sodium wasting

Euvolemic States. These patients are neither dehydrated nor volume overloaded. There is no edema, neither is there orthostasis or decreased skin turgor.

- Psychogenic polydipsia: patients must drink at least 15–20 liters a day of fluid to overwhelm the diluting capacity of the kidney
- Hypothyroidism: mechanism unknown
- Diuretics: can be both hypovolemic and euvolemic

- ACE inhibitors: probably through an increase in ADH
- Endurance exercise
- Syndrome of inappropriate secretion of ADH (SIADH) (see Endrocrine section)

SIADH

Etiology
- CNS diseases: infections, stroke, tumor, trauma, vasculitis, pain
- Pulmonary diseases: pneumonia, TB, PE, asthma
- Neoplastic disease: lung cancer, as well as cancer of the pancreas, duodenum, or thymus

Medications
- SSRIs
- Tricyclic antidepressants
- Haloperidol
- Cyclophosphamide
- Vincristine
- Carbamazepine
- Thiazide diuretics

The presentation of SIADH is similar to all forms of hyponatremia in terms of neurologic symptoms in proportion to the degree of hyponatremia. The diagnosis is based on finding an elevated urine osmolality and urine sodium level. This is inappropriate to find in a patient with hyponatremia. The range on urine osmolality is between 50 and 1,200 mOsm/L. If the urine osmolality is >100 in the presence of hyponatremia, the person most likely has SIADH. The single most accurate test is an elevated ADH level, though it is rarely done and is inferred from the urine osmolarity.

Treatment of SIADH is to restrict fluids for mild disease and give hypertonic saline for severe disease as was previously described. Normal saline with a loop diuretic is also useful to raise the sodium level. For chronic disease in which the underlying cause of the SIADH cannot be corrected, therapy with conivaptan, tolvaptan, or demeclocycline is used. These medications inhibit the effect of ADH on the kidney tubule and lead to water diuresis. Conivaptan and tolvaptan are V2 receptor-antagonists. Demeclocycline and lithium treat SIADH by inducing nephrogenic diabetes insipidus. Lithium, due to toxicity, is rarely used.

Hypernatremia

Etiology
- **Insensible losses:** extrarenal loss without intake of hypotonic fluids; increased skin loss (sweating, burns, fever, exercise) or respiratory infections
- **GI loss:** osmotic diarrhea (e.g., lactulose, malabsorption), some infectious diarrhea
- **Transcellular shift:** rhabdomyolysis or seizures causing muscles to avidly take up water and ↑Na
- **Renal**
  - Nephrogenic diabetes insipidus (NDI), secondary to renal disease, increased calcium, decreased potassium, lithium, demeclocycline, sickle cell disease, and others

- Central DI (CDI)
- Idiopathic, trauma, infectious, tumor, granulomatous, hypoxic brain damage or from neurosurgery. Idiopathic most common.
- Osmotic diuresis: diabetic ketoacidosis (DKA), nonketotic hyperosmolar coma, mannitol, diuretics

Presentation

- Primarily neurologic
- Lethargy, weakness, irritability, seizures, and coma are present with severe hypernatremia of any cause. Diabetes insipidus gives a dilute diuresis of 3–20 L per day.

Diagnosis. Watching for a decrease in urine volume after administering ADH **distinguishes CDI from NDI.**

Treatment. Acute hypernatremia is treated with isotonic fluids intravenously. Correction of sodium should not be >1 mEq every 2 hours or 12 mEq per day. Complications of overly rapid correction include cerebral edema, permanent neurologic damage, or seizures. A rate of correction as fast as 1 mEq per hour is also acceptable if the patient is seizing.

CDI. Correct the underlying cause, if possible.

- Vasopressin (ADH). It can be given subcutaneously, intravenously, intramuscularly, or by nasal spray (all routes except oral).

NDI. Correct underlying cause, if possible.

- Diuretic or NSAIDs. NSAIDs work by inhibiting prostaglandins, which impair concentrating ability. NSAIDs will increase the action of ADH at the kidney.

Hypokalemia

Potassium levels are maintained by transcellular shift and rates of renal excretion. About 95% of potassium is intracellular.

Etiology

- GI losses. This can be from any form of GI loss, such as vomiting, diarrhea, or tube drainage.
- Increased entry into cells (transcellular shift) can be from alkalosis, increased levels of insulin, beta adrenergic activity, and the replacement of vitamin B_{12} in B_{12}-deficient patients. Trauma patients have increased beta adrenergic activity.
- Urinary losses:
  - Diuretics
  - Increased aldosterone states, such as Conn syndrome, excessive licorice ingestion, Bartter syndrome, or Cushing disease. Aldosterone is the most important regulator of potassium levels in the body. Renal artery stenosis results in a high renin/aldosterone state.
  - Low magnesium levels. Magnesium decreases urinary loss of potassium. When you are deficient in magnesium, you start to spill potassium into the urine.

Presentation. The symptoms of hypokalemia predominantly affect muscles and the heart. Patients have weakness, paralysis when it is severe, arrhythmias that can be fatal, and even rhabdomyolysis. Potassium is necessary for ADH effect on the kidney, and hypokalemic patients present with nephrogenic diabetes insipidus.

Diagnostic testing. In emergency cases, the most important diagnostic test is the EKG. EKG abnormalities include T-wave flattening and U-waves. A U-wave is an extra wave after the T-wave that is indicative of Purkinje fiber repolarization.

Treatment. Correction of underlying cause when possible. Replete as follows:

- IV maximum 10–20 mEq/h; do not use dextrose containing fluids, as they increase insulin release and lower potassium.
- Oral: Gut regulates absorption; there is no maximum rate of oral potassium replacement.
- GI tract slows absorption; no dextrose-containing fluids; dextrose brings increased extracellular potassium entry into cells.
- Potential complication of too-rapid repletion is fatal arrhythmia.

Very large amounts of potassium may be necessary to raise the body potassium level by even 1 or 2 points. The total body requirement is to give 4–5 mEq per kg per point. It is important not to use IV fluids that contain dextrose. Dextrose will provide the shift of potassium into the cells and will further lower potassium levels.

Hyperkalemia

Etiology

- Increased intake (orally or by IV)—usually in presence of impaired excretion
- Movement from cells to extracellular fluid (ECF)
  - Pseudohyperkalemia—secondary hemolysis, mechanical trauma during venipuncture, platelet count >1,000,000 (10^6), WBC count >100,000 (10^5)
  - Acidosis—secondary cellular buffering (H^+ moves into cells, K^+ moves out)
  - For every 0.1-point decrease in the pH, the potassium level will increase by 0.7 points because of the transcellular shift
  - Insulin deficiency
  - Tissue breakdown—rhabdomyolysis, tumor lysis after seizures or severe exercise
  - Periodic paralysis—mild, brief episodes of muscle weakness with mild increase in K^+; diagnosis with recurrent attacks and family history
- Decreased urinary excretion
  - Renal failure
  - Hypoaldosteronism: ACE inhibitors, type IV RTA, adrenal enzyme deficiency; heparin inhibits production of aldosterone
  - Primary adrenal insufficiency (Addison disease) or adrenalectomy
  - Potassium-sparing diuretics—amiloride, spironolactone
  - NSAIDs

Presentation

- Muscular weakness can begin usually with K^+ levels >6.5.
- Abnormal cardiac conduction is the most common cause of death, hypoventilation.

Diagnosis. EKG findings: peaked T waves, widened QRS, short QT, or prolonged PR

Treatment

- Calcium chloride—membrane stabilization (most emergent treatment in presence of EKG abnormalities). Effect is immediate and short lived.
- Sodium bicarbonate—alkalosis drives K^+ into cells. Do not give in same IV line as calcium. Forms $CaCO_3$ precipitates.
- Glucose and insulin—drives K^+ intracellular, takes 30–60 minutes to work
- Diuretics, beta agonists
- Cation exchange resin (Kayexalate®)—resin absorbs 1 mEq K^+ per g and releases 1 mEq Na^+. Given with sorbitol to prevent constipation. Kayexalate must be given with the above treatments because they only cause cellular redistribution of K^+ and do not remove it from the body. It can also be given as a retention enema for those who cannot take it orally.
- Dialysis

ACID/BASE DISTURBANCES

Alkalosis (High pH)

Metabolic

For every 1-point increase in the level of serum bicarbonate, there is a 0.7-point increase in the pCO_2. Volume contraction of dehydration results in an increased level of aldosterone, which leads to metabolic alkalosis. Increased levels of aldosterone in volume contraction lead to increased levels of hydrogen ion (H^+) excretion. Increased sodium delivery to the distal tubule leads to increased sodium reabsorption in a segment of the tubule that excretes H^+ and K^+.

H^+ Ion Loss

- Exogenous steroids
- GI loss (vomiting, nasogastric suction)
- Renal loss (Conn syndrome, Cushing, ACTH overproduction, licorice, Bartter syndrome)
- Decreased chloride intake
- Diuretics

HCO_3 Retention

- Bicarbonate administration
- Contraction alkalosis
- Milk-alkali syndrome

H^+ Movement into Cells

- Hypokalemia

Respiratory

Hyperventilation of Any Cause

- Anemia
- Pulmonary embolus
- Sarcoid
- Anxiety
- Pain

Progesterone, catecholamines, hypoxia, cirrhosis, pregnancy, and salicylates are all events or substances that increase the respiratory rate and minute ventilation and lead to respiratory alkalosis.

$$\textbf{Anion gap} = (Na^+) - (HCO_3^- + Cl^-)$$

$$(\text{normal: } 8–12)$$

Acidosis (Low pH)

Metabolic

Low Anion Gap

- Myeloma
- Low albumin level
- Lithium

The anion gap is a gauge of the unmeasured anions in the bloodstream. The majority of the unmeasured anions are usually albumin, which has a significant amount of negative charge. In addition to albumin, which is normal, the other anionic substances are lactate, ketoacids, and the metabolic end products of toxic alcohols.

$$Na^+ \text{ and cations} = HCO_3^- \text{ and } Cl^- \text{ and anions}$$

Hence, if the sodium and cations remain the same and the anions go up, then HCO_3^- must go down. On the other hand, if the amount of cations goes up, this leads to an increase in the amount of HCO_3^- and Cl^-. This is why there is a decreased anion gap in myeloma. Myeloma proteins are cationic. This leads to an increase in the chloride and bicarbonate levels and therefore a decreased anion gap.

A low albumin level does the same thing. For every 1-point decrease in albumin, there is a 2-point decrease in the anion gap. If albumin, the main unmeasured anion, goes down, then the levels of chloride and bicarbonate increase to assure electrical neutrality.

Lithium, magnesium, and calcium are all divalent cations that decrease the sodium level. If the sodium level drops and everything else remains the same, there will be a decreased anion gap. If sodium is lower, but bicarbonate and chloride stay the same, then the anion gap must decrease.

Normal Anion Gap

- Diarrhea
- Renal tubular acidosis
- Ureterosigmoidostomy

Increased Anion Gap

LA MUD PIE (Mnemonic)

Lactate (sepsis, ischemia, etc.)

Aspirin

Methanol

Uremia

Diabetic ketoacidosis (DKA)—*Beta hydroxybutyric acid (BHB) and acetoacetate, which are formed from fatty acids, are an alternate fuel source because the cells cannot absorb glucose because there is a deficiency of insulin*

Paraldehyde, **P**ropylene glycol

Isopropyl alcohol, **I**NH

Ethylene glycol (antifreeze, low calcium)

Respiratory

Hypoventilation of any cause

- Chronic obstructive pulmonary disease (COPD)
- Pickwickian
- Obesity
- Suffocation
- Opiates
- Sleep apnea
- Kyphoscoliosis
- Myopathies
- Neuropathy
- Effusion
- Aspiration

RENAL TUBULAR ACIDOSIS

Distal (Type I)

Etiology

- Usually sporadic
- Also secondary to autoimmune disease (e.g., Sjögren syndrome, SLE)
- Drugs—amphotericin, lithium, analgesics, iphosphamide
- Nephrocalcinosis, sickle cell, chronic infection
- Familial
- Chronic hepatitis

Presentation

- Inability to develop a high H^+ concentration in urine. Urine pH is >5.3.
- Secondary hyperaldosteronism and hypokalemia
- Nephrocalcinosis and nephrolithiasis

Diagnosis. Acid load test; give ammonium chloride, which should lower urine pH secondary to increased H^+ formation. With type I RTA, the urine pH remains elevated. Serum bicarbonate = 10.

Patients with distal RTA develop hypokalemia because patients lose the ability to secrete hydrogen ions or H^+. Instead of excreting H^+, the kidney will excrete K^+.

Diarrhea: Metabolic acidosis with intact ability to excrete acid. The NH_4Cl level will be high in urine. The urinary anion gap will be negative.

RTA: Kidneys cannot excrete acid in the urine. The urine NH_4Cl level will be low. The urinary anion gap will be positive.

Basically, urine anion gap is a way of distinguishing whether a patient with a normal anion gap metabolic acidosis has diarrhea or distal RTA as the etiology.

Treatment. Oral bicarbonate is the treatment because bicarbonate reabsorption in the proximal tubule still works. Also, potassium replacement; potassium citrate will replace both bicarbonate as well as potassium in distal RTA. Further, citrate is an effective calcium stone antagonist.

Proximal (Type II)

Etiology. Fanconi syndrome, Wilson disease, amyloidosis, myeloma, acetazolamide, vitamin D deficiency, secondary hyperparathyroidism, chronic hypocalcemia, heavy metals, chronic hepatitis, autoimmune diseases such as SLE and Sjögren syndrome.

Presentation

- Inability to absorb bicarbonate. The initial urine pH is basic (until the body loses enough bicarbonate that it is within the range of absorption of the distal tubule), then the urine will become acidic (pH <5.4).

- Also with hypokalemia and a serum bicarbonate of 18–20, as well as proximal tubule leak of glucose, phosphate, urate, amino acids
- Patients with type II get bone lesions (osteomalacia and rickets), whereas type I get kidney stones. Both get hypokalemia.

Diagnosis. Patients are unable to absorb bicarbonate loading (sodium bicarb IV) and have a basic urine in the presence of acidemia. Normal individuals do not excrete bicarbonate in their urine until serum bicarbonate is >24.

Treatment. Give potassium; mild volume depletion will enhance proximal bicarbonate reabsorption (a type of contraction alkalosis). Thiazide diuretics and very large amounts of bicarbonates are used. Bicarbonate is generally ineffective and that is why they must be used in such high amounts. Bicarbonate administration increases renal potassium loss.

Hyporeninemic/Hypoaldosteronism (Type IV)
Etiology
- An aldosterone deficiency of any cause or adrenal insensitivity to angiotensin II, which normally stimulates aldosterone release
- Diabetes (50%)
- Addison disease
- Sickle cell disease
- Renal insufficiency

Presentation
- Usually asymptomatic hyperkalemia
- Mild to moderate renal insufficiency
- Hyperchloremic metabolic acidosis (nonanion gap)

Diagnosis. Presence of high urine sodium with oral salt restriction establishes the diagnosis.

Treatment. Administration of fludrocortisone. Fludrocortisone has a high degree of mineralocorticoid effect and is similar to administering aldosterone. Further, loop diuretics will lower potassium.

NEPHROLITHIASIS
Etiology. Occurs in 1–5% of the population.
- Composition of stones
- Calcium oxalate 70%
- Calcium phosphate 10%
- Mg/aluminum/phosphate (Struvite) 5–10%
- Uric acid 5%
- Cysteine 1%
- Indinavir

Hypercalciuria

- *Increased absorption*
  - Vitamin D intoxication
  - Increased vitamin D with sarcoid and other granulomatous disease
  - Familial
- *Idiopathic renal hypercalciuria*
- *Resorptive*
  - Hyperparathyroidism (10–30% of patients present with stones)
  - Multiple myeloma, metastatic disease to bone, hypercalcemia of malignancy

Hyperoxaluria

- Primary familial
- Enteric

With fat malabsorption, the fat binds to calcium, leaving oxalate to be reabsorbed in increased amounts.

Hypocitraturia

Citrate usually binds with calcium and prevents calcium absorption. Low citrate leads to an increase in calcium absorption. Causes of hypocitraturia include any acidotic condition.

Uric acid stones

They form in an acid environment and are associated with diseases like gout, hematologic malignancies, and Crohn's disease. Radiolucent on x-rays.

Cystinuria

Only associated with the genetic disorder.

Infection

Urinary infection with urease-producing organisms such as *Proteus*, *Staphylococcus*, *Pseudomonas*, and *Klebsiella* give a highly alkaline urine that produces struvite stones.

Presentation

- Constant flank pain (not colicky), hematuria, and pain radiating to groin
- Stones <5 mm should pass spontaneously

Diagnosis

- Plain x-ray (80% yield)—x-ray is rarely used
- U/S—high-yield test and most cost-effective
- Strain the urine
- Check serum and urine calcium
- IV pyelogram—always wrong
- Helical (spiral) CT scan—no contrast needed for stones; contrast is to identify masses, abscesses, and tumors; high-yield test

Treatment. Analgesia, hydration, and bed rest are the mainstays of treatment.

- Shockwave lithotripsy for stones <2 cm. Unfortunately, the fragments may cause obstruction themselves.
- Ureteroscopy
- Percutaneous removal (requires more anesthesia and hospital stay)
- Borderline-sized stones 5–7 mm can be expelled by using nifedipine and tamsulosin.

HEREDITARY CYSTIC DISEASE

Adult Polycystic Kidney Disease

Etiology

- Genetic—prevalence of 1:200 to 1:1,000
- Pathogenesis is uncertain

Presentation

- Flank pain, hematuria (micro and gross), infections, and calculi
- May also present as asymptomatic on screening of family members
- Extra-renal manifestations
  - Hepatic cysts (40–60%)
  - Colonic diverticula
  - Hypertension (50%)
  - Intracranial aneurysm (10–20%)—other vascular aneurysms may be seen
  - Mitral valve prolapse (25%)

Diagnosis. U/S and CT scan.

Treatment. Nonspecific; management of complications (UTI, calculi, and hypertension).

Simple Cysts

They are very common, and if they are smooth-walled with no debris in the cyst, they can be managed without any further treatment or need for diagnostic tests. Cysts with irregular walls or debris inside should be closely followed to exclude malignancy. Dialysis causes cysts.

HYPERTENSION

Essential Hypertension

Definition. The most recent guidelines recommend that hypertension be diagnosed when a person's systolic blood pressure is 140 mm Hg or diastolic blood pressure ≥90 mm Hg (or both) on repeated examination.

Systolic blood pressure is particularly important, and is the basis for diagnosis in most patients. These numbers apply to all adults age >18 years, although for patients age ≥80 a systolic blood pressure up to 150 mm Hg is now regarded as acceptable. The goal for treatment of hypertension is to reduce blood pressure to levels below the numbers used for making the diagnosis.

Some recent guidelines have recommended diagnostic values of 130/80 mm Hg for patients with **diabetes or chronic kidney disease**. However, the clinical benefits of this lower target **have not been established**, so these patients should be treated to <140/90 mm Hg.

Patients with very severe hypertension, such as those with a blood pressure >160/100 mm Hg, should receive initial therapy with 2 medications, this is because patients with a blood pressure >160 mm Hg will not be successfully controlled with just one medication.

Table 8-6. Guidelines

Normal	BP 120/80 mm Hg
Hypertension	
Stage 1	Systolic 140–159 Diastolic 90–99
Stage 2	Systolic ≥160 Diastolic ≥100

Etiology/Epidemiology. An estimated 50 million Americans have high blood pressure. Essential hypertension accounts for >95% of all cases of hypertension. Despite multiple theories on the mechanism, there is **no clear understanding** of what causes essential hypertension. It is more common with increasing age and is found in half the population over age 60. It is more common in men than women until after menopause. It is more common in the black population at all ages, and the incidence of end organ damage is more common in blacks as well. Onset is usually between ages 25–55.

Presentation. The most common presentation of essential hypertension is an asymptomatic patient on whom the elevation of blood pressure is found during a routine examination or during evaluation for other medical problems.

When symptoms are associated with hypertension, it is more correct to think of them as:

- Acute symptoms associated with a hypertensive emergency, or
- Complications from end-organ damage

With **hypertensive emergency,** signs and symptoms of cardiac, neurologic, renal, and retinal involvement are the most common. These include evidence of stroke, subarachnoid hemorrhage, encephalopathy, myocardial ischemia, and abnormalities on fundoscopic examination. Requires substantial reduction of blood pressure within one hour to avoid serious morbidity or death. These can acutely and most commonly result in headache, dizziness, chest pain, dyspnea, blurred vision, and palpitations. Malignant HTN is defined as encephalopathy or nephropathy with accompanying papilledema as seen on funduscopic examination.

Long-Term Complications

- **Cardiac**—myocardial ischemia or infarction, CHF, left ventricular hypertrophy, aortic aneurysm, and dissection, on physical exam an S4 gallop, accentuated A2 heart sound, and prominent left ventricular impulse can be present
- **Cerebrovascular**—transient ischemic attack (TIA) or stroke

- **Renal proteinuria**—microscopic hematuria, and elevation of BUN/creatinine, which may lead to the necessity of dialysis
- **Retinopathy**—hemorrhages, exudates, arteriolar narrowing, and papilledema; they result in blurred vision, scotomata, and sometimes blindness

Secondary Hypertension. Less than 5% of patients have secondary hypertension. The presentation depends upon the individual cause. For example: renovascular disease gives an abdominal bruit; Cushing disease gives weight gain, moon-like facies, striae, and ecchymoses; pheochromocytoma gives episodic hypertension associated with headache, palpitations, and sweating; primary aldosteronism (Conns syndrome) gives muscular weakness and polyuria/polydipsia from hypokalemia. These are discussed more fully later in the notes.

Diagnosis. As much as 20–25% of mild office hypertension is artifactual in nature. These initial elevated readings merely represent a manifestation of anxiety on the part of the patient to the doctor and medical environment. This is known as "white coat hypertension." In this case, we are talking about patients who have no evidence of end-organ damage. When these patients are given time to adjust to the environment by being allowed to sit quietly before the reading is taken, their pressure will lower. When these patients are given an ambulatory pressure-monitoring device to measure their own pressure at home or work, many of them will normalize their pressure. In addition, with each subsequent visit to the physician's office, the patient's pressure will often lower toward its true value.

Hence, prior to labeling a patient with a mild elevation as truly hypertensive and initiating therapy, the following steps are necessary:

- Allow the patient to sit quietly for 5 minutes before the pressure is measured
- Never label a patient as hypertensive after only a single reading
- Repeat the reading 3–6 times over several months before confirming the diagnosis and initiating therapy

Laboratory Investigation. Most routine lab testing will generally be normal. Testing is usually kept within the bounds of those done during a routine medical evaluation. The purpose is to evaluate the extent of end-organ damage as well as to exclude some forms of secondary hypertension. The reasons listed are the most common ones, not the only ones.

Basic studies include:

- Urinalysis for protein, glucose, and RBCs
- Hematocrit
- Serum potassium to exclude hyperaldosteronism
- Serum creatinine and BUN
- Electrocardiogram to evaluate for left ventricular hypertrophy
- Glucose and plasma lipid analysis as an indicator of atherosclerotic risk

Treatment. Patients with confirmed mild and moderate hypertension should initially be treated with nonpharmacologic modifications in lifestyle. These include weight reduction in the obese, dietary sodium restriction, aerobic exercise, and avoiding excessive alcohol intake. Dietary modifications such as a low-fat diet with increased dietary fiber can also be effective. Relaxation methods have inconsistent effects. DASH eating plan: increase fruits, vegetables, low-fat dairy, and low-fat diet.

Patients with severe hypertension (diastolic >100 mm Hg) should generally be started immediately on drug therapy. Patients with a blood pressure of >160/100 mm Hg should be started on two medications as part of initial therapy. There is a linear correlation of increasing weight with increasing blood pressure. Obesity further increases cardiovascular risk by increasing LDL cholesterol, decreasing HDL, and decreasing glucose tolerance. There is generally a 0.5–1.0 mm Hg drop in systolic and diastolic blood pressure for every kilogram of weight lost.

Drug Treatment

- **Who to treat?**

  Patients who continue to have a diastolic BP >90 mm Hg despite a 3- to 6-month trial of nonpharmacologic therapy should generally be started on antihypertensive drugs.

  The decrease in end-organ damage, such as myocardial infarction and stroke with drug treatment, is generally greater in those who have a higher baseline BP. In other words, someone who has a diastolic pressure >100 will show a much greater reduction in risk of stroke with drug therapy compared with someone whose diastolic pressure is only 90–95 mm Hg.

- **What to use?**

  There are almost 50 different medications approved for the initial treatment of hypertension, not including combination medications. The major medications with their individual characteristics are listed at the end of this section.

- General principles:

  In the absence of a specific indication or contraindication, diuretics are still recommended as initial treatment. For stage III HTN, BP >160/100, a two-drug combination should be used—diuretic with an ACE/ARB/CCB or beta blocker.

  The mortality benefit of diuretics has been unsurpassed when compared with other medications. If diuretics do not control the blood pressure, then a second medication should be added. The second medication can be a beta-blocker, calcium-channel blocker, ACE inhibitor, or angiotensin-receptor blocker. Beta blockers should be avoided in those with a history of asthma, COPD, heart block, or depression.

  Every attempt should be made to individualize therapy based on the characteristics of each patient. To do this, you must be familiar with the characteristics of each class of drugs.

- **What are the indications for specific hypertensive groups?**

  Diabetics: Should be treated with ACE inhibitors or ARBs, which prevent the development of nephropathy. The blood pressure goal in a diabetic is lower, at <130/80 mm Hg; this is also true in those with renal insufficiency, CHF, retinopathy, or stroke. Patients with microalbuminuria should receive an ACE inhibitor.

  Postmyocardial infarction (ischemic heart disease): Should be treated with beta blockers.

  Diminished left-ventricular systolic function (such as with CHF or postmyocardial infarction): Should receive ACE inhibitors and/or beta blockers.

  African-American patients are least effectively treated with ACE inhibitors.

  Pregnant patients are best treated with alpha-methyldopa, labetalol, hydralazine, or calcium-channel blockers. ACE inhibitors and angiotensin-receptor blockers are absolutely contraindicated in pregnant patients. Diuretics are relatively contraindicated.

Hypertensive Emergencies

Definition. The acute onset of severe hypertension in association with severe and rapidly worsening symptoms of end-organ damage. This usually happens with diastolic pressure >120–130 mm Hg. The terms "malignant" and "accelerated" hypertension are difficult to distinguish clinically, with "malignant" usually referring to the more severe syndrome.

Etiology/Epidemiology. The cause is unknown. Hypertensive emergencies occur in about 1% of hypertensive patients.

Presentation

Neurologic: Encephalopathy, headache, confusion, seizures, and subarachnoid or intracerebral hemorrhage.

Cardiac: Chest pain, myocardial infarction, palpitations, dyspnea, pulmonary edema, jugular venous distension, and gallops.

Nephropathy: Acutely progressive hematuria, proteinuria, and renal dysfunction.

Retinopathy: Papilledema, hemorrhages, and blurred vision.

Diagnosis. The laboratory evaluation is the same as with essential hypertension except that there is no concern of artifactual "white coat hypertension" given the clear symptoms. CT scan of the head may be necessary to exclude hemorrhage. EKG is more important as an initial test to exclude infarction.

Treatment. IV therapy is indicated. Nitroprusside and labetalol are the two best agents. Nitroglycerin is preferable in those who have evidence of myocardial ischemia. Enalaprilat is an IV ACE inhibitor that is now being used as well. Other less commonly used agents include esmolol, diazoxide, and trimethaphan.

The most important point in management is not to lower the pressure too far (e.g., not <95–100 mm Hg diastolic) so as not to compromise myocardial or cerebral perfusion. The initial goal is to reduce BP by no more than 25% within the first 1 to 2 hours.

Secondary Hypertension

Definition. Hypertension in the presence of an identifiable underlying cause.

Etiology/Epidemiology. <5% of cases of hypertension are secondary to an identifiable underlying cause. Renal artery stenosis is the most common of these causes.

The following groups should be screened for secondary hypertension:
- Those who become hypertensive either very young or very old (<25 or >55)
- Those with a key feature of history, physical examination, or laboratory abnormality consistent with a particular form as described below
- Patients who remain hypertensive despite increasing dosages and numbers of antihypertensive medications, i.e., those refractory to what should normally be effective therapy

Renal Artery Stenosis. This is due to atherosclerotic disease in elderly persons and fibromuscular dysplasia in young women.

Presentation: The key feature is an upper abdominal bruit radiating laterally, which is present in 50–70% of patients.

Diagnosis: The best initial screening test is the abdominal U/S. The captopril renogram is a test that measures the uptake of a radioisotope before and after the administration of captopril. A positive test is when there is decreased uptake of the isotope (i.e., decreased GFR) after giving the captopril. The captopril renogram is a noninvasive method of confirming the diagnosis of renal artery stenosis. The accuracy is diminished with renal insufficiency. The arteriogram is still the best method of confirming the diagnosis. Duplex Doppler ultrasonography and magnetic resonance angiography are also used to noninvasively detect stenosis. The accuracy of duplex U/S is operator-dependent.

Treatment: The best initial treatment is percutaneous transluminal angioplasty. If stenosis recurs, then the procedure should be repeated. If angioplasty fails, surgical resection is attempted. Medical therapy with ACE inhibitors should be reserved only for those in whom angioplasty or surgery either fails or is not possible. For unilateral disease it is not clear that angioplasty is superior to ACE inhibitors.

Primary Hyperaldosteronism (Conn Syndrome). This is most commonly due to a unilateral adenoma. Adenomas can also be bilateral. The rest of the cases are from bilateral hyperplasia. Cancer is rare as a cause of hyperaldosteronism.

Presentation: The key features are either:

- Hypertension in association with hypokalemia found on routine screening tests *or*
- Symptoms of hypokalemia such as muscular weakness and polyuria and/or polydipsia from a nephrogenic diabetes insipidus

Diagnosis: Elevated aldosterone levels in urine and blood.

Treatment: Surgical resection in those with an adenoma. Potassium-sparing diuretics such as spironolactone in those with hyperplasia.

Pheochromocytoma. Most often due to a benign tumor of the adrenal gland; 10% are bilateral, 10% are malignant, and 10% are extra-adrenal.

Presentation: The key feature is episodic hypertension in association with headaches, sweating, palpitations, and tachycardia. Pallor or flushing may also occur.

Diagnosis: The best initial tests are urinary vanillylmandelic acid (VMA), metanephines, and free urinary catecholamines. Plasma catecholamine evaluation is helpful as well. CT and MRI scanning is used to localize the site of the tumor.

Treatment: Alpha-adrenergic blockade followed by surgical removal.

Cushing Disease. Most often due to ACTH hypersecretion by a pituitary adenoma.

Presentation: The key feature is hypertension in association with characteristic cushingoid manifestations such as truncal obesity, buffalo hump, menstrual abnormalities, striae and impaired healing, etc.

Diagnosis: Dexamethasone suppression testing and 24-hour urine cortisol are the best initial tests.

Treatment: Surgical resection is best when possible.

Coarctation of the Aorta. The key feature is hypertension markedly greater in the upper extremities compared with the lower extremities.

Miscellaneous. Other causes of secondary hypertension are the use of oral contraceptives, acromegaly, congenital adrenal enzyme deficiencies, and virtually any cause of chronic renal disease such as glomerulonephritis, polycystic disease, diabetic nephropathy, or chronic pyelonephritis.

Antihypertensive Medications

Table 8-7. Antihypertensive Medications

Thiazides	Loop Diuretics	Potassium Sparing
Hydrochlorothiazide	Furosemide	Spironolactone
Chlorthalidone	Bumetanide	Amiloride
Metolazone	Torsemide	Triamterene
Indapamide		

Diuretics

Specific Indications. CHF, edematous states, African-American patients; least expensive.

Major Side Effects. Decreases in potassium and magnesium; increases in calcium, uric acid, glucose, LDL-cholesterol; gynecomastia.

Relative Contraindications. Diabetes, gout, hyperlipidemia.

Angiotensin converting enzyme (ACE) inhibitors

Benazepril	Enalaprilat (only IV form)	Moexipril
Captopril	Fosinopril	Quinapril
Enalapril	Lisinopril	Ramipril

Specific Indications

- Diabetics with hypertension to prevent neuropathy; the blood pressure goal in a diabetic patient is <130/80 mm Hg
- CHF as afterload reduction
- Postmyocardial infarction with left ventricular impairment

Major Side Effects. Cough, angioneurotic edema, neutropenia, hyperkalemia, taste disturbances, anaphylactoid reactions.

Relative Contraindications. Less effective in African-American patients.

Absolute Contraindications. Bilateral renal artery stenosis, pregnancy.

Calcium channel blockers

Amlodipine	Nicardipine
Diltiazem	Nifedipine
Felodipine	Verapamil
Isradipine	

Specific Indications. Angina pectoris, supraventricular arrhythmia, migraine, Raynaud phenomenon, esophageal spasm.

Major Side Effects. Peripheral edema, constipation, heart block, reflex tachycardia.

Relative Contraindications. Atrioventricular conduction defects, CHF from systolic dysfunction.

Angiotensin receptor antagonists

Losartan	Valsartan	Irbesartan
Candesartan	Telmisartan	

Specific Indications. Those intolerant to ACE inhibitors (especially because of cough).

Major Side Effects. Few. This is the newest class of antihypertensives.

Absolute Contraindications. Pregnancy.

The remainder of these medications should be considered second- or third-line agents.

Beta Blockers

Acebutolol	Bisoprolol	Metoprolol	Pindolol
Atenolol	Labetalol (combined alpha/beta)	Nadolol	Propranolol
Betaxolol		Penbutolol	Timolol

Metoprolol and atenolol are the most commonly used.

Specific Indications

- Myocardial infarction or ischemic heart disease
- Supraventricular arrhythmias
- Migraine headaches, glaucoma, anxiety (resting tachycardia)
- Congestive failure from diastolic dysfunction

Major Side Effects. Bronchospasm, heart block, bradycardia, Raynaud phenomenon, depression, impotence, fatigue, decreased HDL, increased triglycerides, hyperglycemia.

Relative Contraindications. Asthma or COPD, atrioventricular conduction defects, CHF from systolic dysfunction, diabetes because of masking signs of hypoglycemia.

Central-acting sympatholytics

Clonidine	Guanabenz
Guanfacine	Methyldopa

Specific Indications. Clonidine can be useful in opiate detoxification.

Major Side Effects. Depression, fatigue, dry mouth, impotence, bradycardia, heart block, memory loss. Methyldopa gives hepatitis and Coombs-positive hemolytic anemia.

Relative Contraindications. Elderly or depressed patients.

Direct vasodilators

Hydralazine	Minoxidil

Specific Indications

- Hydralazine is used in eclampsia
- Minoxidil is used locally to treat baldness

Major Side Effects

- Minoxidil gives marked fluid retention, pericardial effusion, and hirsutism
- Hydralazine gives a lupus-like syndrome

Relative Contraindications. Angina pectoris.

Alpha-adrenergic blockers

Doxazosin	Prazosin	Terazosin

Specific Indications. Patients with lipid disorders (they reduce LDL and increase HDL), prostatic hypertrophy (to reduce obstructive symptoms).

Major Side Effects. Syncope after the first dose, dizziness, headache.

Relative Contraindications. None.

NEPHROLOGY PROBLEMS

1. What acid-base disorders are represented by the following sets of arterial blood tests?

	pH	P_{CO_2}, mm Hg	HCO_3^-, mEq/L
(A)	7.32	28	14
(B)	7.47	20	14
(C)	7.08	49	14
(D)	7.51	49	38

Answers:

(A)   Metabolic acidosis (low pH, low HCO_3^- concentration, compensatory reduction in P_{CO_2}).

(B)   Respiratory alkalosis (high pH, low P_{CO_2}, compensatory reduction in HCO_3^- concentration). Note that a low HCO_3^- concentration does not necessary imply a primary metabolic acidosis.

(C)   Combined respiratory and metabolic acidosis (low pH, high P_{CO_2}, low HCO_3^- concentration).

(D)   Metabolic alkalosis (high pH, high HCO_3^- concentration, compensatory increase in P_{CO_2}).

2. Match the clinical histories with the appropriate arterial blood values.

	pH	P_{CO_2}, mm Hg	HCO_3^-, mEq/L
(A)	7.37	65	37
(B)	7.22	60	26
(C)	7.35	60	32

1.   A 60-year-old man with chronic bronchitis develops persistent diarrhea

2.   A markedly obese 24-year-old man

3.   A 14-year-old girl with a severe acute asthmatic attack

4.   A 56-year-old woman with chronic bronchitis is started on diuretic therapy for peripheral edema, resulting in a 3-kg weight loss

Answers:

It is easiest to answer this problem by first determining the acid-base disorders represented by the 3 sets of blood values.

(A)   The low pH and high P_{CO_2} indicate respiratory acidosis. In chronic respiratory acidosis, a P_{CO_2} of 65 mm Hg (25 mm Hg greater than normal) should be associated with a plasma HCO_3^- concentration of approximately 33 mEq/L (3.5 mEq/L increase in the plasma HCO_3^- concentration for each 10 mm Hg elevation in the P_{CO_2}). Thus, the HCO_3^- concentration of 37 mEq/L represents a superimposed metabolic alkalosis.

(B)   At a P_{CO_2} of 60 mm Hg, the HCO_3^- concentration should be roughly 26 mEq/L in acute respiratory acidosis (1 mEq/L increase per 10 mm Hg elevation in the P_{CO_2}) and 31 mEq/L in chronic respiratory acidosis. Therefore, these values may represent acute respiratory acidosis or metabolic acidosis (lower the HCO_3^- concentration from 31 to 26 mEq/L) superimposed on chronic respiratory acidosis.

(C)   Chronic respiratory acidosis or metabolic acidosis (raising the HCO_3^- concentration from 26 to 32 mEq/L) superimposed on acute respiratory acidosis.

From the history:

1.   Chronic bronchitis plus diarrhea suggests combined chronic respiratory acidosis and metabolic acidosis, or B.

2.   Marked obesity suggests chronic hypercapnia, or C.

3.   Severe acute asthma suggests acute respiratory acidosis, or B.

4.   Chronic bronchitis plus diuretics suggests chronic hypercapnia with superimposed metabolic alkalosis, or A. The metabolic alkalosis in this case is on the basis of volume contraction from the use of the diuretic.

DIAGNOSTIC TESTS

Pulmonary Function Tests

Pulmonary function tests (PFTs) are used mainly for (*1*) the categorization of different types of lung processes (restrictive versus obstructive), (*2*) the assessment of disease severity (in overall prognosis and preoperative evaluation), and (*3*) post-treatment evaluation of lung function.

Spirometry can be done in the office setting and allows the determination of most lung volumes and capacities, as well as expiratory flows and bronchodilator response. Complete PFTs are done in the pulmonary lab and allow the measurement of TLC, DLco, and methacholine challenge testing.

PFTs consist of different tests: static lung compartments are measured by lung volumes (total lung capacity [TLC], residual volume [RV]); airflow is measured by expiratory flow rate (ratio of forced expiratory volume in 1 second to forced vital capacity [FEV_1/FVC] or forced expiratory flow between 25 and 75% of expiration [FEF_{25-75}, also called midmaximal flow rate: MMFR]); and alveolar membrane permeability is measured by the diffusing capacity of a gas (DLco). The methacholine challenge test may be used to evaluate bronchial hyperreactivity.

Remember that generally <80% of predicted in any lung volume or flow rate is considered abnormal, while >120% of predicted is consistent with air trapping.

Table 9-1. Types of Pulmonary Function Tests

PFT	Normal Range
TLC	80–120% predicted
RV	75–120%
FEV_1/FVC Ratio	80%
DLco	75–120%
FEV_1	80–120%

Lung volumes

Ventilatory function is measured under static conditions for the determination of lung volumes (*see* Figure 9-1) and thus allows for the diagnosis of restrictive lung disease.

Clinical Pearl

Perform PFTs in all patients before they undergo lung resection surgery.

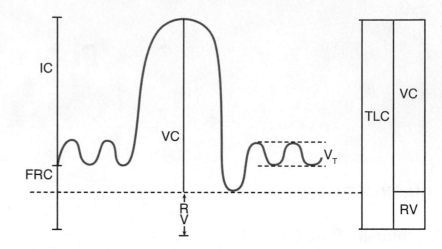

IC = inspiratory capacity

FRC = functional residual capacity

V_T = tidal volume

Figure 9-1. Determination of Lung Volumes

Table 9-2. Pulmonary Indices

Index	Acronym	Description
Total lung capacity	TLC	Volume of gas in the lungs after maximal inspiration
Residual volume	RV	Volume of gas remaining in the lungs after forced maximal expiration (unused space)
Vital capacity	VC	Volume of gas exhaled with maximal forced expiration TLC = RV + VC or VC = TLC − RV

Forced expiratory volumes (FEVs)

Forced expiratory volumes measure air movement in and out of the lungs (airflow measurement under dynamic conditions). FEVs can determine the degree of obstruction by comparing the forced volume expired at 1 second (FEV_1) to the forced vital capacity (FVC). In patients with no obstruction, the ratio is 0.80 (80% of predicted). It is decreased in patients with chronic obstructive disease (emphysema and chronic bronchitis) and asthma.

The FEVs are normal or elevated in patients who have restrictive disease because there is no problem with airflow. Also, asthmatic patients may have a normal FEV_1/FVC because they may have normal airflow (no bronchoconstriction) when asymptomatic.

Forced expiratory flow (FEF_{25-75}) is another measurement that can be done during the FEVs and is another way to express airflow. Generally consider the FEF_{25-75} equivalent to the FEV_1/FVC, but the FEF_{25-75} usually detects obstructive disease earlier.

FEVs can be determined during spirometry or full pulmonary function testing.

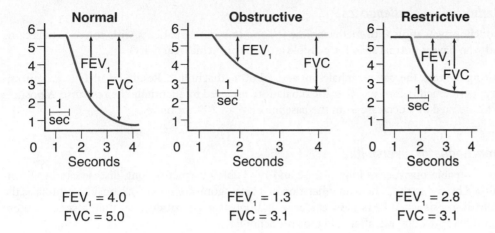

Figure 9-2. Forced Expiratory Volumes

Carbon monoxide diffusing capacity (DLco)

Lung diffusion testing is used to determine how well oxygen passes from the alveolar space of the lungs into the blood. Whereas spirometry measures the mechanical properties of the lungs, the lung diffusing capacity test (DLco) measures the ability of the lungs to perform gas exchange. The single-breath DLco test requires the patient to inhale DLco gas consisting of helium, carbon monoxide, and room air. Generally, diffusing capacity is reduced when alveolar walls are destroyed and pulmonary capillaries are obliterated by emphysema, or when the alveolar-capillary membrane is thickened by edema, consolidation, or fibrosis (as in interstitial lung disease).

PFTs with an obstructive pattern and decreased DLco should prompt the consideration of emphysema. PFTs with a restrictive pattern and decreased DLco are likely to be some type of interstitial lung disease (intrapulmonary restriction) or mild left heart failure.

Increased DLco may be seen in pulmonary hemorrhage, e.g., Goodpasture syndrome.

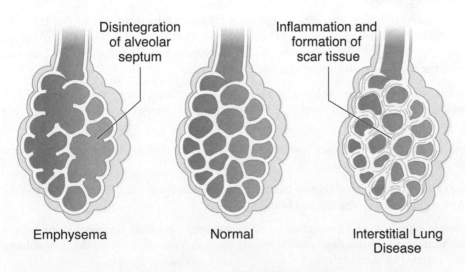

Figure 9-3. Alveolar Diffusing Capacity

Methacholine challenge test

Bronchoprovocation with methacholine is done to evaluate patients with cough or wheezing and who have a normal PFT, for possible asthma (bronchial reactivity).

During the test, the patient inhales an aerosol of methacholine. Results of PFTs (e.g., spirometry) performed before and after the inhalations are used to quantitate the response. A positive test is defined as a decrease from the baseline FEV_1 of 20% or more.

Bronchodilator reversibility

Nonreversible obstructive lung disease and reversible obstructive lung disease can be distinguished by giving the patient an inhalation of a beta-agonist (albuterol). Consider asthma as the likely diagnosis when PFTs show evidence of an obstructive pattern, but then reverse by more than 12% and 7,200 mL after using the bronchodilator.

Table 9-3. PFT Questions

PFT Indices	Patient 1	Patient 2
TLC	110%	55%
RV	120%	50%
VC	90%	50%
FEV_1/FVC	80%	90%
FEF_{25-75} (MMFR)	50%	90%
DLco	Patient 1a: 90% Patient 1b: 40%	Patient 2a: 90% Patient 2b: 40%
What is your diagnosis?		

Flow Volume Loops

Flow volume loops diagrams also express airflow in different lung diseases and give the relationship between flow rates compared with lung volumes. On the y-axis is flow rate and on the x-axis is volume. Lung volumes increase to the left on the abscissa. The shape of the loop can characterize the type and distribution of airway obstruction.

When comparing a normal flow volume loop with one of restrictive lung disease, the restrictive lung disease alters the size of the loop (a shift to the right of the x-axis), which is related to a reduction in lung volumes.

On the other hand, obstructive lung disease alters the shape of the loop by causing a reduction of airflow (alterations on the y-axis).

In the case of a fixed airway-obstruction (tracheal stenosis after prolonged intubation), the flow volume loop is flattened on the top and bottom.

With dynamic extrathoracic airway obstruction (vocal cord paralysis), the obstruction occurs mostly with inspiration while expiration is mostly normal. This effect causes the flow volume loop to be flattened only on bottom.

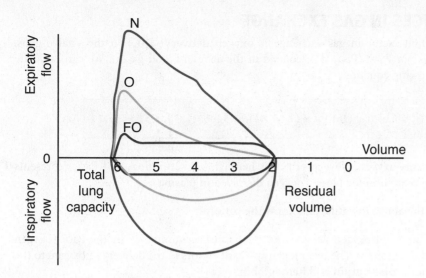

N = normal
O = obstructive
FO = fixed obstruction

Figure 9-4. Flow Volume Loops

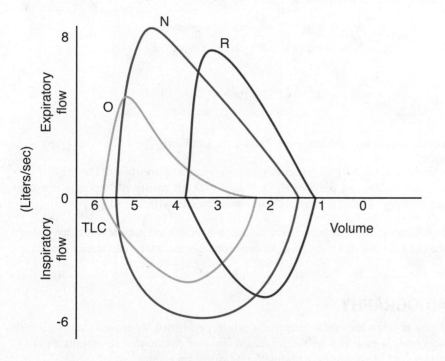

N = normal
R = restrictive
O = obstructive

Figure 9-5. Flow Volume Loops

Clinical Pearl

FEO may occur in the setting of a tracheal tumor or foreign object aspiration or tracheal stenosis after prolonged intubation.

DISTURBANCES IN GAS EXCHANGE

The most important factor in gas exchange is **oxygen delivery (Do_2)** to the vital organs. Remember, Do_2 is not Pao_2 (Pao_2 is calculated in the arterial blood gases). We can calculate Do_2 from the following equation:

$$Do_2 = \text{Cardiac Output} \times (1.34 \times Hb \times HbSat) + 0.0031 \times Pao_2$$

where Do_2 represents oxygen delivery, HbSat is hemoglobin saturation, and Pao_2 represents partial pressure of oxygen in the blood (oxygen dissolved in plasma).

Don't memorize the above formula, just know the concept.

Notice that the amount of oxygen delivered to the tissues accounted for by the Pao_2 (oxygen dissolved in blood) is minimal. The two most important factors in the delivery of oxygen to the vital organs are the **cardiac output** and **hemoglobin**.

In a critically ill patient, it is most important (the next step) to keep the hemoglobin and cardiac output near normal. There will be minimal change in Do_2 if you increase the Pao_2 from 60 to 100 mm Hg by giving the patient 100% oxygen.

The **alveolar–arterial gradient** (PAo_2–Pao_2 gradient) is useful in the assessment of oxygenation and is calculated by the following formula:

$$PAo_2\text{–}Pao_2 \text{ gradient} = (150 - 1.25) \times Pco_2 - Pao_2$$
$$\text{or}$$
$$A - a = [150 - (1.25 \times PaCO_2) - PaO_2]$$

Know this formula and how to calculate the PAo_2–Pao_2 gradient.

The above formula is valid only in patients who are breathing room air. This gradient is 5–15 mm Hg in normal young patients. It increases with all causes of hypoxemia except hypoventilation and high altitude. The gradient also increases with age.

Clinical Problem. Can you think of any clinical condition in which the patient would have severe hypoxemia but a normal gradient? Hint: You will commonly see this in the emergency room.

CHEST RADIOGRAPHY

Chest radiography is often the initial diagnostic study performed to evaluate patients with respiratory symptoms. It may also be the initial evidence of pulmonary disease in a patient without symptoms, e.g., the pulmonary nodule found on an incidental x-ray.

Note

The answer to this clinical problem can be found at the end of this chapter.

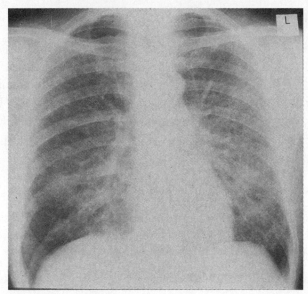

Dr. Conrad Fischer

Figure 9-6. Bilateral Interstitial Infiltrates on Chest X-ray

Pulmonary Nodule

A 26-year-old man is found to have a 2.5-cm calcified nodule in the right middle lung on a routine chest x-ray before starting his residency. He has never smoked and otherwise feels well. The physical examination is unremarkable. What will you recommend for this patient?

The solitary pulmonary nodule that is found incidentally on an x-ray poses a specific problem for the clinician. Almost one-third of all solitary nodules are malignant.

Calcification of the nodule points toward a benign diagnosis, e.g., popcorn calcifications usually are caused by hamartomas, whereas bull's-eye calcifications are caused by granulomas.

The *first step* in the evaluation of a pulmonary nodule is to look for a *prior x-ray*. Finding the same pulmonary nodule on an x-ray done years ago may save you from doing any further workup. If no prior x-ray is available, then consider whether this patient is high or low risk for lung cancer.

In *low-risk patients*, <35 years of age and nonsmokers with calcified nodules, you may follow the patient with chest x-rays or chest CT every 3 months for 2 years. Stop the follow-up if after 2 years there is no growth.

High-risk patients >50 years of age with a smoking history and a nodule are likely to have bronchogenic cancer. The best diagnostic procedure is open-lung biopsy and removal of the nodule at the same time.

Bronchoscopy will *not* reach peripheral lesions and will mislabel 10% of central cancers by finding only nonspecific inflammatory changes. Bronchoscopy is performed blindly and the specimen obtained can be limited, hence the nonspecific findings (inflammation, etc.). If you suspect cancer in a patient and the bronchoscopy returns with a negative result, open lung biopsy and lung nodule resection must be considered.

Clinical Pearl

In all patients with a pulmonary nodule, first try to obtain an old chest x-ray.

Pleural Effusion

A 67-year-old man presents with complaints of dyspnea and pleuritic chest pain that has worsened over the past month. He has also noticed weight loss of 20 pounds and low-grade fever over this time period. On physical examination his respiratory rate is 24/min, and you find decreased air entry in the right lower lobe with dullness to percussion. Chest x-ray shows a pleural effusion involving about one-third of the lung field. A decubitus x-ray shows layering of the fluid.

Definition. The accumulation of fluid in the pleural cavity. It is either transudative or exudative.

Transudative effusion is caused by systemic factors: either increased hydrostatic pressure (e.g., CHF) or decreased oncotic pressure (e.g., nephrotic syndrome or cirrhosis). Because these diseases are systemic, they usually cause bilateral and equal effusion.

A transudative effusion needs no further evaluation. It resolves by adequate treatment of the primary disease.

Exudative effusion is caused by local processes: pneumonia, cancer, and tuberculosis.

An exudative effusion will cause unilateral effusions. This type of effusion needs further investigation.

How do we make the distinction between these two?

Thoracentesis should be performed for new and unexplained pleural effusion when sufficient fluid is present to allow a safe procedure. It is reasonable to observe pleural effusion when there is overt CHF (especially if bilateral), viral pleurisy, or recent thoracic or abdominal surgery. However, it is important not to assume that new effusions in a patient with a history of CHF are solely due to the CHF. Have a low threshold for performing diagnostic thoracentesis in any new or unexplained effusions.

Table 9-4. Causes of Pleural Effusion

Transudative	Exudative
Heart failure	Parapneumonic effusions (pneumonia)
Nephrotic syndrome	Malignancy (lung, breast, lymphoma)
Liver disease	Tuberculosis
Pulmonary embolism	Pulmonary embolism
Atelectasis	Collagen vascular disease (rheumatoid arthritis, systemic lupus erythematosus)
	Drug induced
	Pancreatitis

Get 2 tests from the thoracocentesis fluid—lactate dehydrogenase (LDH) and protein—and get 2 tests from the serum—LDH and protein. Do the ratios of effusion to serum for these measurements, and you have a diagnosis (Table 9-5).

Table 9-5. Light Criteria for Exudative Pleural Effusion

	Transudative	Exudative
LDH effusion	<200 IU/mL	>200 IU/mL
LDH effusion/serum ratio	<0.6	>0.6
Protein effusion/serum ratio	<0.5	>0.5

If at least one criterion is not met, then this is an exudative effusion; in that case, further evaluation has to be done.

One of the few conditions that can cause a transudate or exudate is pulmonary embolism (PE). The clinical significance of this is that if a patient has a transudative effusion but no apparent cause, consider PE.

Parapneumonic effusion is caused by bacterial pneumonia. A thoracocentesis is mandatory also in this setting to rule out a complicated parapneumonic effusion (because of the possibility of progression to an empyema). An empyema (or complicated effusion) needs chest-tube drainage to resolve, while an uncomplicated parapneumonic effusion responds to antibiotics alone.

The most common causes of malignant pleural effusion are lung cancer, breast cancer, and lymphoma. When considering a malignant pleural effusion, make sure to send the thoracocentesis fluid for *cytologic examination*.

Hemorrhagic pleural effusion may be seen in mesothelioma, metastatic lung or breast cancer, pulmonary thromboembolism (with infarction), and trauma.

In patients with lymphocytic predominant exudative pleural effusions, consider tuberculosis. The pleural effusion is thought to be due to a hypersensitivity reaction to the tuberculosis mycobacterium and its antigens. The adenosine deaminase is elevated, and the polymerase chain reaction (PCR) for tuberculous DNA is positive. The acid-fast stain and culture for tuberculosis are positive in <30% of the cases. A pleural biopsy confirms the diagnosis and is the most sensitive and specific test for pleural tuberculosis.

Always perform thoracocentesis under the guidance of ultrasonography. If ultrasonography is not available, then perform a decubitus chest x-ray before the thoracocentesis. If the decubitus chest x-ray detects 1 cm or more of *free-flowing fluid*, the thoracocentesis can be performed with a minimal risk of complications. If the decubitus detects non-free fluid (loculated), it would be safer to perform an U/S-guided thoracocentesis.

Evaluating patients with acute respiratory compromise and distress

Respiratory compromise may result from airway obstruction (asthma, COPD, foreign object), but it also accompanies parenchymal lung disease (bacterial or viral pneumonia, lung injury), heart failure, pulmonary embolism, neurogenic processes (respiratory depression from opiates), and neuromuscular disease (myasthenia gravis).

Respiratory distress is usually the presenting complaint or sign. Complaints of shortness of breath or signs of tachypnea or labored breathing are the most common. The patient may also develop neurologic symptoms: agitation, confusion, and a depressed level of consciousness. Stridor indicates upper airway obstruction.

The physician's first task is to ensure that the patient's airway is patent and that breathing is adequate. Supplemental oxygen should be provided immediately to ensure adequate oxygen saturation. The resources to perform endotracheal intubation and assisted ventilation should be made available.

The history should focus on the quickness of onset, as well as associated symptoms (cough, fever, etc.). Acute presentations accompanied by cough, fever, and sputum production suggest an infectious etiology. Sudden onset of dyspnea without systemic symptoms should raise the possibility of airway obstruction, cardiac disease, or thromboembolic disease. Chronic and progressive dyspnea (with or without recent exacerbation) is usually associated with a chronic pulmonary process, like interstitial lung disease or COPD.

The physical examination should focus on finding the cause, as well as assessing the degree of respiratory compromise. A respiratory rate >30/min in an adult suggests severe respiratory compromise. Wheezing on auscultation accompanies asthma and COPD. Localized wheezing usually suggests a foreign object or mass. Rales on examination may accompany pneumonia, interstitial lung disease, or heart failure. Consolidative changes may accompany pneumonia or atelectasis. Normal lung examination may be seen in thromboembolic disease, infections like *Pneumocystis carinii*, and disorders of the central respiratory drive.

An arterial blood-gas (ABG) measurement is the most important initial laboratory test in determining the presence and severity of respiratory compromise.

The **hallmark** of acute respiratory failure is a rise in P_{CO_2} accompanied by a drop in pH. The bicarbonate level will initially be normal, but will increase over 24–48 hours with the appropriate renal compensation. Hypercapnia may accompany hypoxemia or may be absent if ventilation is adequate. The presence of metabolic acidosis (lactic acidosis) in the presence of hypercapnia should prompt the consideration of mechanical ventilation.

In the setting of acute-on-chronic respiratory failure, the administration of supplemental oxygen is often associated with a rise in Pa_{CO_2}. Although attributed to a decreased respiratory drive, the pathophysiology of this is more complex. For the clinician, fear of a rising Pa_{CO_2} should **never** preclude the administration of enough supplemental oxygen to ensure adequate oxygen delivery. The target range of 88–92% oxygen saturation usually allows for adequate oxygen delivery while minimizing the potential increase in Pa_{CO_2}.

Other diagnostic tests

- **B-type natriuretic peptide (BNP)** appears useful as an adjunct to clinical assessment in determining the cause of acute dyspnea in patients presenting emergently. An elevated BNP is seen in almost all patients with left heart failure. It is important to remember that cor pulmonale and acute right ventricular failure (thromboembolism) may also cause a rise in the BNP. Thus, although the BNP is a very sensitive test for heart failure, it is not specific.

- The **chest x-ray** is particularly helpful in determining the cause of respiratory failure. A chest x-ray without parenchymal infiltrates accompanies respiratory failure due to thromboembolism, central respiratory depression, neuromuscular disease, and upper airway obstruction. Airway obstruction that accompanies asthma and COPD is usually associated with evidence of hyperinflation (large lung volumes and hyperlucency). The chest x-ray is diagnostic in cases of respiratory compromise caused by large pleural effusions or tension pneumothorax. Focal infiltrates suggest bacterial, viral, or fungal pneumonia; aspiration; or pulmonary hemorrhage. Unusual causes of localized infiltrates may be Churg-Strauss or Wegener granulomatosis. Heart failure and ARDS present with a diffuse edema pattern.

Treatment. New, persistent hypoxemia is generally an indication for admission to the hospital. The need for mechanical ventilation and close monitoring of a patient with respiratory compromise is an indication for admission to the ICU. Also, ICU admission should be considered for all patients with increasing oxygen demands, as well as those requiring continuous nursing.

The presence of respiratory acidosis and hypercapnia in a patient presenting with asthma exacerbation is an ominous sign and should prompt consideration for intubation and mechanical ventilation. Indications for intubation (with or without ventilation) also include upper-airway injury (burns, laryngeal edema, trauma) and airway compromise, often in the setting of neurologic depression with loss of protective reflexes, including gag and cough.

Acute respiratory failure presenting during hospitalization deserves a specific mention. The immobility which accompanies the hospitalized patient puts him at significant risk for pulmonary thromboembolic disease, so that should be considered in any patient who develops dyspnea, tachypnea, and/or hypoxemia. Inpatients are also at risk for developing aspiration, which may precipitate respiratory failure directly or through the development of pneumonia or acute respiratory distress syndrome (ARDS). The risk factors for aspiration include impaired consciousness and upper airway instrumentation (nasogastric tubes). Iatrogenic causes must also be considered, especially respiratory depression from opiates causing respiratory arrest.

ARDS is a frequent cause of respiratory failure in patients suffering from other serious illnesses. ARDS represents a diffuse inflammatory response of the lung and develops within 24–72 hours of the onset of illness or injury. The clinical presentation is increasing respiratory distress with tachypnea and hypoxemia. The chest x-ray reveals diffuse pulmonary infiltrates, consistent with pulmonary edema (noncardiogenic pulmonary edema).

OBSTRUCTIVE DISEASES

Asthma

A 26-year-old woman with a history of asthma presents to the emergency room with 3 days of progressive wheezing and shortness of breath after an upper respiratory tract infection. She is taking inhaled albuterol and an over-the-counter medication for her cold symptoms. Her respiratory rate is 28/min and pulse 110/min; she is afebrile. Her right nasal turbinate is edematous and erythematous. There is evidence of wheezing throughout both lungs, but no crackles are noted. Supplemental oxygen by nasal cannula is administered. What should be the next appropriate treatment?

Definition. A disease characterized by inflammatory hyperreactivity of the respiratory tree to various stimuli, resulting in *reversible* airway obstruction. A combination of mucosal inflammation, bronchial musculature constriction, and an excessive secretion of viscous mucus-causing mucous plugs which produce bronchial obstruction. The bronchial hyperreactivity occurs in an episodic pattern with interspersed normal airway tone. Asthma can occur at any age but is usually seen in young persons, 50% of whom "outgrow" their asthma by adulthood.

Etiology

Intrinsic or idiosyncratic asthma occurs in 50% of asthmatics who are nonatopic (nonallergic). A bronchial reaction occurs secondary to nonimmunologic stimuli, such as infections, irritating inhalants, cold air, exercise, and emotional upset. The asthma attacks are severe, and prognosis is less favorable.

Extrinsic (allergic, atopic) asthma results from sensitization. Specific immunoglobulins (IgE class [type 1]) are produced, and the total serum IgE concentration is elevated. There is a positive family history of allergic disease. Extrinsic asthma is precipitated by allergens and accounts for 20% of asthmatics. Other symptoms include allergic rhinitis, urticaria, and eczema. Prognosis is good.

Many patients have features of both types.

Respiratory infections are the most common stimuli to cause asthma exacerbations; studies have documented that viruses (respiratory syncytial virus in young children, rhinoviruses in adults) are the major causes.

Pharmacologic stimuli are very important in some cases, and the most common etiologic agents associated with asthma exacerbation are aspirin, coloring agents such as tartrazine, and β-adrenergic antagonists.

The typical aspirin sensitivity–nasal polyposis syndrome affects adults. It starts usually with perennial vasomotor rhinitis; later, asthma occurs with minimal ingestion of aspirin. The prevalence of this type of asthma is approximately 10%. There is significant cross-reactivity between aspirin and other NSAIDs. Patients can be desensitized by daily administration of aspirin; cross-tolerance also develops to other NSAIDs. The mechanism by which aspirin and similar drugs cause asthma appears to be chronic overexcretion of leukotrienes, which activate the mast cells. This is the reason why leukotriene inhibitors are considered to be so effective.

Pathophysiology. There is a narrowing of large and small airways caused by hypertrophy and spasm of bronchial smooth muscle, edema and inflammation of the bronchial mucosa, and production of viscous mucus. The mediators released by the lung during an acute asthmatic attack are histamine, bradykinin, leukotrienes (LTs) C, D, and E, and prostaglandins (PGs) E_2, $F_{2\alpha}$, and D_2, which cause an intense inflammatory process leading to bronchoconstriction and vascular congestion. The cells thought to play an important role in the inflammatory response are the mast cells, lymphocytes, and eosinophils.

Signs and Symptoms. In a mild attack, slight tachypnea, tachycardia (increased respiratory rate), prolonged expirations, and mild, diffuse wheezing are seen. In a severe attack, use of accessory muscles of respiration, diminished breath sounds, loud wheezing, hyper-resonance (increased vocal fremitus), and intercostal retraction are noted.

Poor prognostic factors include fatigue, diaphoresis, pulsus paradoxus (>20 mm Hg), inaudible breath sounds, decreased wheezing, cyanosis, and bradycardia.

Variants of asthma include asthma presenting primarily with *nocturnal cough* and *exercise-induced asthma* (both presentations of asthma are commonly tested).

In the acute phase, **arterial blood gas (ABG)** abnormalities will be consistent with a decrease in arterial carbon dioxide tension ($Paco_2$), increase in pH, and normal or low Pao_2. In severe asthma or status asthmaticus there will be a decreased PaO_2, increased $PaCO_2$, and decreased pH (bicarbonate level usually will not be elevated in an acute setting, but it becomes elevated in chronic obstructive pulmonary disease). A normal $PaCO_2$ may indicate respiratory muscle fatigue in an acute asthmatic patient.

Chest x-ray findings are nonspecific in an asthmatic attack. The chest x-ray may be helpful in ruling out acute infection as the cause of an acute attack.

Diagnosis. PFTs show an obstructive pattern that typically reverses with bronchodilation (FEV_1 must show 12% and 200 mL reversibility at 5 and 20 min with the use of a β_2-adrenergic agonist). Sometimes the PFTs may be entirely normal because asthma is reversible and episodic; in this case a provocative challenge may be performed with methacholine or cold air, which typically shows a decrease in FEV_1/FVC or FEF_{25-75} of 20%.

Treatment. β-adrenergic agonist inhalers like albuterol (salbutamol) and terbutaline are the mainstay of treatment in acute and chronic asthma. Inhaled (metered-dose inhalers [MDIs]) β-adrenergic agonists are the preferred route of administration because they allow maximal bronchodilation with minimal side effects. Their most common side effect is tremor. β-adrenergic agonists alone terminate approximately 70% of asthmatic attacks.

Salmeterol is a long-lasting (12 h) type of albuterol that is effective in nocturnal cough variant and exercise-induced asthma. Salmeterol has no benefit in acute episodes.

β-adrenergic agonists must be used with caution in patients who have coexisting cardiovascular disorders, hypothyroidism, diabetes mellitus, hypertension, and coronary insufficiency.

Other adrenergic stimulant drugs like the *catecholamines* (isoproterenol, epinephrine, and isoetharine) are given orally or intravenously and are *not* routinely used.

Aminophylline (ethylenediamine salt of theophylline) and *theophylline* are only modest bronchodilators. They are sometimes of benefit in chronic management, especially in patients with nocturnal cough. Their mechanism of action is by improving contractility of the diaphragm as well as other respiratory muscles. Generally, aminophylline and theophylline are *not* routinely used in asthma because they appear to add no benefit to optimal inhaled beta-agonist therapy.

Anticholinergic drugs (ipratropium bromide and tiotropium) have particular benefit in patients with heart disease, in whom the use of β-adrenergic agonists and theophylline may be dangerous. Their major disadvantages are that they take *significant time* to achieve maximal bronchodilation *(~90 min)* and they are only of medium potency.

Supplemental oxygen, by nasal cannula or mask, should be given immediately when a patient presents with acute asthma exacerbation. Always maintain an oxygen saturation above 90%.

The use of "routine" *antibiotic treatment* in asthma exacerbation has not been established. Two recent prospective trials have not showed a benefit. Antibiotic treatment should be considered in patients with symptoms (purulent sputum) and chest x-ray findings (infiltrates) consistent with bacterial pneumonia.

Treatment of asthma in the **outpatient setting** consists of looking for and removing environmental irritants and allergens. The goal is to remove or minimize contact with precipitating factors of asthma (such as pets).

Inhaled corticosteroids are the cornerstone of chronic asthma therapy in adults. They work by reducing airway inflammation. Inhaled corticosteroids have been shown in studies to reduce asthma exacerbations and hospitalizations. Side effects of inhaled corticosteroids include oral candidiasis, glaucoma, cataracts, diabetes, muscle weakness, and osteoporosis.

Systemic steroids are used only in acute exacerbations (for 10–14 days) and in the treatment of chronic severe asthma. Systemic corticosteroids should not be used before inhaled corticosteroids.

Inhaled short-acting beta 2 agonists such as albuterol are the mainstays of treatment of chronic asthma and are usually in conjunction with inhaled corticosteroids. Use of short-acting beta-2 agonists for 3 days/week indicates poor control of symptoms, and treatment should be intensified.

Inhaled long-acting beta 2 agonists like salmeterol and formeterol have a sustained effect on bronchial smooth muscle relaxation. Long-acting beta-2 agonists are indicated for the treatment of moderate to severe persistent asthma (after initial therapy with short-acting beta 2 agonist plus inhaled corticosteroids) and especially when the patient has a significant nocturnal component. Long-acting beta-2 agonists should not be used for mild asthma or the acute exacerbation of asthma; moreover, they should never be used alone and always in conjunction with inhaled corticosteroids. Studies have shown that when long-acting beta 2 agonists are used as a single agent, patients may have increased mortality.

Remember that neither short-acting nor long-acting beta 2 agonists address the inflammatory component of asthma.

The leukotriene modifiers are approved for severe asthma resistant to maximum doses of inhaled corticosteroids and as a last resort before using chronic systemic corticosteroids. Leukotriene modifiers inhibit 5-lipoxygenase, the enzyme involved in leukotriene production (LTC4, LTD4, LTE4), or competitive antagonist the principal moiety (LTD4). Zileuton is a typical leukotriene inhibitor that is available. The receptor antagonists are zafirlukast and montelukast.

MAST cell stabilizers (cromolyn and nedochromil) have been used in the treatment of chronic asthma. In terms of preventing asthma exacerbations and reducing inflammation in adults, they are not as effective as inhaled corticosteroids. They may be used also in exercise-induced asthma and allergic asthma. Cromolyn and Nedocromil are used extensively in the chronic treatment of pediatric asthma.

Theophylline is generally not preferred for the treatment of asthma. In chronic treatment of asthma, it is indicated only as a possible adjunct to inhaled corticosteroids for difficult-to-control asthma. In an acute exacerbation of asthma, a combination of long-acting beta agonist and inhaled corticosteroids has been shown to have better efficacy.

Let's go back to the patient.

She is likely having an acute exacerbation of asthma.

Note

Answers to these questions can be found at the end of this chapter.

What is the treatment of choice in this patient? (Only one drug.)

What are bad prognostic indicators in this patient?

Which one of the ABGs below is considered ominous for this patient (as well as all asthmatic patients)?

7.32/45/60 or 7.45/30/50

Three days after hospitalization the patient is improving, and you decide to send her home. What is her drug regimen likely to be at this time?

She comes to you 3 months later for follow-up. She needs documentation of asthma for her work. What will you do now? What medications is she likely to be taking now?

Outpatient Setting. Clinical guidelines have classified asthma as "mild intermittent," "mild persistent," "moderate," or "severe" on the basis of the frequency and severity of symptoms and the requirement for medications. This classification provides general guidelines for therapy.

For testing purposes, we will *simplify the above guidelines:*

- **Mild asthma:** symptoms ~2 times/week and rare night symptoms (1–2 nights/month); FEV_1 is "normal" (>80%).
  Treatment—no medications for long-term control (this patient should not be on inhaled steroids). What do these patients do when they have symptoms? Inhaled, short-acting bronchodilators as needed (albuterol inhaler).
- **Moderate asthma:** symptoms are frequent (most of the week or daily) and night symptoms occur at least 5 nights out of the month; FEV_1 is decreased between 60–80%.
  Treatment—daily inhaled steroids are the mainstay treatment (some patients with milder symptoms in this category may benefit from cromolyn, which is less effective in adults, but works well in children), along with inhaled beta-agonists as needed to control breakthrough symptoms. Some patients in this category who have nocturnal symptoms, despite short-acting beta agonists, will benefit from daily long-acting beta agonists, like salmeterol.
- **Severe asthma:** daily symptoms with frequent symptoms at night; frequent emergency room admissions and hospitalizations are also common in this group; FEV_1 is <60%.
  Treatment—inhaled steroids daily, inhaled long-acting beta agonists (like salmeterol), inhaled short-acting agonists for breakthrough symptoms, *along with* antileukotriene drugs (montelukast) and oral steroids (lowest dose possible).

Chronic Obstructive Pulmonary Disease (COPD)

A 67-year-old woman with COPD is evaluated for dyspnea that occurred the prior day. She denies fever and chills but has noted productive cough. Her medications include ipratropium MDI. Her respiratory rate is 32/min and pulse 106/min; she is afebrile. She looks cachectic and is breathing fast. You note an increased anteroposterior diameter, distant heart sounds, and expiratory wheezing.

Definition. COPD includes patients with emphysema and chronic bronchitis. Emphysema and bronchitis must be identified as separate entities, but most patients with COPD have characteristics of both conditions. Patients with chronic bronchitis have productive cough for most days of a 3-month period for at least 2 consecutive years. In emphysema patients have abnormal permanent dilation of air spaces distal to the terminal bronchioles with destruction of air space walls.

Both of these processes are defined by *nonreversible obstruction* of the airways. This is the pathognomonic differentiating finding on PFTs when compared with asthma.

Cigarette smoking is a cause of COPD, with 10–15% of smokers developing COPD (80–90% of COPD patients are cigarette smokers). COPD symptoms usually begin after at least 20 pack-years of tobacco exposure. The number of pack-years of smoking correlates to the reduction of FEV_1. The fact that a small percentage (10–15%) of smokers develops COPD suggests that other factors may be involved in the pathogenesis. Air pollution, airway infections, and allergies can lead to bronchitis.

α_1-*antitrypsin deficiency* is a rare hereditary autosomal recessive disease that can cause emphysema and liver abnormalities.

Pathogenesis. After long-term exposure to cigarette smoke, inflammatory cells are recruited in the lung. These inflammatory cells in turn secrete proteinases, which may lead to air space destruction and permanent enlargement. Eventually, decreased elastic recoil (mainly in emphysema) and increased airway resistance (mainly with chronic bronchitis) occur.

Physical Examination. In emphysema, distant breath sounds will be heard on auscultation. In chronic bronchitis, there may be evidence of rhonchi and wheezes to auscultation. Signs and symptoms of right heart failure (cor pulmonale) and clubbing can also be seen on physical examination in COPD.

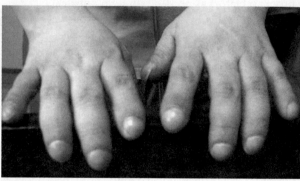
wikipedia.com

Figure 9-7. Clubbing of the Fingers Seen with Chronic hypoxemia

Chest X-Ray Findings. In chronic bronchitis, increased pulmonary markings can be seen. In emphysema, hyperinflation of bilateral lung fields with diaphragm flattening, small heart size, and increase in retrosternal space can be seen on x-ray.

Cor pulmonale in COPD is associated with chronic pulmonary hypertension.

Diagnosis. *Pulmonary Function Testing.* On PFT, a reduction in FEV_1/FVC ratio and FEF_{25-75} occurs. RV and TLC are usually increased in COPD. Emphysema will have a decreased DLco, whereas chronic bronchitis will generally have a normal DLco.

After a bronchodilator is given, you would expect the FEV_1/FVC to _____.

PFTs are the diagnostic test of choice.

Complications. Hypoxemia with *nocturnal desaturation* is sometimes seen. Secondary *erythrocytosis* can result from chronically low Po_2. Pulmonary hypertension is a complication that can lead to *cor pulmonale* and subsequent right heart failure. Chronic ventilatory failure and CO_2 retention are seen in chronic bronchitis early and at the end stages of emphysema.

Management of Stable Phase COPD. The goal in treatment is to treat airway inflammation and bronchospasm, reduce airway resistance and work of breathing, and improve gas exchange and ventilation-perfusion (V̇/Q) mismatching.

Anticholinergic agents (ipratropium bromide [Atrovent®] and tiotropium) are the first-line drugs in COPD. These agents are given via MDI and control airway caliber and tone. Anticholinergic agents can be used synergistically with β_2-adrenergic agonists in patients with COPD.

β_2-adrenergic agonists (albuterol) are used after anticholinergic agents. The inhaled route is the preferred administration.

Beta agonists are not first-line agents in the management of COPD because many of the patients have underlying heart disease and the tachycardia commonly associated with these agents may precipitate heart failure.

Note

The answer to this question can be found at the end of this chapter.

Chronic **inhaled corticosteroids** are reserved for severe cases of COPD.

Theophylline, a xanthine derivative, may be added to the regimen if beta-2 agonists and anticholinergics are not effective in managing the symptoms of chronic obstructive lung disease. Remember that theophylline has significant toxicity. Symptoms include nausea and vomiting, palpitations, and tremulousness. Death can occur from theophylline toxicity from cardiac arrhythmias.

The list of drug interactions with theophylline is significant. Theophylline levels increase with fluoroquinolones, clarithromycin, H2-blockers (cimetidine, ranitidine), certain beta blockers and calcium channel blockers. Theophylline levels decrease (due to increased clearance) with rifampin, dilantin, phenobarbital, and smoking.

Despite the above treatments, the only interventions which have been shown to decrease mortality in patients with COPD are home oxygen and smoking cessation.

Home oxygen therapy is given to patients with hypoxemia (PaO_2 <55 mm Hg or saturation <88%), and the goal is to try to keep the O_2 saturation >90% as much as possible, especially at night when patients generally desaturate. Patients with cor pulmonale will benefit from home oxygen when PaO_2 <59 mm Hg. A special category is the patient who desaturates with exercise; she or he will benefit from intermittent oxygen.

All patients with COPD must have the pneumococcal vaccine (Pneumovax®) every 5 years and the influenza vaccine yearly. They should also receive the *H. influenzae* vaccine if they were not previously immunized.

Several trials have failed to find a beneficial effect for the regular chronic use of inhaled corticosteroids in patients with COPD.

Management and Treatment of COPD Exacerbation (Acute Setting Treatment). Acute exacerbation of COPD is considered acute worsening of the patient's respiratory symptoms (increased dyspnea, increased sputum volume, production of purulent sputum) that necessitates a change in medications.

The most common causes of COPD exacerbation are viral lung infections. Other precipitating causes that should be sought out are bacterial infections, heart failure, myocardial ischemia, pulmonary embolism, lung cancer, esophageal reflux disease, and medications (e.g., beta-blockers).

Initial Management

1. **Measure O_2 saturation** via pulse oximetry (on the spot) to determine oxygen saturation.
2. **ABG determination** is very useful to identify the level of hypercapnia and thus the severity of exacerbation.
3. **Chest x-ray** is expected in all patients with COPD exacerbation to identify pulmonary infiltrates consistent with pneumonia. It may also show evidence of pulmonary edema, indicating possible heart failure as the cause of the exacerbation.
4. Spirometry (and other PFT evaluation) is **not** helpful in COPD exacerbation because measurements (FEV_1, etc.) have not been shown to correlate well with the severity of the exacerbation.
5. Always check levels in patients taking theophylline for chronic treatment. Remember, drugs like erythromycin, cimetidine, and ciprofloxacin may decrease theophylline clearance and cause theophylline toxicity.
6. Other tests as part of the initial evaluation of COPD exacerbation might include *CBC* (looking for elevated WBCs and polycythemia); *ECG* (looking for new arrhythmias, e.g., atrial fibrillation that may precipitate heart failure and exacerbate COPD).

7. Any significant changes of hypercapnia or hypoxemia from baseline should prompt consideration for *admission to the hospital*. Also, patients on home O_2 who have exacerbation, and those with severe symptoms, should be hospitalized.

8. Consider *intubation and mechanical ventilation* in patients with decreased levels of consciousness, cyanosis, or hemodynamic instability and in those with persistent hypoxemia despite adequate oxygen supplementation.

Specific Therapy

1. *Oxygen supplementation* should be titrated to ~90% saturation on the pulse oximeter. The first and foremost concern is to deliver adequate oxygenation. In COPD exacerbation, we should be concerned about CO_2 retention as a secondary issue.

2. *Inhaled bronchodilators* are the *most effective* medications to improve airway diameter (the drugs of choice). In acute COPD exacerbations, use both beta-agonists (albuterol) and anticholinergics (ipratropium) *simultaneously*. Trials have shown that administration of these drugs by a nebulizer or metered dose inhaler (MDI) with a spacer is equally efficacious. Patients with severe exacerbations are unable to hold their breath for more than a few seconds and are thus initially treated with nebulizers and then switched to the MDIs.

3. *Systemic corticosteroids* have now been shown in multiple trials to shorten the recovery time of lung function and decrease the length of stay in patients with COPD exacerbation. Corticosteroids may be given intravenously or orally because the *efficacy is similar* in both modes of administration. The equivalent of 60 mg prednisone appears to be the sufficient starting dose and is usually continued for 2 weeks. It makes sense clinically to start patients who have a severe exacerbation with IV methylprednisolone (it is difficult for these patients to take oral meds), then change to oral prednisone as they improve. Inhaled corticosteroids have *not* been shown to improve outcomes in patients with COPD exacerbation and cannot be substituted for systemic corticosteroids.

4. *Antibiotics* seem to be beneficial in COPD exacerbations despite "normal" chest radiograms. Patients with productive, purulent cough benefit the most because they are more likely to have an underlying bacterial infection. Antibiotics commonly used are second-generation macrolides (clarithromycin, azithromycin), extended-spectrum fluoroquinolones (levofloxacin, moxifloxacin), cephalosporins (second- and third-generation), and amoxicillin clavulanate.

5. There is no real benefit to using IV aminophylline. However, if the patient is using theophylline on a chronic basis (in outpatient setting), it should be continued during the exacerbation because abrupt discontinuation may worsen symptoms.

6. Always avoid opiates and sedatives because they may suppress the respiratory system.

7. Although specific chest physiotherapy (postural drainage, etc.) has not been shown to benefit patients with exacerbation, they should be encouraged to increase activities as tolerated to prevent deconditioning.

8. Counseling the patient on smoking cessation in the hospital setting is the single most important intervention.

9. Teaching the patient optimal use of MDIs has been shown to reduce readmission rates.

Prognosis. FEV_1 is the best predictor of survival (the higher the FEV_1, the better the survival and the less symptomatic the patients). The rate of FEV_1 decline may also predict survival because patients with a faster decline will have increased morbidity. Patients that have a FEV_1 $\leq 25\%$ will usually complain of dyspnea at rest.

Tobacco cessation is the only means of slowing progression of COPD and the decrease in FEV_1.

It is very important that patients with COPD have vaccinations against *Pneumococcus* with a booster at 5 years and yearly for influenza. Some experts consider the *H. influenzae* vaccine mandatory.

Let's go back to our patient.

What are you likely to find on her PFTs? How will you treat this patient in the acute exacerbation? What are your treatment options after she goes home?

She asks you to inform her about "how bad her disease is." What will you consider now?

Note

The answers to these questions can be found at the end of this chapter.

Bronchiectasis

A 17-year-old girl is admitted to the hospital with a right lower lobe pneumonia. She gives you a history of recurrent pneumonias, some of which have kept her in the hospital for weeks, and of chronic productive cough that occurs every day. Her parents inform you that she has had "loose stools" since childhood. On the examination she is thin and in distress. There are diminished breath sounds on the right lower lobe with rhonchi.

Definition and Etiology. Bronchiectasis is the permanent dilation of small- and medium-sized bronchi that results from destruction of bronchial elastic and muscular elements. Eventually the bronchi become fibrotic. Bronchiectasis can occur secondary to repeated pneumonic processes such as tuberculosis (TB), fungal infections, lung abscess, and pneumonia (focal bronchiectasis) or when the defense mechanisms of the lung are compromised as in cystic fibrosis and immotile cilia syndrome (diffuse bronchiectasis).

About 50% of patients with primary ciliary dyskinesia will have situs inversus and sinusitis—Kartagener syndrome.

Bronchiectasis should be suspected in any patient with chronic cough, hemoptysis, foul-smelling sputum production, and recurrent pulmonary infections, sinusitis, and immune deficiencies.

Signs and Symptoms. Patients will have persistent cough with purulent copious sputum production, wheezes, or crackles. There is a significant history of recurrent pneumonias that commonly involve gram-negative bacteria, especially Pseudomonas species.

Hypoxemia may occur causing secondary polycythemia.

Diagnosis. Early chest x-ray findings may be normal in patients with bronchiectasis. Chest x-ray in advanced cases may show 1- to 2-cm cysts and crowding of the bronchi (tram-tracking). High-resolution computed tomographic (CT) scan of the chest is the best noninvasive test to detect bronchiectasis.

Treatment. Bronchodilators, chest physical therapy, and postural drainage are used to control and improve drainage of bronchial secretions. Patients should be treated with antibiotics such as trimethoprim sulfamethoxazole, amoxicillin, and amoxicillin/clavulanic acid (Augmentin®) when sputum production increases or they have mild symptoms. This is referred to as "rotating antibiotics" because a different antibiotic is chosen each time to diminish resistance of microorganisms. Chronic prophylaxis with antibiotics is not recommended.

If the patient exhibits significant symptoms or pneumonia they should be treated with IV antibiotics that cover gram-negative bacteria, e.g., quinolones, ceftazidime, or aminoglycosides.

Clinical Pearl

- 5–7% of patients with cystic fibrosis initially present in early adulthood.

- Consider cystic fibrosis in adult patients with chronic productive cough (symptoms of bronchiectasis), especially if they have history of recurrent sinusitis, nasal polyps, and weight loss. Most males are infertile.

Surgical therapy should be considered for patients with localized bronchiectasis with adequate pulmonary functions or in massive hemoptysis.

All patients with bronchiectasis require yearly vaccination for influenza and vaccination for pneumoccocal infection with a single booster at 5 years.

Specific considerations for the treatment of CF include:

- Aggressive percussion and lung exercises
- Pancreatic enzymes
- Supplemental vitamins
- Recombinant human DNAse
- Inhaled hypertonic saline

Complications include massive hemoptysis, amyloidosis, cor pulmonale, and visceral abscesses.

Let's go back to our patient.

How would you treat this patient?

What investigations will you consider based on her history?

Note

The answers to these questions can be found at the end of this chapter.

INTERSTITIAL LUNG DISEASE

Interstitial lung disease (ILD) is a group of heterogeneous diseases and includes >100 disorders. ILD is characterized by chronic inflammation and fibrosis of the interstitium and lung parenchyma. The worst prognosis is with idiopathic pulmonary fibrosis and usual interstitial pneumonitis.

The interstitium of the lung (supporting structure) is the area in and around the small blood vessels and alveoli where the exchange of oxygen and carbon dioxide takes place. Inflammation and scarring of the interstitium (and eventually extension into the alveoli) will disrupt normal gas exchange. Although the progression of ILD may be variable from one disease to another, they have common clinical, radiographic, and spirometric findings.

All patients with ILD develop exertional dyspnea (the most common complaint that brings them to the physician) and nonproductive cough. The examination shows the typical coarse crackles, evidence of pulmonary hypertension (increased pulmonic sound, right heart failure), and clubbing (not always). The chest x-ray is consistent with reticular or reticulonodular pattern ("ground-glass" appearance). PFTs show evidence of intrapulmonary restrictive pattern.

Causes include:

- Idiopathic pulmonary fibrosis
- Sarcoidosis
- Pneumoconiosis and occupational lung disease
- Connective tissue or autoimmune disease–related pulmonary fibrosis
- Hypersensitivity pneumonitis
- Eosinophilic granuloma (a.k.a. Langerhan cell histiocytosis)
- Chronic eosinophilic pneumonia
- Wegener granulomatosis

- Idiopathic pulmonary hemosiderosis
- Bronchiolitis obliterans
- Lymphangioleiomyomatosis

Diagnostic evaluation should include high-resolution CT scan and, eventually, biopsy via bronchoscopy or open lung biopsy.

Idiopathic Pulmonary Fibrosis (IPF)

A 55-year-old man comes for evaluation of exercise intolerance over the past 6 months. He has no significant past medical history. He informs you that over the past week he cannot walk across the room without getting "short of breath." He takes no medications and has never smoked. The physical exam is significant for a respiratory rate of 24/min, jugular venous distention ~8 cm, coarse crackles on auscultation, clubbing, and trace pedal edema on both legs. The chest x-ray reveals diffuse reticular disease.

Definition. IPF is an inflammatory lung disease of unknown origin that causes lung fibrosis and restrictive lung disease. This disease characteristically involves only the lung and has no extrapulmonary manifestations except clubbing.

Prevalence. IPF occurs in patients in the fifth decade of life, with an equal distribution between men and women.

Clinical Manifestations. Progressive exercise intolerance and dyspnea are seen most commonly. There are coarse dry crackles on auscultation.

The chest x-ray reveals reticular or reticulonodular disease. High-resolution CT scan may show ground-glass appearance. As IPF progresses, there is evidence on imaging of extensive fibrosis with honeycomb pattern. A restrictive intrapulmonary process is evident on PFTs.

Bronchoalveolar lavage will show nonspecific findings, specifically increased macrophages.

A lung biopsy is done to exclude other causes that may have similar findings, e.g., vasculitis, infections, cancer.

Treatment.

Pharmacologic treatment includes pirfenidone, a new small-molecule compound that has antifibrotic effects. A recent trial showed that pirfenidone significantly reduced decline in lung function and IPF disease progression.

Drugs no longer used in the treatment of IPF include corticosteroids, anticoagulants, interferon, and bosentan.

Non-pharmocologic treatment includes lung transplantation and is suitable for those patients physically eligible to undergo a major transplant operation. In IPF patients, lung transplant has been shown to reduce the risk of death by 75% as compared with those who remain on the waiting list.

Sarcoidosis

A 27-year-old woman comes to your office with painful erythematous papules that occurred yesterday. She has no other complaints except joint swelling and pain that occurred 3 days ago. Physical examination discloses low-grade fever, symmetric swelling of the knees, PIP (proximal interphalangeal) and MCP (metacarpophalangeal) joints, and well demarcated, 3- to 4-cm papules over the anterior aspect of her legs. What is the next step in confirming the likely diagnosis?

Definition. Sarcoidosis is a systemic disease of unknown cause, characterized histologically by the presence of nonspecific noncaseating granulomas in the lung and other organs.

Prevalence. There is an increased incidence of sarcoidosis among blacks and patients age 20–40 years.

Clinical Manifestations. Sarcoidosis can involve almost any organ system, but pulmonary involvement is most common. Ocular, skin, myocardial, rheumatologic, GI, and neurologic manifestations can also occur.

Commonly, sarcoidosis is discovered in a completely asymptomatic patient, usually in the form of hilar adenopathy on a chest x-ray.

There are 2 distinct sarcoid syndromes with acute presentation:

- *Löfgren syndrome* includes erythema nodosum, arthritis, and hilar adenopathy.
- *Heerfordt-Waldenstrom syndrome* describes fever, parotid enlargement, uveitis, and facial palsy.

Lung involvement in sarcoidosis occurs in 90% of patients at some time in their course. Hilar and left paratracheal adenopathy is the most common presentation.

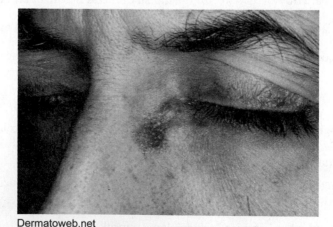

Dermatoweb.net

Figure 9-8. Lupus Pernio Sometimes Seen with Sarcoidosis

Chest X-Ray. Chest x-ray findings can show 4 stages of disease (the stages are not progressive), which include bilateral hilar adenopathy, hilar adenopathy with reticulonodular parenchyma, reticulonodular parenchyma alone, or honeycombing of bilateral lung fields with fibrosis.

Laboratory Findings. Hypercalcemia or hypercalciuria caused by increased circulation of vitamin D produced by macrophages.

Elevation in angiotensin-converting enzyme (ACE) can be seen in 60% of patients with sarcoidosis. ACE levels are *nonspecific* but can be used to follow the course of the disease.

Abnormalities in liver function tests are seen in 30% of patients with liver involvement, with 90% of patients being symptomatic.

Other findings on diagnosis of sarcoidosis include skin anergy, and PFTs may be normal or show a restrictive pattern. All patients with suspected sarcoidosis should have an ophthalmologic examination because uveitis and conjunctivitis are found in >25% of the cases.

Diagnosis. The definitive diagnosis of sarcoidosis rests on biopsy of suspected tissues, which show noncaseating granulomas.

Prognosis. Eighty percent of patients with lung involvement from sarcoidosis remain stable, or the sarcoidosis spontaneously resolves. Twenty percent of patients develop progressive disease with evidence of end-organ compromise.

Treatment. There is no evidence that any therapy alters the course of disease. Generally in the setting of organ impairment, a trial of steroids may be used, giving a high dose for 2 months followed by tapering the dose over 3 months. There are certain scenarios in which *steroids are mandatory:* uveitis, sarcoidosis involving the CNS, and hypercalcemia.

Pneumoconiosis

Definition. The pneumoconioses are occupational lung diseases in which inhalation of certain fibers initiates an inflammatory process that eventually leads to fibrosis of the lung.

Usually, pneumoconiosis appears 20–30 years after constant exposure to offending agents (metal mining of gold, silver, lead, copper) but can develop in <10 years when dust exposure is extremely high.

History is of primary importance in assessing possible occupational lung diseases.

Pathology. Alveolar macrophages engulf offending agents, causing inflammation and fibrosis of the lung parenchyma in pneumoconiosis. Respiratory insufficiency is the ultimate consequence of the pneumoconioses.

Diagnosis. Signs and symptoms include dyspnea, shortness of breath, cough, sputum production, cor pulmonale, and clubbing.

PFTs show a restrictive pattern with a decreased DLCO.

Hypoxemia is evident with an increased PAO_2-PaO_2 gradient.

Chest x-ray findings include small irregular opacities, interstitial densities, ground glass appearance, and honeycombing.

Clinical Pearl

Don't use ACE levels to diagnose sarcoidosis.

Clinical Pearl

If a patient is asymptomatic and has bilateral hilar adenopathy on a routine chest x-ray, assume this is sarcoidosis and follow with imaging.

Asbestosis

Definition. Asbestosis is an occupational lung disease caused by prolonged inhalation of asbestos dust. The result is lung parenchymal fibrosis which results in respiratory compromise.

Epidemiology. Asbestos fiber exposure may be seen in mining, milling, foundry work, shipyards, or the application of asbestos products to pipes, brake linings, insulation, and boilers.

History of exposure to asbestos is needed to consider the diagnosis.

Signs and Symptoms. These include exertional dyspnea and reduced exercise tolerance, cough and wheezing (especially among smokers), chest wall pain, and ultimately respiratory failure.

On chest x-ray, diffuse or local pleural thickening, pleural plaques, and calcifications at the level of the diaphragm are seen. Pleural effusions are commonly seen, and the interstitial lung process associated with asbestosis usually involves the lower lung fields.

The most common cancer associated with asbestosis is bronchogenic carcinoma (adenocarcinoma or squamous cell carcinoma).

Pleural or peritoneal mesotheliomas are also associated with asbestos exposure but are not as common as bronchogenic cancer.

Diagnosis. A lung biopsy is usually necessary for the diagnosis of asbestosis, in which the classic barbell-shaped asbestos fiber is found.

Treatment. No specific treatment is offered. It is important that patients with asbestos exposure stop smoking since the risk of lung cancer is 75 times higher than that of the normal population.

Silicosis

Definition. Silicosis is an occupational lung disease caused by inhalation of silica dust.

Epidemiology. Silicosis is seen in individuals who work in mining, quarrying, tunneling, glass and pottery making, and sandblasting.

Signs and Symptoms. Silicosis will cause similar symptoms to asbestosis (or any other pneumoconiosis) except the acute form of silicosis, which is caused by massive exposure that causes lung failure in months.

Pathology. Silica causes inflammatory reactions with pathologic lesions being the hyaline nodule.

Chest X-Ray. In silicosis there are nodules (1–10 mm) seen throughout the lungs that are most prominent in the upper lobes. A characteristic finding is eggshell calcifications (rare). In progressive massive fibrosis, densities are 10 mm or more and coalesce in large masses.

Diagnosis. Same as asbestosis.

Treatment. There is no effective therapy for silicosis. Death occurs usually because of progressive respiratory insufficiency.

There is an association of silicosis with pulmonary TB. Patients with silicosis should have yearly purified protein derivative (PPD) tuberculin testing; a patient with positive reactive PPD (>10 mm) should get isoniazid (INH) prophylaxis for 9 months.

Coal miner's lung/coal worker's pneumoconiosis (CWP)

Epidemiology. The risk of development and progression of CWP is related to the amount of coal dust exposure, higher rank (hardness) of coals, and increased silica content of inhaled dust. Simple CWP is seen in 12% of all miners.

Signs and Symptoms. CWP clinically presents as any other occupational lung disease.

Chest X-Ray. Small round densities are seen in the parenchyma, usually involving the upper half of the lungs. Complicated or progressive massive fibrosis is diagnosed by the presence of larger densities from 1 cm in diameter to the entire lobe.

Associated Immunologic Abnormalities. Increased levels of IgA, IgG, C3, antinuclear antibodies (ANA), and rheumatoid factor are abnormalities seen in CWP.

In *Caplan syndrome* there are rheumatoid nodules in the periphery of the lung in a patient with rheumatoid arthritis and coexisting pneumoconiosis (usually CWP).

PULMONARY THROMBOEMBOLISM

A 32-year-old woman is brought to the emergency department with an acute onset of shortness of breath and pleuritic chest pain that occurred while she was shopping. She has never been sick and takes no medications other than oral contraceptives. Her respiratory rate is 26/min and pulse 107/min. Auscultation is clear, and the rest of the examination is normal. ABG shows evidence of mild hypoxemia (7.52/70/25/93%). Chest x-ray is normal.

Overview. Thromboembolic disease is a common cause of morbidity and mortality in the hospital and outpatient setting and poses a diagnostic challenge even for seasoned clinicians.

Clinically significant pulmonary emboli, for the most part, arise from proximal (above-the-knee) deep vein thrombi (DVT). In turn, most proximal DVT are a consequence of propagation of distal (below-the-knee) DVT. Studies have shown that distal DVT, by themselves, do not pose a risk for the development of a pulmonary embolus. In one-third of the cases, they extend to the proximal veins and thus become a source of pulmonary emboli.

Pulmonary embolism can infrequently occur with upper extremity, subclavian, and internal jugular vein thrombosis. This type of thromboembolic disease occurs in patients when IV catheters are placed in the associated veins. Also, in the pregnant patient, thrombosis may occur initially in the pelvic veins rather than follow the usual course of starting in the distal and then extending to the proximal veins.

- Pulmonary embolism and DVT are considered one disease.

- Be concerned about (and treat) proximal vein thrombosis because this may result in pulmonary embolism.

- In pregnant patients and those with IV catheters, look for the source of the thromboembolism in uncommon places (pelvic veins, upper extremity veins, etc.).

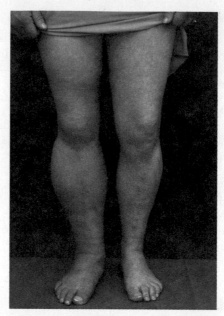

Biomedical Communications 2007—Custom Medical Stock Photo.

Figure 9-9. Unilateral Right Leg Swelling Due to Deep Venous Thrombosis

Natural Course. After a proximal DVT dislodges, it travels through the vena cava and into the right side of the heart. It usually breaks off into multiple thrombi as it goes into the pulmonary circulation, obstructing parts of the pulmonary artery. This results in increased alveolar dead space, vascular constriction, and increased resistance to blood flow. When ~50% of the lung vasculature is involved, significant pulmonary hypertension may occur. This is followed by an increase in right ventricular workload and may lead to right-sided heart failure. A massive pulmonary embolus occurs when >70% of one lung is involved.

About 10% of patients with pulmonary embolus will die within 1 hour of the event, most from a massive pulmonary embolus or significant comorbid conditions (e.g., preexisting CHF or COPD).

When to Consider Pulmonary Embolism and DVTs:

1. *High-risk patients:*

   - Recent surgery, especially orthopedic surgery (knee replacement surgery carries a 70% risk for DVT)

   - Cancer history (prostate, pelvic, abdominal, and breast). *Note:* Studies following patients with unexplained DVT found that 15–20% of these patients developed cancer within the first 2 years after the diagnosis of a DVT.

   - Immobile patients (especially those hospitalized); patients with significant heart failure; long travel

   - Acquired thrombophilia, especially lupus anticoagulant, nephrotic syndrome (loss of antithrombin III in the urine), and oral contraceptives (the risk increases further if the patient is a current smoker)

   - Inherited thrombophilia, of which the most common is *factor V Leiden mutation* (protein C resistance); others include protein C and S deficiency and antithrombin III deficiency

   - Pregnancy, for which increased risk for thromboembolism will continue until 2 months after the delivery

2. *Consistent symptoms and signs:*

- Sudden onset of dyspnea (shortness of breath) and tachypnea
- Thigh or calf swelling with or without dyspnea
- Pleuritic chest pain
- Hemoptysis (occurs only with infarction, which is rare because of the dual circulation [bronchial and pulmonary] that supports lung parenchyma)
- On exam, always increased respiratory rate with tachycardia; increased pulmonic sound (P_2)

Tests for the Diagnosis of Thromboembolic Disease

General tests. These tests are nonspecific, although they may provide important clues for the diagnosis. They are done routinely in the emergency department in the evaluation of patients with dyspnea.

Arterial blood gas (ABG) tests usually show evidence of hypoxemia with an elevated A-a gradient. In ~10% of patients with documented pulmonary thromboembolism, the A-a gradient may be normal and the hypoxemia mild.

Chest x-rays are very important in finding other causes that may account for the patient's symptoms. The most common chest x-ray finding associated with pulmonary thromboembolism is a "normal" chest x-ray. Other nonspecific findings include atelectasis and pleural effusion (transudative and exudative).

- Westermark sign is the lack of vascular markings that occur distal to the pulmonary embolus.
- Hampton hump is a wedge-shaped infiltrate (just above the diaphragm) and is due to pulmonary infarction

The ECG may show evidence of right heart strain (due to the development of acute pulmonary hypertension), which manifests as large S waves in lead I and deep Q waves in lead III with T-wave inversion in the same lead (mnemonic: S_1, Q_3, T_3). The most common finding on the ECG is sinus tachycardia. The ECG is also an important tool in excluding other causes with similar symptoms, specifically acute pericarditis and myocardial ischemia.

Specific Tests. These tests are more specific for the evaluation of thromboembolic disease (do them when considering the diagnosis).

Clinical Pearl

Generally speaking, **high-risk patients** are considered those with 1 risk factor and consistent symptoms and *no* alternative diagnosis. **Low-risk patients** have no risk factors, somewhat atypical symptoms, and possibly an alternative diagnosis (e.g., an infiltrate on the x-ray consistent with pneumonia).

There are clinical scoring systems that assess the risk for thromboembolism, but it is not necessary to know them for the USMLE.

Clinical Pearl

Consider pulmonary embolus in all patients with dyspnea and *normal* chest radiography.

1. Pulmonary embolism:

   - CT pulmonary angiogram (CT-PA) is the most frequently performed initial test for the diagnosis of pulmonary embolism. It allows direct visualization of the pulmonary embolus, and it also allows for the diagnosis of alternative diseases involving the lung parenchyma (pneumonia, pneumothorax, etc.). The older generation of CT-PAs may miss pulmonary emboli that involve the smaller (peripheral) pulmonary arteries.

   - *Ventilation-perfusion (V̇/Q̇) scan* is a pair of nuclear scan tests that use inhaled and injected material to measure breathing (ventilation) and circulation (perfusion) in all areas of the lung. A pulmonary embolus will typically cause perfusion defects with normal ventilation. The V̇/Q̇ scan, depending on the number of defects, is classified as normal, low probability, intermediate probability, or high probability. Patients that have any preexisting lung disease (COPD) will have at least intermediate scans, which make this test less helpful. A *normal* V̇/Q̇ scan rules out pulmonary embolus.

   - *Pulmonary angiogram* is the gold standard procedure for the diagnosis of pulmonary embolus. Its risk of complication (e.g., pulmonary artery rupture) is <1%. With the new generation of CTs able to visualize the smallest peripheral vessels, the invasive pulmonary angiogram is becoming obsolete.

2. DVT:

   - Compression on duplex U/S (US)
   - Venogram is rarely done.
   - MRI

3. Both pulmonary embolism and DVT:

   - *D-dimer* is the most sensitive test for thromboembolic disease. Elevated D-dimer indicates the presence of an abnormally high level of fibrin degradation products, possibly because of thrombus formation and breakdown. An elevated D-dimer may be due to a thromboembolism, but it may also be due to a recent surgery, infection, trauma, pregnancy, and DIC. Normal D-dimer tests mean that there is no thrombus formation or breakdown. For the above reasons, a D-dimer can only be used to *rule out* PE or DVT if the levels are normal. Trials have shown that the D-dimer is most useful when the test is done on patients considered to be low-risk and is recommended as an adjunct test (i.e., a negative D-dimer and a normal CT-PA scan rule out thromboembolism 98% of the time).

   There are many types of D-dimer tests with different sensitivities. The ELISA assay is the best test overall, whereas the latex agglutination test is less sensitive.

General diagnostic concepts in patients suspected of pulmonary embolism:

   - It makes sense to start with a CT-PA after a chest x-ray is completed.
   - Normal CT scan and normal D-dimer test in low-risk patients excludes pulmonary embolism.
   - Normal CT scan and normal Doppler U/S in low-risk patients excludes pulmonary embolism.
   - Even if all tests are negative for pulmonary embolism but the patient is high risk, go for the angiogram.
   - If a V̇/Q̇ scan is completely normal (not near normal or low probability), the chance of pulmonary embolism is almost 0%.
   - Know how to use Doppler U/S in the evaluation of pulmonary embolism. For example, if a V̇/Q̇ scan is reported as low probability, still be concerned about pulmonary

Clinical Pearl

- Order CT-PA as the primary test to diagnose pulmonary embolus.

- Use V̇/Q̇ scan in patients with iodine allergy, renal insufficiency, or morbid obesity.

embolism. An angiogram is not preferred unless absolutely necessary because it is an invasive procedure. Therefore, do an U/S of both lower extremities to look for a DVT (remember that most pulmonary emboli are complications of DVTs arising in the proximal veins).

- All patients (especially high risk) should be on anticoagulation while completing diagnostic evaluations, so start heparin before sending that patient off to the radiology department for the CT or the V̇/Q̇ scan.

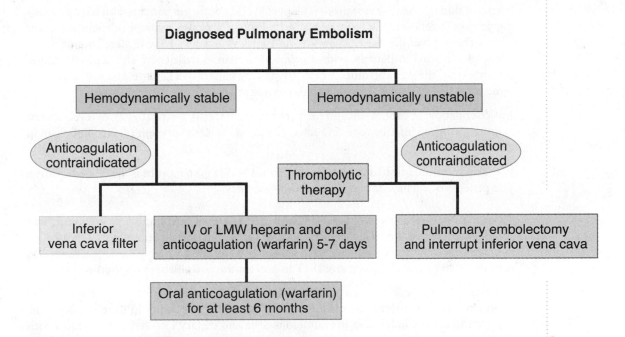

Figure 9-10. Management of Diagnosed Pulmonary Embolism

Treatment. Give oxygen and start heparin immediately before the diagnosis is confirmed and while the diagnostic workup is being completed. Once the diagnosis is confirmed:

- Heparin—LMWH or unfractionated for 5–7 days (or until INR is therapeutic)

    In most institutions, LMWH has supplanted the use of unfractionated heparin as the primary heparinoid in the treatment of PE and DVT.

- Warfarin (Coumadin®)—should be *started with heparin* and continued for 6 months for both pulmonary emboli and DVT.

1. LMWH or fractionated heparin inactivates factor Xa but has no effect on thrombin (no need to follow PTT). Dosing is based on patient's weight, and the effect is very predictable. The long half-life makes it ideal for a 1× or 2×/day dosing interval. Trials have shown that LMWH is as good as unfractionated heparin in the treatment of DVT and pulmonary emboli; also, LMWH is less likely to cause hemorrhage or heparin-induced thrombocytopenia (HIT).

HIT is a common complication of heparin treatment and occurs 5–7 days after starting treatment in about 5% of patients. Paradoxically, it is associated more with thrombotic events than bleeding diathesis. Always stop heparin when platelets decrease by a significant amount. Also, consider HIT in a patient with recurrent pulmonary embolism or DVT despite heparin treatment. HIT is treated with the new anticoagulants (argatroban, lepirudin).

2. Warfarin works by inhibiting the vitamin K–dependent factors (II, VII, IX, and X). Because factor VII has the shortest half-life of all the affected factors, prothrombin time (PT) is monitored to assess the warfarin anticoagulant effect. International normalized ratio (INR) is a way to report PT and is used to control for variability in PT between different laboratories. The warfarin dose should be titrated to an INR of 2–3 for effective anticoagulation.

Warfarin skin necrosis is a rare procoagulant effect that occurs in patients who have preexisting protein C deficiency and receive warfarin. Protein C is also a vitamin-dependent factor with a shorter half-life than factor VII. A "transient hypercoagulable state" occurs when warfarin is started in patients with subclinical protein C deficiency. This leads to diffuse thrombosis of the skin and other organs. By starting patients on heparin and warfarin at the same time, you minimize the risk for this complication.

Anticoagulation is contraindicated in patients with recent neurosurgery or eye surgery. Consider using an inferior vena cava filter (Greenfield filter) to prevent further embolism in these patients.

Warfarin is contraindicated in pregnant patients. LMWH for 6 months is the best alternative. The patient should have injections once or twice a day.

3. Thrombolytics (tPA, streptokinase) are not used routinely in pulmonary embolism and should be reserved for patients that become hemodynamically unstable (indicated by hypotension, right heart failure, etc.). In clinical practice, thrombolytics are sometimes also considered in patients with massive DVT to prevent the postphlebitic syndrome.

Although the available vitamin K antagonists are highly effective for the prevention and treatment of most thrombotic disease, significant patient variability in dose response, the narrow therapeutic index, and the numerous drug and dietary interactions associated with these agents have led clinicians to search for alternative agents. These new anti-thrombotic drugs have relatively discrete targets within the coagulation pathway. Two new classes of orally administered anticoagulants, inhibitors of factor X and thrombin inhibitors, have been approved for the management and prevention of venous thromboembolic disease. Rivaroxaban is a direct factor Xa inhibitor. Dabigatran is a direct thrombin inhibitor that has been approved for venous thromboembolism prophylaxis.

The postthrombotic syndrome (postphlebitic syndrome) is the most common complication of DVT, occurring in up to two-thirds of patients. It may result from some obstructions that remain in the vein or backflow of blood due to destruction of the valves or both. Signs and symptoms include pain, edema, hyperpigmentation, and skin ulceration. The use of compression stockings has been shown to prevent the postthrombotic syndrome.

Other Concepts in Treatment

- Noncomplicated proximal DVTs are usually treated for a total of 6 months.
- In patients with thrombophilias (hypercoagulable states), lifelong anticoagulation is considered with warfarin (usually reserved for at least two episodes of thrombosis).
- Do not check for protein C or protein S deficiency during acute thrombosis. Both warfarin (which the patient should be on) and acute clot formation *lower* protein C and S.
- In patients that develop recurrent thrombosis while on anticoagulants, consider HIT or cancer-related thrombosis (very resistant). Consider placing an inferior vena cava (IVC) filter or using some of the newer anticoagulant classes (e.g., hirudin derivatives). IVC

filters are associated with clot formation around the filter site and may cause pulmonary thromboembolism.

- **Limited distal DVT** (below-the-knee DVT) are not themselves a cause of pulmonary embolism, unless they extend to the proximal veins. Management of distal DVT includes 2 options: monitor for possible extension to the proximal veins by using serial U/S or treat with anticoagulation for 3 months.

Fat embolism is a rare type of embolism that occurs 3 days after long bone fracture (most commonly seen with femur fracture). It may occur, although rarely, after CPR. The clinician should consider this entity with presence of acute dyspnea, petechiae (neck and axilla), and confusion. Treatment is supportive (no anticoagulation).

ACUTE RESPIRATORY DISTRESS SYNDROME (ARDS)

A 32-year-old man is admitted to the intensive care unit with the presumed diagnosis of gram-negative sepsis. He is placed on double gram-negative antibiotic coverage and remains stable for 24 hours. The blood cultures grow pseudomonas sensitive to both ceftazidime and ciprofloxacin, which the patient has been started on. The patient seems to improve but suddenly during day 2 of hospitalization develops severe dyspnea. The examination reveals diffuse crackles; an ABG shows hypoxemia and hypercarbia. Diffuse alveolar densities are seen on chest x-ray (the admission chest x-ray was unremarkable).

Definition. ARDS is defined as an acute lung injury that is characterized by increased permeability of the alveolar-capillary membrane and pulmonary edema. It eventually leads to severe hypoxemia and decreased pulmonary compliance.

Etiology. Etiology of ARDS includes sepsis, trauma, disseminated intravascular coagulation, drug overdose, inhalation of toxins, Goodpasture syndrome, systemic lupus erythematosus, drowning, and the period after bypass surgery.

ARDS usually occurs within 5 days of the initiating event, and >50% will develop it within the first 24 hours. A major component of ARDS seems to be accumulation of inflammatory cells and their mediators.

Signs and Symptoms. Signs and symptoms of ARDS are dyspnea, increased respiratory rate, and diffuse rales and rhonchi on auscultation.

Chest x-ray findings include diffuse interstitial or alveolar infiltrates; whiteout of both lung fields may be seen. **ABGs** reveal decreased Pao_2 and increased or normal $Paco_2$. Swan-Ganz catheter findings will reveal normal cardiac output and normal capillary wedge pressure but increased pulmonary artery pressure.

Treatment. Treat underlying disorder. Mechanical support with increased positive end-expiratory pressure and permissive hypercapnea. Studies have shown that conservative fluid replacement decreased ICU and ventilatory time but mortality remained unchanged. Steroid use is controversial.

Prognosis. Mortality rates are approximately 50%.

SLEEP APNEA

Sleep apnea is defined as the cessation of airflow (>10 s) that occurs at least 10–15x per hour during sleep. Oxygen saturation decreases during these apneic episodes, and pulmonary pressures increase.

Daytime somnolence is mandatory for the diagnosis of sleep apnea. Systemic hypertension also occurs. When severe, sleep apnea will cause pulmonary hypertension and cor pulmonale.

There are 2 main classes of sleep apnea:

- **Obstructive** sleep apnea (OSA) occurs because of floppy airways despite adequate ventilatory effort. These people are usually obese and have abnormal airways. The treatment is weight loss and nasal continuous positive airway pressure (CPAP).
- **Central** sleep apnea occurs in <5% of patients with sleep apnea and is caused by inadequate ventilatory drive. Treatment is acetazolamide, progesterone, and supplemental O_2.

The diagnosis of sleep apnea syndromes is confirmed by polysomnography (sleep studies).

LUNG CANCER

Bronchogenic Carcinoma

A 65-year-old man is admitted because of headache and blurry vision the past few days. In the emergency room the physicians also notice that he has neck vein distension and darker coloration over his face and neck. He is confused. Chest x-ray reveals a right upper lobe lung mass, and blood tests indicate significant hypercalcemia.

Bronchogenic carcinoma is the leading cause of death because of malignancy in men and women. The overall 5-year survival rate for small cell cancer is 5% and non-small cell cancer is 8%.

Etiology. Ninety percent of cases of bronchogenic carcinoma are directly related to cigarette smoking in both men and women. The occasional nonsmoker who has lung cancer develops adenocarcinoma.

Smoking is the major cause of lung cancer. Active smokers have a 10× greater risk compared with nonsmokers. The risk is directly related to the number of pack-years (40-pack-year history increases risk 60–70×). Asbestos exposure increases the risk of bronchogenic carcinoma 75× that in the nonexposed normal patients.

All lung cancers are associated with smoking.

There is no available screening test for lung cancer at this time.

Pathology. The most common lung cancers are adenocarcinoma (~40% in some studies) and squamous cell carcinoma.

- **Adenocarcinoma.** Adenocarcinoma is a peripherally located lesion. This lesion metastasizes widely to essentially the same sites as small-cell carcinoma. Bronchioalveolar carcinoma is a subtype of adenocarcinoma; it is a low-grade carcinoma that can occur in single or multiple nodules. Asbestos exposure can be an underlying causative agent, usually after a latent period of 30 years. Adenocarcinoma is usually associated with pleural effusions that have high hyaluronidase levels. Diagnosis often requires thoracotomy with pleural biopsy.

- **Squamous Cell Carcinoma.** Squamous cell carcinoma is a centrally located lesion. It is associated with cavitary lesions. Squamous cell carcinoma usually metastasizes by direct extension into the hilar node and mediastinum. These lesions are associated with hypercalcemia from the secretion of a parathyroid hormone–like substance.

- **Small-Cell Carcinoma.** Small-cell carcinomas are centrally located lesions. These tumors are rapidly growing with early distant metastasis to extrathoracic sites such as liver, adrenal glands, brain, and bone. Prognosis does not improve with early diagnosis. Small-cell carcinoma is associated with Eaton-Lambert syndrome, syndrome of inappropriate antidiuretic hormone, and other paraneoplastic syndromes. Small-cell carcinoma is also the most common cause of venocaval obstruction syndrome.

- **Large-Cell Carcinoma.** Large-cell carcinoma is a peripherally located lesion. This carcinoma can metastasize to distant locations late in the course of disease. Large-cell carcinoma in early stages is associated with cavitation.

Symptoms. The most common symptom at the time of diagnosis is cough (74%). Weight loss is seen in 68% of patients. Dyspnea is seen in 58% of patients. Other associated symptoms of bronchogenic carcinoma include hemoptysis, chest wall pain, and repeated pneumonic processes (caused by postobstructive pneumonia).

Hoarseness when seen indicates a nonresectable bronchogenic carcinoma.

Diagnosis. The diagnosis of bronchogenic carcinoma can be made by sputum cytology, with the highest yield in patients with squamous cell carcinoma (>80%) because it is intraluminal and centrally located. Bronchoscopy is best for centrally located lesions (yield of 90%) and is helpful in staging. For the 10% of centrally located lesions not detected by bronchoscopy, a needle aspiration biopsy should be performed if carcinoma is highly suspect. In other words, if there is a high degree of suspicion for carcinoma and the bronchoscopy results are nonspecific, a biopsy must be requested. Needle aspiration biopsy is also good for peripheral nodules with pleural fluid aspirate (positive in 40–50% of cases). Mediastinoscopy is useful in diagnosing and staging mediastinal tumors.

- **Workup of solitary pulmonary nodule on chest x-ray:** 75% of solitary pulmonary nodules are benign. This percentage is reduced to 25% if the patient has a history of cancer. Features that indicate a benign solitary pulmonary nodule include patients age <35 years; nonsmokers; lesion <2 cm, smooth distinct margins, calcification typical of benign lesions; and a nodule that has not changed in size compared with old x-ray studies.

   If a patient is at low risk for carcinoma, follow-up CT scans are indicated; in a high-risk patient the lesion should be removed and tissue diagnosis confirmed. Bull's-eye lesions are seen in granulomas, whereas popcorn-ball lesions are seen in hamartomas.

- **Workup of a chest x-ray with an effusion and a nodule:** 90% of tumors with malignant effusions are unresectable. These tumors are usually adenocarcinomas. Atelectasis on chest x-ray suggests central airway obstruction.

Treatment. Symptoms that suggest an unresectable lesion include weight loss >10%, bone pain or other extrathoracic metastases, CNS symptoms (treated by radiation or chemotherapy), superior vena cava syndrome, hoarseness, mediastinal adenopathy on the contralateral side, split-lung test tidal volume <800 ml, tumor classification of M1 within 3 months, and tumor involving the trachea, esophagus, pericardium, or chest wall.

Resectable lesions of small-cell carcinoma are treated with chemotherapy; VP16 (etoposide and platinum) is the treatment of choice. Surgery is not indicated for these lesions. Non-small-cell lesions that are resectable are treated with chemotherapy and radiation therapy or CAP (cyclophosphamide, adriamycin, and platinum). Effusions can be sclerosed with tetracycline. Complications are treated with radiation therapy, which in most cases is palliative.

Prognosis. Prognosis is best after surgical resection of squamous-cell carcinoma (30–35%). Large-cell carcinoma and adenocarcinoma have a prognosis of 25%. Prognosis is poorest for small-cell carcinoma.

ATELECTASIS

A 62-year-old man is dyspneic 24 h after cholecystectomy. His respiratory rate is 22/min and pulse 112/min. He has a mild fever, and decreased breath sounds are noted in the left lower lobe. Complete blood count shows leukocytosis 27,000/mm³.

Definition. A collapse of part or the entire lung. It is seen most commonly in the immediate postoperative period. It occurs secondary to poor inspiration or lack of coughing during this time. A mucous plug, tumor, or foreign body can also lead to atelectasis.

Signs and Symptoms. Acute symptoms include tachycardia, dyspnea, fever, and hypoxemia. In the chronic phase patients may be asymptomatic with only x-ray abnormalities. On x-ray, upper lobe atelectasis can appear as tracheal deviation to the affected side. This phenomenon occurs secondary to volume loss from atelectasis. Lower lobe atelectasis may cause an elevation of the corresponding part of the diaphragm. In massive atelectasis, a mediastinal shift to the involved side can be seen. The atelectatic lobe will appear to be densely consolidated and smaller than the normal lobe on x-ray.

Treatment. In the postoperative phase, it is important to induce deep breathing and stimulate coughing. Incentive spirometry and pulmonary toilet are effective. Bronchoscopy with subsequent removal of mucous plugs is highly effective for spontaneous atelectasis.

ANSWERS TO QUESTIONS THROUGHOUT CHAPTER

Pg. 276   *Patient 1a*—chronic bronchitis or asthma

Patient 1b—emphysema

Patient 2a—extrapulmonary restriction (e.g., kyphoscoliosis, morbid obesity)

Patient 2b—interstitial lung disease

Pg. 278   *Clinical problem*—overdose from opiates (any scenario in which the respiratory rate is decreased)

Pg. 286
- *What is the treatment of choice in this patient?* bronchodilator; albuterol
- *What are bad prognostic indicators in this patient?* cyanosis, silent lung, increase in CO_2
- *Which one of the ABGs below…?* The first ABG with CO_2 of 45 is the worst.
- *Three days after hospitalization…What is her drug regimen…?* oral prednisone taper, albuterol inhaler, steroid inhaler
- *What will you do now? What medications is she likely to be taking now?* She should have a PFT to document asthma, and her basic asthma regimen should be inhaled steroids daily and albuterol inhaler as needed.

Pg. 288   After a bronchodilator is given, you would expect the FEV_1/FVC to <u>remain the same or improve minimally</u>.

Pg. 291
- *What are you likely to find…?* decreased DLco
- *How will you treat…?* systemic steroids, antibiotics, and bronchodilators; O_2 as needed
- *What are your treatment options…?* ipratropium inhaler, home O_2
- *She asks you to…what will you consider now?* measure FEV_1

Pg. 292
- *How would you treat this patient?* antipseudomonal antibiotics (ciprofloxacin, ceftazidime)
- *What investigations will you consider…?* chloride test to diagnose cystic fibrosis

Emergency Medicine 10

BASIC LIFE SUPPORT (CARDIOPULMONARY RESUSCITATION)

A 54-year-old man is at the opera when he suddenly jumps up and clutches his chest. He falls to his side into the lap of the woman sitting next to him.

Definition. The initial management algorithm of any patient who seems to have become unresponsive.

Etiology. A cardiac, neurologic, or toxicologic event leading to markedly diminished responsiveness or loss of pulse. Most causes of cardiac arrest are related to ventricular rhythm disturbance. The most common etiology of serious cardiac dysrhythmia is ischemia-related, particularly with coronary artery disease or another cardiac anatomic abnormality (especially cardiomyopathy).

Clinical Presentation. Any patient with diminished responsiveness that is usually sudden in onset.

Diagnosis. This is a clinically determined diagnosis at first. The initial step is, in fact, to assess the responsiveness of the patient to make sure that he is truly unresponsive and not just asleep. This is accomplished by calling to or gently shaking the patient. Be careful about shaking a patient who might have serious traumatic injury, particularly of the cervical spine.

Treatment. After determining that the patient is truly unresponsive, the next step is to call for help (dial 911). Although it is natural to reach down to check a pulse, this is not the action that the USMLE or the American Heart Association (AHA) wants you to build as a reflex. Without the EKG, defibrillator, and cardiac medications you need, there is very little that one or even two rescuers can do for a patient with a serious dysrhythmia beyond chest compressions and opening the airway.

If a patient has a serious dysrhythmia such as asystole or ventricular fibrillation, there is virtually no survival if the heart has not been restarted within 10 minutes. Chest compressions just perfuse vital organs; they will not convert the arrhythmia back to normal sinus.

AHA guidelines emphasize the following:

- High-quality CPR with uninterrupted chest compressions of adequate depth (5 cm, 2 in.) at a rate of 100/min
- Decreased intervals between stopping the chest compression and shock delivery

Avoid excessive ventilation because it can be detrimental. ABC, according to new guidelines is now **CAB** (excluding newborns). Removing the 2 rescue breaths allows chest compressions to be delivered sooner. Earlier chest compressions and defibrillation are critical elements of CPR.

- Do look, listen, feel for breathing.
- Do check for pulse (for 10 seconds); if you establish that there is no pulse, start chest compressions (after calling 911).
- Do not give rescue breaths first, as that has been shown to delay vital chest compressions, which leads to an increase in mortality.
- Do not perform jaw thrust, which just delays chest compression.

After calling for help, position the patient on a firm, flat surface, and roll the patient so that he or she is face up. Check to see if there is a pulse by feeling for at least 5-10 seconds at the carotid artery. If there is no pulse, perform chest compressions at a rate of 100 per minute, "push hard and push fast." In adults, provide 30 compressions and then 2 ventilations, regardless of whether one or two rescuers is present. In children, perform 30 compressions and 2 ventilations if one rescuer is present, and give 15 compressions and 2 ventilations if two rescuers are present. Depth of chest compression 2 in. or 5 cm.

Advanced Cardiac Life Support Algorithms

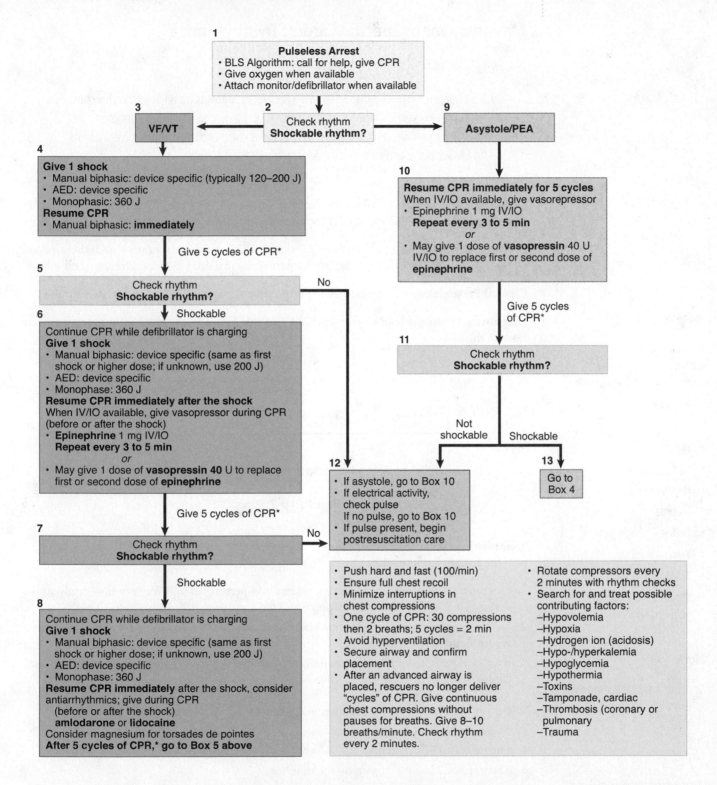

Figure 10-1. ACLS Pulseless Arrest Algorithm

CARDIAC DYSRHYTHMIAS

Management of Specific Cardiac Dysrhythmias

Asystole

> A 54-year-old man is at the opera when he suddenly jumps up and clutches his chest. He falls to his side into the lap of the woman sitting next to him. After confirming that he is unresponsive, a nearby physician performs chest compressions and ventilations. An EKG is done and reveals no evidence of electrical activity.

Definition. The complete absence of electrical activity in the heart. This does not necessarily mean a completely flat line on an EKG because there may be slight variability on the rhythm strip.

Etiology. Ischemia and severe underlying cardiac disease most commonly underlie asystole. Other possible etiologies include metabolic derangements, drug overdose, trauma, and others.

Clinical Presentation. An unresponsive person with asystole on EKG; person has no pulse.

Diagnosis. Asystole should always be confirmed by observing the rhythm in more than one lead on the EKG.

Note

For asystole and other arrhythmias in this chapter, remember the "Hs and Ts":

- **H**ypoxia
- **H**yper/Hypokalemia
- **H**ypothermia
- **H**ypoglycemia
- **H**ypovolemia
- **T**rauma
- **T**oxins (including overdose)
- **T**amponade
- **T**ension pneumothorax
- **T**hrombosis (coronary and pulmonary)

Note

Atropine is no longer indicated in asystole.

Note

Transcutaneous pacemaker is not useful for asystole.

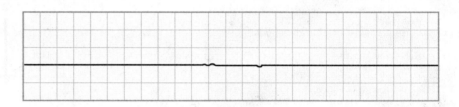

Figure 10-2. Asystole

Treatment. As you continue cardiopulmonary resuscitation (CPR), obtain IV access and prepare the patient for intubation.

1. Transcutaneous pacing should be considered and performed only for very slow bradycardia. Perform it as early as possible. Pacing is not for asystole.
2. Next, administer 1 mg epinephrine via IV push every 3–5 minutes. (**Atropine is no longer recommended for asystole.**)
3. If asystole persists, withhold resuscitative efforts in order to evaluate the presence of atypical clinical features or cease-effort protocol.

When you see asystole on the monitor, make sure of the following:

1. There are no loose or disconnected leads
2. The power to ECG machine and monitor is on
3. There is not a low signal gain on the monitor

Note: Bicarbonate is useful if the cause of asystole is attributed to a preexisting acidosis (except hypercarbic acidosis), tricyclic antidepressant overdose, aspirin overdose, hyperkalemia, or diabetic ketoacidosis.

Ventricular fibrillation

A 54-year-old man is at the opera when he suddenly jumps up and clutches his chest. He falls to his side into the lap of the woman sitting next to him. He is not breathing. After confirming that he is unresponsive, a nearby physician performs chest compressions and ventilations. An EKG is done and reveals ventricular fibrillation. He has no spontaneous respirations.

Definition. Significant electrical activity on EKG with no signs of an organized pattern.

Etiology. Ischemia, myocardial infarction, cardiomyopathy, and severe underlying cardiac disease most commonly underlie ventricular fibrillation. Remember the "Hs and Ts."

Clinical Presentation. A dead person with ventricular fibrillation on EKG.

Diagnosis. Entirely based on the EKG.

Treatment. The differences between defibrillation and cardioversion are very important.

- **Defibrillation** is a nonsynchronized delivery of shock at any phase of cardiac cycle. It is used in VF and pulseless VT. During defibrillation you depolarize all of the myocytes simultaneously, hoping that the SA node will start up normal sinus rhythm.

- **Cardioversion** means that the shock that is synchronized with the QRS complex. When performing cardioversion, the defibrillator will not shock until the QRS complex appears. You will be able to see spikes over the QRS complexes on the monitor. If you shock on the T wave, when ventricular repolarization is taking place, you may induce VF.

Make sure that the SYN button is pushed when performing cardioversion. Use UNsynchronized shock (defibrillation) for VF or pulseless VT only.

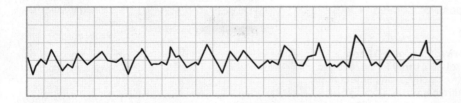

Figure 10-3. Ventricular Fibrillation

Post-Resuscitation Care. Most patients who survive resuscitation have anoxic brain injury. Hypothermia protocol reduces the risk of this type of severe neurologic injury. If a patient is not following commands or showing purposeful movements, the hypothermia protocol should be used. The goal of protocol is to reach core temperature 32–34° C (90–93° F) within 6 hours and maintain for 12–24 hours. Absolute contraindications for induced hypothermia are active bleeding and do-not-resuscitate order.

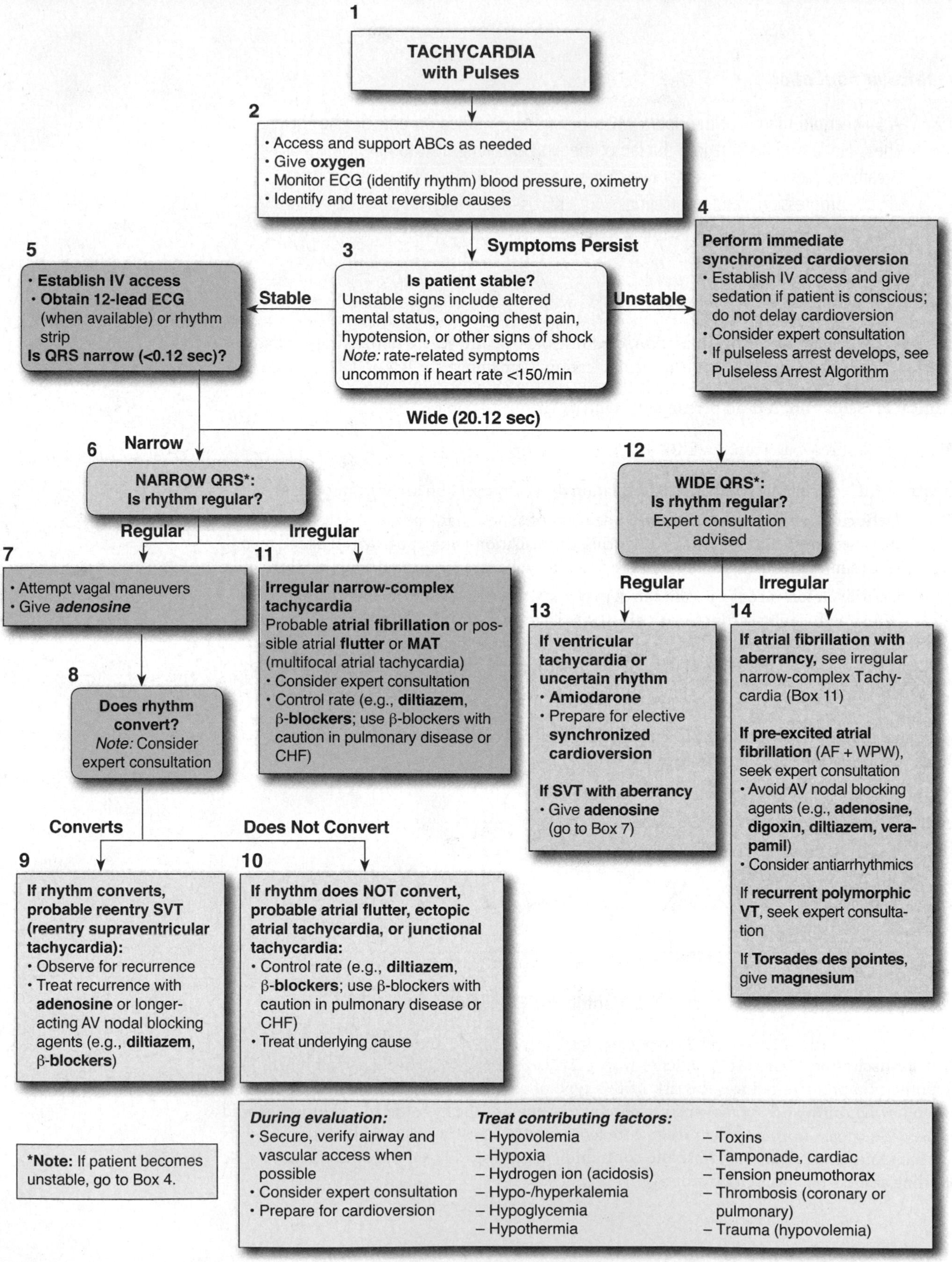

1

> **TACHYCARDIA**
> **with Pulses**

2

> - Access and support ABCs as needed
> - Give **oxygen**
> - Monitor ECG (identify rhythm) blood pressure, oximetry
> - Identify and treat reversible causes

Symptoms Persist

4

> **Perform immediate**
> **synchronized cardioversion**
> - Establish IV access and give sedation if patient is conscious; do not delay cardioversion
> - Consider expert consultation
> - If pulseless arrest develops, see Pulseless Arrest Algorithm

5

> - **Establish IV access**
> - **Obtain 12-lead ECG** (when available) or rhythm strip
> **Is QRS narrow (<0.12 sec)?**

Stable

3

> **Is patient stable?**
> Unstable signs include altered mental status, ongoing chest pain, hypotension, or other signs of shock
> *Note:* rate-related symptoms uncommon if heart rate <150/min

Unstable

Wide (20.12 sec)

Narrow

6

> **NARROW QRS*:**
> **Is rhythm regular?**

12

> **WIDE QRS*:**
> **Is rhythm regular?**
> Expert consultation advised

Regular   **Irregular**

7

> - Attempt vagal maneuvers
> - Give *adenosine*

11

> **Irregular narrow-complex tachycardia**
> Probable **atrial fibrillation** or possible atrial **flutter** or **MAT** (multifocal atrial tachycardia)
> - Consider expert consultation
> - Control rate (e.g., **diltiazem**, **β-blockers**; use **β-blockers** with caution in pulmonary disease or CHF)

Regular   **Irregular**

13

> **If ventricular tachycardia or uncertain rhythm**
> - **Amiodarone**
> - Prepare for elective **synchronized cardioversion**
>
> **If SVT with aberrancy**
> - Give **adenosine** (go to Box 7)

14

> **If atrial fibrillation with aberrancy,** see irregular narrow-complex Tachycardia (Box 11)
>
> **If pre-excited atrial fibrillation** (AF + WPW), seek expert consultation
> - Avoid AV nodal blocking agents (e.g., **adenosine, digoxin, diltiazem, verapamil**)
> - Consider antiarrhythmics
>
> **If recurrent polymorphic VT**, seek expert consultation
>
> **If Torsades des pointes**, give **magnesium**

8

> **Does rhythm convert?**
> *Note:* Consider expert consultation

Converts   **Does Not Convert**

9

> **If rhythm converts, probable reentry SVT (reentry supraventricular tachycardia):**
> - Observe for recurrence
> - Treat recurrence with **adenosine** or longer-acting AV nodal blocking agents (e.g., **diltiazem**, **β-blockers**)

10

> **If rhythm does NOT convert, probable atrial flutter, ectopic atrial tachycardia, or junctional tachycardia:**
> - Control rate (e.g., **diltiazem**, **β-blockers**; use **β-blockers** with caution in pulmonary disease or CHF)
> - Treat underlying cause

> ***During evaluation:***
> - Secure, verify airway and vascular access when possible
> - Consider expert consultation
> - Prepare for cardioversion

> ***Treat contributing factors:***
> – Hypovolemia
> – Hypoxia
> – Hydrogen ion (acidosis)
> – Hypo-/hyperkalemia
> – Hypoglycemia
> – Hypothermia
> – Toxins
> – Tamponade, cardiac
> – Tension pneumothorax
> – Thrombosis (coronary or pulmonary)
> – Trauma (hypovolemia)

> ***Note:** If patient becomes unstable, go to Box 4.

Figure 10-4. Algorithm for Tachycardia with Pulses

Ventricular tachycardia

A 54-year-old man is at the opera when he suddenly jumps up and clutches his chest. He falls to his side into the lap of the woman sitting next to him. He is awake but disoriented and confused. He is complaining of dyspnea and lightheadedness. His exam reveals jugulovenous distention and a blood pressure of 114/80. The EKG shows ventricular tachycardia at a rate of 180.

Definition. A wide complex tachycardia with an organized, uniform pattern on the EKG. There are no P-waves visible.

Etiology. Ischemia, myocardial infarction, and anatomic cardiac disease most commonly underlie VT. Other possible etiologies include quinidine, tricyclics, and phenothiazines. Long QT syndromes also cause VT. The dysrhythmia originates from an ectopic focus in the myocardium or from the AV node. When the impulse originates from around the AV node, this is from reentry. The electrical impulses must travel throughout the myocardium from myocyte to myocyte without the benefit of the more rapidly conducting normal pathways, such as the bundle branches or the His-Purkinje fibers.

The slowness of the conduction produces the slower and therefore wider complexes on the EKG. The rate most often varies 160–240/min. Torsade de pointes is a form of VT in which the morphology varies with an undulating amplitude, making it seem that it "twists around a point." Torsade may be associated with hypomagnesemia and preceded by long QT interval.

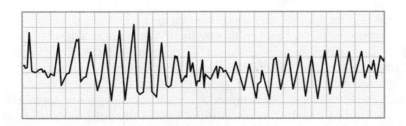

Figure 10-5. Torsade

Clinical Presentation. Symptoms are often related to duration of the dysrhythmia. Short bursts of a few seconds may produce no symptoms at all. VT lasting >30 seconds is referred to as sustained VT. Symptoms include lightheadedness, hypotension, CHF, syncope, and death.

Diagnosis. The EKG shows the VT. For those patients presenting with syncope suspected to be of cardiac origin and in whom an arrhythmia is not visible on the initial EKG, an electrophysiologic study can be done to try to elicit the VT.

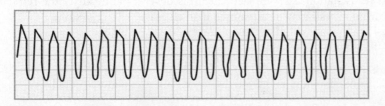

Figure 10-6. Ventricular Tachycardia

Treatment. For those with sustained VT and a pulse who are hemodynamically unstable, immediate synchronized cardioversion is required. Signs of hemodynamic instability requiring cardioversion include hypotension, chest pain, altered mental status, and CHF. A lower dose of electricity, starting at 100 J, can be used at first for monomorphic VT. The cardioversion should be synchronized. Conscious patients should be sedated with midazolam, fentanyl, or morphine before cardioversion.

VT in those patients without a pulse should be managed in the same way as ventricular fibrillation (unsynchronized shock). Stable VT (wide, monomorphic, regular) without serious hemodynamic compromise can be treated medically with adenosine initially and then with antiarrhytmics if no response. In stable patients with pulse, procainamide and sotalol are preferred drugs. If there is no response to procainamide, then amiodarone may be tried, followed by lidocaine and finally electrical cardioversion.

Magnesium may be useful in general but it is most useful for Torsade de pointes. If magnesium fails to treat Torsade, then isoproterenol or lidocaine can be attempted. Overdrive pacing can be used if pharmacologic treatment fails. Patients undergoing cardioversion should be sedated first with midazolam, fentanyl, or morphine. Long-term therapy is most effective with beta-blockers. VT that produces sudden death or VT that is sustained through initial drug therapy may require the placement of an implantable cardiac defibrillator (ICD). All patients with ejection fraction <35% should have ICD, due to increased risk of VT and VF.

Pulseless electrical activity

Definition. Hypotension to the point of losing one's pulse; there is still some type of electrical activity on the EKG that may even be normal or a simple tachycardia.

Etiology. More than the other dysrhythmias, knowing the etiology of pulseless electrical activity (PEA) is the key to the therapy because the specific therapies are so divergent. Essentially, the heart may still be beating, but there is no blood in the heart, and therefore there is no cardiac output. Examples of this type of PEA are severe hypovolemia, cardiac tamponade, tension pneumothorax, massive pulmonary embolism, and a massive myocardial infarction. Other types of PEA in which there may not be actual muscular contraction are hypoxia, hypothermia, potassium disorders, acidosis, and drug overdoses with tricyclics, digoxin, beta-blockers, or calcium-channel blockers.

Clinical Presentation. The patient appears to be dead with no pulse. Other symptoms are based on the specific nature of what led to the PEA, such as those described above.

Diagnosis. A pulseless patient who has significantly organized, and occasionally normal, activity on the EKG.

Treatment. The most important action is to maintain CPR while determining the specific origin of the PEA. General therapy includes CPR, IV access, intubation, and epinephrine. Do not shock PEA arrest. The most important therapy is repair of the cause (possibilities described above). Bicarbonate is useful if a known acidosis has caused the arrest; it can also be used in a prolonged resuscitation if severe lactic acidosis develops and causes the refractory state of arrest. Pericardiocentesis may be attempted if all else fails.

Atrial dysrhythmias

A 24-year-old medical student is brought to the emergency department because of palpitations. He has been studying vigorously for the USMLE Step 2 exam and has been up for the last 24 hours. He has had 5 cups of coffee, 4 beers, 3 stimulant tablets, 2 cheeseburgers, and 1 Viagra. An electrocardiogram reveals an atrial dysrhythmia.

Definition. A-fib, atrial flutter, and SVT are all characterized by either an ectopic focus in the atrium or re-entry at the AV node. All have normal conduction in the ventricular myocardium once the impulse successfully passes the AV node and travels down the normal ventricular conduction system. They all have a normal or narrow QRS complex and the absence of a normal P-wave.

Etiology. A-fib is most commonly caused by chronic hypertension, but it can be caused as well by valvular heart disease (most often mitral valve pathology), left ventricular hypertrophy, cardiomyopathy, atrial fibrosis, atrial dilation, CAD, and CHF. Another cause is toxicity causing overstimulation of the heart, i.e., hyperthyroidism, pheochromocytoma, caffeine, theophylline, alcohol, and cocaine. Drug toxicity (such as digoxin), pericarditis, pulmonary embolism, surgery, chest wall trauma, or ischemia can also cause atrial dysrhythmias.

SVT is caused by a re-entrant mechanism around or within the AV node.

Clinical Presentation. Symptoms vary on the basis of the duration of the disorder, the ventricular rate, and the underlying health of the heart. With a normal heart, only 10-20% of cardiac output is directly derived from the contribution of atrial systole. With a dilated or postinfarction heart, or with significant valvular disease, this contribution may rise to 30-40%, in which case more severe symptoms arise. Symptoms range from complete absence to palpitations to lightheadedness, hypotension, disorientation, CHF, and syncope. Rate-related symptoms are unlikely in those with heart rate <150 per minute in atrial dysrhythmias.

Narrow complex tachycardia is always atrial in origin (QRS <0.12). Wide complex tachycardia can be atrial or ventricular. For example, it is very difficult to distinguish A-fib in the presence of LBBB and VT. The key is that in A-fib with LBBB, the rate is irregular on EKG, whereas in VT it is regular. If in doubt, treat as VT.

Diagnosis. Initially, the diagnosis is based entirely on the EKG. Other patients may need a 24-72 hour Holter monitor to detect brief paroxysms of the dysrhythmia not seen on the initial brief EKG.

Note

For Step 2, you will need to know atrial fibrillation (A-fib), atrial flutter, and supraventricular tachycardia (SVT). They are discussed as a group because the initial management has considerable overlap.

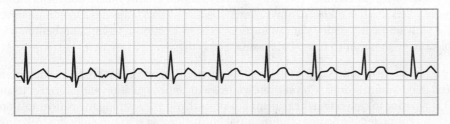

Figure 10-7. Normal Sinus Rhythm

Note

- Narrow complex tachycardia is *always* atrial in origin (QRS <0.12).

- Wide complex tachycardia can be atrial or ventricular in origin.

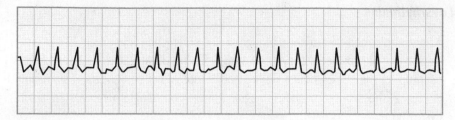

Figure 10-8. Atrial Tachycardia

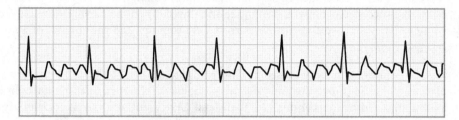

Figure 10-9. Atrial Flutter

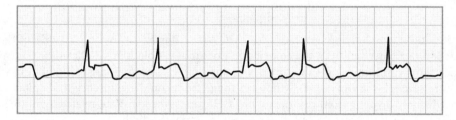

Figure 10-10. Atrial Fibrillation

Treatment. Initial therapy is based on whether there are signs or symptoms of severe hemodynamic compromise, such as hypotension, confusion, CHF, or chest pain. If these are present, then immediate synchronized cardioversion is performed. Palpitations and lightheadedness are not signs of hemodynamic compromise. If the patient is hemodynamically stable, then the first step is to control the ventricular rate. Vagal maneuvers such as carotid sinus massage, Valsalva, or ice water immersion are most effective in SVT. Do not do carotid sinus massage bilaterally. Avoid carotid massage in those with carotid bruits. If vagal maneuvers do not work, SVT is initially treated with several rapid IV infusions of adenosine. For atrial fibrillation, atrial flutter, and in SVT after the failure of adenosine, several therapies are available to slow the heart rate. These include calcium-channel blockers (such as diltiazem or verapamil), beta-blockers, or digoxin. Do not use verapamil in those with severe left ventricular dysfunction and low ejection fractions and beware of using beta-blockers in those with a history of reactive airway disease.

After the rate has been lowered to <110 beats/min, conversion of the rhythm to normal sinus does not need to be routinely done. Chronic rate control with anticoagulation with warfarin to an INR of 2–3 is superior to converting the patient into sinus rhythm. Returning the patient to a normal sinus rhythm is preferable because chronic atrial fibrillation can result in embolic stroke in 5-7% of patients per year.

Amiodarone, ibutilide, propafenone, and dofetilide can all convert a minority of patients to sinus rhythm. At the level of Step 2, you will not need to know much about the specific indications for each. You do, however, need to know that elective cardioversions should be preceded and followed by several weeks of anticoagulation with coumadin.

Rate Control vs. Rhythm Control. When patients present in A-fib with rapid ventricular response, hemodynamic stability must first be determined. If they are hemodynamically stable, they should be rate-controlled with AV nodal blocking agents. If they are unstable, immediate synchronized cardioversion is required. With long-term management, rate control and anticoagulation are preferred over rhythm control. **Rhythm control** should be considered in the following situations:

1. Symptomatic patients on rate control (poor exercise tolerance)
2. Younger patients with normal heart structure and function
3. Patients that are unable to be rate controlled with AV nodal blocking agents

It is very difficult to keep patients with structural heart disease in normal sinus rhythm. Several studies have shown an increase in overall mortality with rhythm control. Catheter-directed ablation of the AV node or accessory pathway may also be used when pharmacological treatment fails to control rate.

The rate control goal is 60–80 bpm at rest and 90–115 bpm with moderate exercise. Medications that might be used for **rate control** are diltiazem, beta-blockers, verapamil, or digoxin. Most patients require combined therapy. B-blockers with digoxin have been shown to be the best combination. Digoxin should be used for rate control in patients with CHF first; amiodarone can be used as second-line therapy. B-blockers should be started with caution in CHF patients once they are euvolemic on exam.

Agents for chemical cardioversion in A-fib: amiodarone, dofetilide, flecainide, ibutilide, propafenone. In CHF patients, use amiodarone and dofetelide.

Agents for maintaining sinus rhythm: flecainide, propafenone, sotalol, dofetilide, and amiodarone. To maintain normal sinus rhythm in CHF patients, use only amiodarone or dofetilide. In patients with coronary artery disease, dofetilide and sotalol are superior to amiodarone.

- The CHADS$_2$ score is used to determine if a patient with non-valvular A-fib needs anticoagulation.

CHADS$_2$ Score	Treatment
0	Give aspirin
1	Give aspirin or anticoagulation
≥2	Give anticoagulation

Dabigatran is an oral direct thrombin inhibitor that has been shown to reduce the incidence of ischemic stroke compared to warfarin, with similar rates of bleeding. Rivaroxaban is an oral factor Xa inhibitor. For anticoagulation, you can use coumadin, dabigatran, or rivaroxaban. Apixaban, another oral factor Xa inhibitor, may be used instead of coumadin for stroke prophalaxis in patients with atrial fibrillation and a high risk of stroke (CHADS$_2$ score of 2 or higher). All 3 drugs—dabigatran, rivaroxaban, and apixaban—lead to similar or lower rates both of ischemic stroke and major bleeding compared to coumadin; there is no need for monitoring INR.

Note

Atrial fibrillation and flutter are routinely rate-controlled with anticoagulation with aspirin, warfarin, dabigatran, or rivaroxaban.

Note

CHADS$_2$ RISKS:
- **C**HF
- **H**TN
- **A**ge >75
- **D**iabetes mellitus
- **S**troke (gives 2 points)

Important additional advantages of these newer agents include convenience (no requirement for routine testing of the international normalized ratio), a small reduction in the risk of intracranial hemorrhage, and less susceptibility to dietary and drug interactions.

Disadvantages include lack of an antidote and the potential that new side effects may be seen over time.

For patients undergoing elective cardioversion, first determine if they have been in A-fib for >48 hours. If they have, there are 2 options:

- Transesophageal echo can be done to exclude a clot; then, cardioversion (electrical or chemical). Cardioversion should be followed by 6 weeks of coumadin.
- Coumadin can be administered for 3 weeks before electrical or chemical cardioversion. Cardioversion should be followed by another 6 weeks of coumadin.

> **Note**
>
> Patients with A-fib and thyrotoxicosis always get anticoagulation until euthyroid and back in NSR.

It is very difficult to maintain patients with structural heart disease in NSR, and most convert back into atrial fibrillation. Atrial flutter is managed the same way as atrial fibrillation.

For patients in A-fib with Wolff-Parkinson-White syndrome, administration of drugs which slow AV node conduction (Ca-channel blockers, digoxin) is strongly contraindicated as they can induce VT. Procainamide, ibutilide, flecanide, or amiodarone can be used in such cases.

If none of the medications described above can successfully convert the patient to a normal sinus rhythm, then elective electrical cardioversion can be attempted. This too must be preceded and followed by several weeks of anticoagulation if the A-fib has been present for >48 hours. Transesophageal echo can be done to exclude a clot and allow the cardioversion without preconversion anticoagulation. Neither medical nor electrical cardioversion can permanently maintain the majority of patients on sinus rhythm. Most convert back into atrial fibrillation.

Bradycardia

> A 48-year-old manager comes for advice about vaccinations and travel medicine before traveling to a far-off land. He feels well and has no symptoms. He takes no medications. On examination you find a blood pressure 118/76 mm Hg and pulse 40/min.

Definition. A slow heart with a rate <60 beats/min.

Etiology. Sinus bradycardia can be a normal phenomenon, particularly in trained athletes. Medications such as beta-blockers can also give a sinus bradycardia without serious sequelae. Symptomatic sinus bradycardia from sinus node disease can be from degeneration of the node or from ischemia. More serious types of bradycardia can be from Mobitz type II second-degree heart block and third-degree (complete) heart block. These can occur secondary to ischemic damage of the AV node. Other causes are myocarditis, infiltrative disease, such as amyloidosis or sarcoidosis, or neoplasms.

Clinical Presentation. This can range from the lifelong absence of symptoms to severe symptoms of hypotension and decreased cardiac output.

Diagnosis. EKG

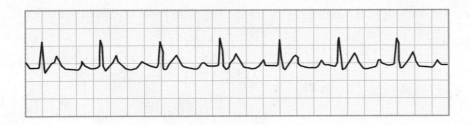

Figure 10-11. First-Degree Heart Block

Note

Mobitz type I second-degree block is characterized by *progressive* P-R lengthening, whereas in Mobitz-type II, the P-R interval remains constant.

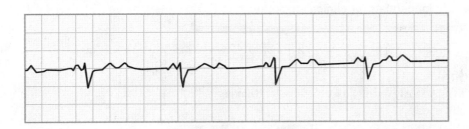

Figure 10-12. Second-Degree Heart Block

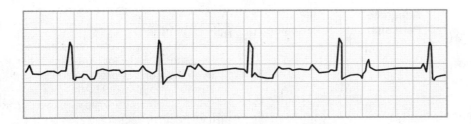

Figure 10-13. Complete Heart Block

Note

Transcutaneous pacing is always preferred over transvenous pacing in the acute setting.

Treatment. Asymptomatic sinus bradycardia, first-degree AV block, and Mobitz type I (Wenckebach) second-degree AV block often need no specific therapy. Any form of severe symptomatic bradycardia is treated initially with atropine and then a pacemaker, if there is no improvement in symptoms.

Mobitz type II second-degree block and third-degree block require the placement of a pacemaker, even in the absence of symptoms. Dopamine or epinephrine is used to improve blood pressure if there is still hypotension after the use of atropine.

For symptomatic sinus bradycardia, treatment is atropine. If atropine fails, then use transcutaneous pacing.

Note

- If the patient is on a beta blocker, give glucagon.

- If the patient is on a calcium channel blocker, give calcium.

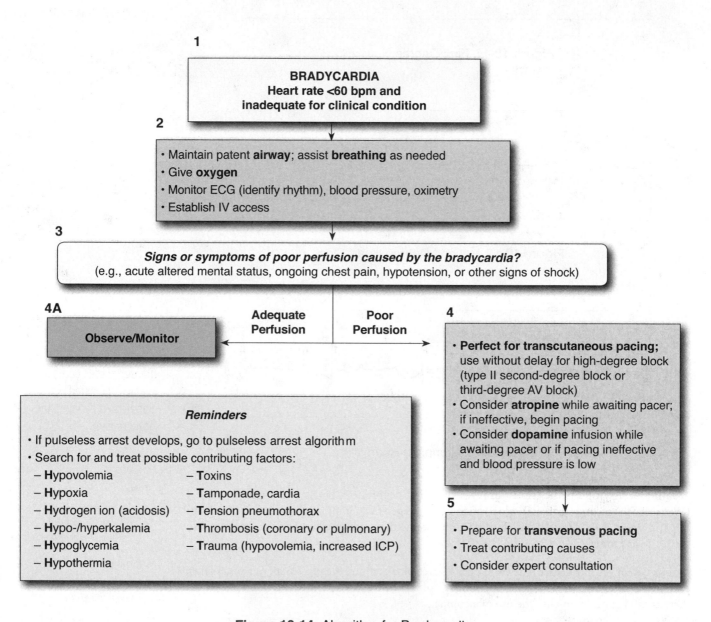

Figure 10-14. Algorithm for Bradycardia

TOXICOLOGY: GENERAL PRINCIPLES/INITIAL EVALUATION

A 25-year-old medical student goes home after class and finds no messages on the answering machine from his girlfriend. In a fit of despair he takes a full bottle of pills in an attempt to commit suicide. He takes the label off the bottle to prevent any attempt to reverse the poisoning through the identification of the specific agent. Immediately after doing this, his girlfriend calls, after which he runs to the nearest emergency department and states that he has changed his mind and wants to live after all. He walks into the emergency department 30 minutes after the ingestion. He won't tell you the specific name of what he took and wants to know what is the next best thing to do.

Management. The initial evaluation of a patient who has been poisoned involves attempting to find out the nature of the toxin ingested. At the same time, history and physical examination can give clues to the nature of the toxin. In this patient, the key issue is the short time between the ingestion and his arrival in the emergency department. He is awake.

Toxidromes

Associated physical findings in specific toxidromes

- Miosis: clonidine, barbiturates, opiates, cholinergics, pontine stroke
- Mydriasis: sympathomimetics, anticholinergics
- Dry skin: anticholinergics
- Wet skin: cholinergics, sympathomimetics
- Blisters: barbiturates, carbon monoxide poisoning

Management of Toxic Ingestions or Overdose

Gastric emptying is rarely, if ever, utilized. In ingestions of an unknown type, a urine or blood toxicology screen should be performed, but this should not delay the administration of antidotes, charcoal, or gastric emptying in the rare circumstances in which emptying is indicated.

- **Induced vomiting.** Ipecac can only be used within 1-2 hours after ingestion, so it has no use in the hospital setting. Very few people arrive within the first hour. In addition, ipecac can delay the use of oral antidotes such as charcoal or N-acetyl cysteine because of the vomiting it induces. Ipecac is more useful for ingestions in the home, in which the time period since ingestion is short and there are no other effective modalities immediately available. Ipecac decreases absorption by 60% at 5 minutes after ingestion, 32% at 30 minutes, and 30% at one hour. Ipecac is never recommended for use in children.
- **Lavage.** Gastric emptying with a large-bore (37-42 French) oropharyngeal hose (e.g., an Ewald tube) should only be used in those with an altered mental status and in whom ipecac is dangerous because of possible aspiration. Lavage should therefore be preceded by endotracheal intubation. Lavage is also only useful within the first hour after ingestion, and is therefore very rarely, if at all, useful any more. Both ipecac and lavage are contraindicated with the ingestion of caustic substances such as acids or alkalis. Lavage decreases absorption by 52% at 5 minutes, 26% at 30 minutes, and 16% at 60 minutes. The exact indications for lavage are not clear, however, the contraindications are very clear.

Note

- Ipecac is never used by physicians.

- Lavage has almost no utility.

Note

Charcoal does not bind to some substances (**PHAILS**):

- **P**esticides
- **H**eavy metals
- **A**cid/alkali/alcohol
- **I**ron
- **L**ithium
- **S**olvents

Note

Substances/drugs that may require hemodialysis for removal include (**I STUMBLE**):

- **I**sopropanol
- **S**alicylates
- **T**heophylline
- **U**remia
- **M**ethanol
- **B**arbiturates
- **L**ithium
- **E**thylene glycol

- **Charcoal.** After gastric emptying or if, as in most cases, the patient arrives >1-2 hours after the ingestion, the mainstay of therapy is activated charcoal administration. Repeated doses every 2-4 hours are recommended to both block further absorption of the substance and to accelerate the removal of already absorbed toxins from the body. Charcoal is safe for all patients.

- **Whole bowel irrigation.** For large-volume pill ingestions in which the pills can be seen on an x-ray, whole bowel irrigation can be effective. A gastric tube is placed and high-volume (1-2 liters per hour) GoLYTELY (polyethylene glycol) is administered until the bowel movements run clear.

- **Dialysis.** Dialysis is rarely necessary because the time delay to its initiation limits its efficacy. If it is necessary, hemodialysis is 20x more efficacious at removing drugs from the body than peritoneal dialysis. Dialysis is your answer when there are profoundly serious symptoms such as coma, hypotension, or apnea, especially when renal or hepatic failure limits the usual means of excreting substances from the body.

- **Cathartics.** Cathartics are useful when used with charcoal administration. Otherwise, they are almost never helpful. When you see cathartics in the answer, it is generally the wrong answer.

- **Forced diuresis.** Alkaline diuresis can help eliminate salicylates and phenobarbital. Otherwise, simply making patients urinate in high volumes does not help the patient. Except for salicylates and phenobarbital, forced diuresis is generally the wrong answer.

- **Naloxone/dextrose/thiamine.** These agents should be given first to any patient who presents with altered mental status or coma. They are particularly useful in any toxin ingestion that produces confusion. Naloxone has almost no adverse effects and works instantly. Because of its rapid response, naloxone is both therapeutic and diagnostic. Dextrose is also very effective at preventing permanent brain damage from hypoglycemia. It does not matter whether the dextrose or thiamine is given first.

Remember: Any toxin-related seizure should be treated with benzodiazepines as first-line therapy. When benzodiazepines are not effective, barbiturates should be used next. Phenytoin and fosphenytoin are not indicated or even effective for this type of seizure.

ACETAMINOPHEN

A 38-year-old man comes to the emergency department 4 days after the ingestion of a full bottle (60 tablets) of acetaminophen (500 mg each). He complains of vomiting and right upper quadrant pain. He has an elevated bilirubin, AST, and prothrombin time.

Definition. Acetaminophen is one of the few toxins about which precise toxicity levels are known; the ingestion of approximately 140 mg per kg is usually sufficient to cause serious toxicity. In other words, in an average-sized, 70-kg person, about 7–10 grams is enough to produce toxicity, and fatalities can occur >12–15 grams. In those patients with liver disease or concomitant alcohol abuse and thus depleted glutathione stores, the hepatotoxic dose is less (4 grams/day).

Clinical Presentation. As with most large-dose pill ingestions, the initial symptoms are nausea and vomiting, caused mostly from a gastritis caused by irritation from the pills over the first 12-24 hours (Stage I). Between 24-72 hours (Stage II), there often follows an asymptomatic period as the acetaminophen is metabolized and part of the drug is converted to a toxic metabolite. Starting at

24-48 hours, subclinical elevation of the transaminases and bilirubin develops. This is followed at 48-72 hours after ingestion by clinically symptomatic signs of liver damage: more nausea, jaundice, abdominal pain, and signs of hepatic encephalopathy, renal failure, and death.

Diagnosis. A clear history of a large volume of acetaminophen ingestion is initially sufficient to establish a diagnosis that warrants therapy with N-acetyl cysteine (NAC). Starting at 4 hours after ingestion, when most of the drug has been absorbed, drug levels are reliable. A nomogram based on relating the drug level to the time of ingestion is necessary to determine who will develop toxicity. In other words, a level by itself is not enough to determine who will develop toxicity. A certain level at 5 or 6 hours may not be toxic; however, the same level at 10–12 hours after ingestion may lead to the development of liver failure.

Elevated AST is more common than elevated ALT. If a patient is known for alcohol abuse and presents with AST and ALT >500 U/L, the diagnosis is more likely to be acetaminophen toxicity than alcoholic hepatitis. NAC should be given in such cases. Elevated bilirubin and prothrombin time indicates severe toxicity and hepatic necrosis. Studies show that NAC administration within the first 8 hours of severe drug poisoning improves liver microcirculation and prevents the need for liver transplant.

Treatment. Gastric emptying should not be used because it will delay the administration of NAC as a specific antidote. Activated charcoal is given in repeated doses. NAC is preferably given within 8 hours of the ingestion, when it is most efficacious. When >24 hours have elapsed since ingestion, there is no specific therapy that can prevent or reverse the toxicity, but still give NAC always. NAC and charcoal are superior to any form of gastric emptying.

ALCOHOLS (METHANOL AND ETHYLENE GLYCOL)

At the opera, you go to see the Three Tenors, who exhibit confusion, ataxia, lethargy, drowsiness, and slurred speech; which is to say, you have really gone to see the Three *Drunken* Tenors. How would you distinguish between the tenors drunk on methanol or ethylene glycol from those drunk on simple ethanol?

Etiology. Methanol (wood alcohol) is found in paint thinner, sterno, photocopier fluid, solvents, and windshield washer solution. Ethylene glycol is most often found in automotive antifreeze. All of the alcohols are metabolized by alcohol dehydrogenase. Alcohol dehydrogenase metabolizes methanol to formaldehyde and formic acid. Ethylene glycol is metabolized partially to oxalic acid and oxalate, which leads to kidney damage.

Clinical Presentation. Ethanol, methanol, ethylene glycol, and isopropyl alcohol can all produce intoxication. Methanol is more characteristically associated with visual disturbances up to and including blindness from the production of formic acid. Ethylene glycol is distinguished by the development of renal failure and oxalate crystals and stones in the urine. Isopropyl alcohol ingestion can only be distinguished before a specific drug level is done by the history or by the development of acidosis in the absence of an elevated anion gap.

Diagnosis. Determining specific levels of each alcohol is the most specific test. Ethylene glycol is characterized by oxalate crystals in the urine, increasing BUN/creatinine, or by adding fluorescein to the urine and then observing for urine fluorescence with an ultraviolet Wood's lamp. Ingestion of methanol and ethylene glycol will be characterized by an increased serum osmolar gap and metabolic acidosis with an elevated anion gap. Isopropyl alcohol will produce an osmolar gap without an increased anion gap. Remember this difference when differentiating them. Ethylene glycol intoxication may also be characterized by hypocalcemia.

Note

Ingestion of methanol, ethylene glycol, and isopropyl alcohol will all result in an osmolar gap.

Note

Charcoal will not inhibit the absorption of alcohols.

Treatment. Ethylene glycol and methanol intoxication were previously treated with an ethanol infusion (to prevent the production of the toxic metabolites) followed by hemodialysis to remove the substance from the body. Fomepizole (alcohol dehydrogenase inhibitor) is the drug of choice. Fomepizole inhibits the production of toxic metabolites without leading to intoxication. Dialysis can be used in patients with severe anion gap metabolic acidosis or signs of end-organ damage (coma, seizures, renal failure).

CARBON MONOXIDE (CO)

> You are the chief resident at a great metropolitan training program at the time of a fire at a large office building. A total of 2,500 people come to your emergency department at the same time to be treated for smoke inhalation. Among them is a 68-year-old man with a history of aortic stenosis who had to walk down 90 flights of stairs. What is the most important initial test for this man?

Note

In the winter of Northern climates, space heaters are a common cause of carbon monoxide poisoning. Headache is the most common symptom. Nausea is also very common.

Source. Poisoning with CO occurs with exposure to various forms of burning materials, such as gasoline, wood, and natural gas, and with entrapment in fires and smoke inhalation. Low levels of CO poisoning are present in most tobacco smokers. CO itself is odorless and tasteless.

Metabolism. CO binds to hemoglobin 200 times more avidly than oxygen. Carboxyhemoglobin decreases release of oxygen to tissues and inhibits mitochondria. This results in tissue hypoxia and anaerobic metabolism similar to what would occur with anemia.

Clinical Presentation. Pulmonary symptoms include dyspnea, tachypnea, and shortness of breath. Cardiac symptoms include chest pain, arrhythmia, and hypotension.

Early neurologic symptoms include headache (most common), nausea, blurry vision, and dizziness, while late symptoms include confusion, seizures, impaired judgment, and syncope.

Laboratory. Carboxyhemoglobin levels can give an indication of the severity of the exposure.

<10%:	Levels up to 10% may occur in city dwellers who are smokers
20-30%:	Mild symptoms
30-50%:	Moderate to severe symptoms
>50-60%:	May be fatal

Note

CO poisoning initially presents just like hypoglycemia. When a fingerstick glucose is normal, this should raise your suspicions.

Influenza is the most common misdiagnosis because most people present during wintertime. When an entire family presents with "flu" symptoms without fever, think CO poisoning.

- Arterial blood gases or venous blood gases. Metabolic acidosis is present from the failure of carboxyhemoglobin to release oxygen to tissues. The pO_2 will be normal.
- CPK may be elevated.
- Pulse oximetry is not helpful.

Treatment

- Removal from source of exposure
- 100% oxygen administration
- Hyperbaric oxygen in severe cases
  - COHb levels >25%
  - Myocardial ischemia

- EKG changes
- CNS abnormalities other than headache or chest pain
- Pregnant women when carboxyhemoglobin levels >15%

In room air, carbon monoxide has a half-life of 4-6 hours, which decreases to 40-80 minutes on 100% oxygen and to 15-30 minutes with hyperbaric oxygen.

CAUSTICS/CORROSIVES (ACIDS AND ALKALI)

Definition. The oral ingestion, inhalation, or cutaneous or ocular contact with a wide variety of corrosive substances.

Etiology. The most common household acids are various toilet, drain, swimming pool, and metal cleaners. The most common alkali ingestions or exposures are from liquid and crystalline lye, dishwasher detergents, hair relaxers, and oven cleaners. The most common serious injury is from the oral ingestion of liquid drain cleaner.

Clinical Presentation. The most common symptoms from ingestion injury are oral pain, drooling, odynophagia, and abdominal pain. Esophageal injury with subsequent stricture formation may occur from either acid or alkali ingestion. Gastric perforation may occur. In most circumstances, alkali exposures are more serious than acid exposures. Alkaline substances are more destructive to tissues.

Diagnosis. The history of exposure with subsequent characteristic injury is sufficient to establish the diagnosis. Upper endoscopy is critical for determining the extent of the injury.

Treatment. The management of both acid and alkali caustic ingestions is essentially the same. Immediately wash out the mouth with large volumes of cold water. Irrigate ocular exposures with large volumes of either saline or water, followed by fluorescein staining to determine if there is significant corneal injury. **Do not induce emesis** with either acids or alkaline ingestion because it can worsen the injury. Simply give water. **Do not try to neutralize the acid** with a base or a base with an acid because a heat-producing reaction can occur, which would destroy more tissue. Charcoal is not useful, nor are steroids or prophylactic antibiotics.

DIGOXIN

Epidemiology. Poisoning occurs from a suicide attempt or accidentally during therapeutic use. Poisoning is more common with renal failure because 60% of digoxin is normally excreted renally, and it will accumulate. **Hypokalemia** predisposes to toxicity because potassium and digoxin bind to the same site on the sodium-potassium ATPase pump, leading to increased intracellular calcium → increased cardiac contractility.

Presentation. GI symptoms are most common: nausea, vomiting, diarrhea, and anorexia. Neurologic and visual symptoms include blurred vision, color vision abnormality, hallucinations, and confusion. Cardiac disturbance is predominantly secondary to arrhythmia.

Laboratory. EKG abnormalities are most common. Bradycardia, premature contractions, ventricular tachycardia, and any other type of arrhythmias may be seen. Paroxysmal atrial tachycardia is the most common arrhythmia. Hyperkalemia occurs acutely from inhibition of Na^+/K^+ ATPase by digoxin. A serum digoxin level should be ordered in patients you suspect of being toxic (history, etc.).

Treatment

- GI decontamination with repeated doses of *charcoal* is effective.
- Digoxin-specific antibodies (Digibind®) are useful for life-threatening toxicity, particularly with arrhythmias.
- Electrolyte abnormality correction: *Potassium correction* is most important.
- Antiarrhythmic medications, such as phenytoin and lidocaine, are used as necessary with ventricular arrhythmias.
- Pacemaker placement may be necessary for bradycardia or third-degree AV block refractory to atropine.

DRUGS OF ABUSE

Opiates

Opiate toxicity is predominantly respiratory related, via depressant effects upon the respiratory centers in the brain stem. Death can occur through acute respiratory acidosis. In addition to their analgesic and euphoric effects, opiates also cause pupillary constriction, constipation, bradycardia, hypothermia, and hypotension. Opiates can be rapidly reversed by naloxone. Although withdrawal of opiates is uncomfortable, it is not fatal. It is usually treated with methadone or buprenorphine. Opiate withdrawal symptoms are the following.

- 3–4 hours: fear, anxiety, and drug craving
- 8–14 hours: insomnia, yawning, rhinorrhea, diaphoresis, mydriasis, anxiety
- 1–3 days: tremor, muscle spasms, vomiting, diarrhea, tachycardia, chills, piloerection

Cocaine

Pathophysiology. Cocaine blocks the reuptake of norepinephrine and other catecholamines at the synapse. This leads to a wide variety of euphoric and toxic effects. Amphetamines work in a similar way but are less likely to produce severe toxicity or death. Severe toxicity from cocaine is far more likely with smoked ("crack") or injected cocaine rather than snorted (inhaled).

Clinical Presentation. Toxic effects of cocaine are related to a very significant alpha-adrenergic stimulatory effect, resulting in very high blood pressure, hemorrhagic stroke, subarachnoid hemorrhage, myocardial infarction, arrhythmia, and seizures. These may lead to death. Metabolic acidosis, rhabdomyolysis, and hyperthermia may also occur with cocaine toxicity. Pulmonary edema is specific to smoked cocaine. Cocaine withdrawal results in depression from norepinephrine depletion. There is limited physiologic withdrawal from cocaine.

Treatment. Benzodiazepines such as diazepam are used to control acute agitation. Combined alpha/beta agents such as labetalol or alpha-blockers such as phentolamine are useful to control hypertension. Pure beta-blockers should be avoided because they lead to unopposed alpha stimulatory effects. There is no specific drug to reverse cocaine.

Benzodiazepines

These drugs produce somnolence, dysarthria, ataxia, and stupor. Benzodiazepines very rarely result in death from respiratory depression. Most deaths from benzodiazepine ingestion are in association with ethanol or barbiturate ingestion. Benzodiazepine withdrawal can be similar to the symptoms of alcohol withdrawal. Flumazenil is the specific antidote but should be only occasionally used. Acute withdrawal from flumazenil use can result in seizures.

Barbiturates

This is a class of drugs with a large variety of long- and short-acting agents. Massive overdose can result in death from respiratory depression or CNS depression. Barbiturates can cause hypothermia, loss of deep tendon reflexes, and loss of corneal reflexes, and could result in a coma simulating brain death. Barbiturates may lead to absent EEG activity. Barbiturate withdrawal may result in seizures similar to alcohol or benzodiazepine withdrawal. Although there is no specific antidote for any of the barbiturates, you can increase the urinary excretion of phenobarbital by the use of bicarbonate. This is similar to the treatment for salicylate intoxication.

Hallucinogens

This includes a wide variety of agents such marijuana, LSD, mescaline, peyote, and psilocybin. Although they may cause delirium and bizarre behavior, the adverse effects are often limited to their anticholinergic effects, such as flushed skin, dry mouth, dilated pupils, and urinary retention. The only hallucinogen associated with a potentially fatal outcome is the artificially created, dissociative, anesthetic phencyclidine (PCP or "angel dust"), which may cause seizures. Treatment for severe hallucinogen intoxication is with benzodiazepines.

HEAVY METALS

Lead

Epidemiology/Source. Up to 12 million preschool children per year may be affected in the United States. Lead is ingested from paint, soil, dust, drinking water, and in the past from gasoline.

Metabolism. Lead can be absorbed from the GI tract, the skin, or by inhalation. GI absorption is increased by deficiencies of zinc, iron, and calcium.

Excretion is primarily through the urine (80–90%), with the remainder through the stool. Lead poisoning is primarily a chronic condition, not acute.

Clinical Presentation

- Adults: Abdominal pain, anemia, renal disease, and neurologic manifestations, such as headache and memory loss. Hypertension can occur as well.
- Children: Acute: abdominal pain, anemia, lethargy, seizures, and coma; chronic: irreversible neurologic damage, such as mental retardation and poor cognitive and behavioral function.

Laboratory. *Blood lead levels* are the key to diagnosis and <10 µg/dL is considered acceptable. "Lead lines" are densities seen at the metaphyseal plate of the long bones of children. They indicate long-term exposure. Anemia and azotemia occur.

Treatment

- Chelation with calcium EDTA, dimercaprol (BAL), penicillamine, or succimer (oral therapy)
- In acute lead poisoning, patients should undergo GI decontamination with charcoal. Urine output should be maintained at a rate of 1–2 mL/kg/hr to aid in maximal excretion.

Note

Think *lead* in patients with microcytic anemia and abdominal pain.

Mercury

Source. A variety of inorganic and organic sources, such as thermometers, sphygmomanometers, cathartic medicines, paints, and cosmetics. Industrial exposure can lead to significant inhalation injury.

Metabolism. Mercury is absorbed through the skin, GI tract, and lungs. The majority of cases are due to industrial inhalation in manufacturing plants. It easily *crosses the blood-brain barrier.* It is concentrated in the brain, kidneys, and RBCs.

Presentation

- Pulmonary symptoms of interstitial pneumonitis occur from inhalation.
- Neurologic symptoms can be irreversible. These are tremors, excitability, memory loss, delirium, and insomnia—collectively known as *"erethism."*
- GI symptoms such as nausea, vomiting, pain, and bleeding occur from oral ingestion.

Treatment

- Removal from source
- Oral chelation with succimer or dimercaprol is preferred

SALICYLATES

An elderly woman with osteoarthritis comes to the emergency department with dyspnea, intractable nausea, vomiting, and tinnitus. She is fully alert and able to give a good history. Her only other problem is hypertension. She is on a wide variety of medications to reduce her pain. Her husband says she was in so much pain lately that she took half a bottle of extra pills 30 minutes ago.

Definition. Salicylate intoxication results from the ingestion of a large amount of aspirin and other salicylate-containing medications, resulting in a complex, systemic toxicity.

Clinical Presentation. The most common presentation is GI distress, such as nausea, vomiting, and gastritis. Salicylates are complex metabolic poisons. Tinnitus is one of the more specific complaints and is one of the best ways to identify the case, so as to answer the question: "Which of the following is the most likely diagnosis?" Salicylates affect respiratory function in 2 ways: They directly stimulate the respiratory centers in the brainstem to cause a centrally mediated hyperventilation and hyperpnea; in addition, they are directly toxic to the lungs themselves and can cause a noncardiogenic pulmonary edema similar to ARDS. Hyperthermia is possible. CNS toxicity such as confusion, coma, seizures, and encephalopathy can also occur. This can cause death. Salicylates also interfere with Krebs cycle and lead to a metabolic acidosis through the reversion to anaerobic glycolysis as a method of energy production in the body. In other words, salicylates lead to significant lactic acid production with metabolic acidosis and an elevated anion gap. This ultimately results in a compensatory respiratory alkalosis.

Diagnosis. The most specific test is an *aspirin level.* Suggestive findings are an *elevated anion gap* with *metabolic acidosis.* However, a respiratory alkalosis may be the predominant defect, especially early on. Hence the blood gas can show a low pH, a high pH, or a normal pH. An elevated prothrombin time and hypoglycemia may also occur. The chest x-ray may be normal or occasionally show pulmonary edema.

Treatment. If the patient comes within the first hour after ingestion, gastric decontamination may be attempted. Charcoal is also useful, as it is in many types of ingestions. The mainstay of therapy, however, is by trying to *increase urinary excretion by alkalization of the urine* along with aggressive fluid resuscitation to maximize urinary output. When the urinary pH rises, this will charge the salicylate molecule, which is a weak acid. This will block the reabsorption of the substance at the kidney tubule. Dialysis is sometimes necessary.

Indications for dialysis:

- Renal failure
- CHF
- ARDS
- Persistent CNS symptoms (confusion/seizures)
- Hemodynamic instability
- Severe acid/base or electrolyte imbalance
- Hepatic failure with coagulopathy
- Salicylate level >100 mg/dL

TRICYCLIC ANTIDEPRESSANTS

A 28-year-old man with a history of depression comes to the emergency department one hour after a suicide attempt with his tricyclic antidepressants and benzodiazepines. He is stuporous with a respiratory rate of 7/min. An EKG shows a wide QRS. What would you do next?

Etiology/Pathophysiology. Tricyclic antidepressants (TCAs) are characterized by a number of anticholinergic and sodium channel blocker side effects. This is the predominant cause of their cardiac and CNS toxicities.

Clinical Presentation. The most common adverse effects are *anticholinergic*-mediated findings of dry mouth, tachycardia, dilated pupils, and flushed skin. A quick onset with rapid deterioration is common. The most serious effects are cardiac dysrhythmia with *widening of the QRS complex*, resulting in ventricular tachycardia and first-degree conduction blocks. CNS effects include altered mental status, confusion, and seizure.

Diagnosis. Serum drug levels are the most specific test, but an EKG showing abnormalities is more important to determine who will have serious toxicity. The EKG may be normal or show any range of ventricular or atrial arrhythmias or conduction delays.

Treatment. TCA overdose has anticholinergic side effects, which include impaired peristalsis and delayed gastric emptying. Charcoal is the primary treatment in the acute setting. Any sign of cardiac toxicity should lead to the immediate use of bicarbonate. *Bicarbonate protects the heart from the TCAs.* Bicarbonate is not to increase urinary excretion (as opposed to the treatment of aspirin overdose). This case also shows why patients with benzodiazepine ingestions should generally not be treated with flumazenil. Flumazenil would reverse the effects of the benzodiazepines and therefore lead to a seizure.

ANTICHOLINERGIC POISONING

A 65-year-old man is brought to the emergency department by his wife with lethargy and confusion. She says that he has had a cold and has taken over-the-counter cold preparations for the last few days. On examination he is confused and does not recognize his wife. His temperature is 39.2° C (102.5° F), pulse 130/min and blood pressure 100/60 mm Hg. The skin is flushed, dry, and warm. The eyes are dilated.

Definition. Anticholingeric overdose may occur in any age group with high dose, but most commonly presents in the elderly. Anticholinergic drugs competitively inhibit binding of the neurotransmitter acetylcholine to muscarinic acetylcholine receptors, and are commonly called "antimuscarinic agents." Muscarinic receptors are found on peripheral postganglionic cholinergic nerves in smooth muscle (intestinal, bronchial, and cardiac), in secretory glands (salivary and sweat), on the ciliary body of the eye, and in the central nervous system (CNS). Anticholinergic agents do not antagonize the effects at nicotinic acetylcholine receptors, such as at the neuro-muscular junction.

The onset of anticholinergic toxicity varies depending on the particular toxin, but usually occurs within 1–2 hours of oral ingestion. Some drugs may take up to 12 hours to have an effect. Be aware with patients on psychotropic agents.

The following medications may cause anticholinergic effects:

- Diphenhydramine
- Scopolamine and hyoscyamine
- TCAs
- Cyclobenzaprine
- Benztropine
- Belladonna

Clinical Presentation. Patients will present with the following characteristics:

- "Red as a beet": flushed, red skin due to cutaneous vasodialation
- "Dry as a bone": dry skin (anhydrosis) due to inability to sweat
- "Hot as a hair" anhydrotic hyperthermia
- "Blind as a bat": mydriasis
- "Mad as a hatter": delirium, psychosis, hallucinations, and seizures
- "Full as a flask": urinary retention and absent bowel sounds
- Tachycardia

Treatment. ABCs, supportive care, EKG monitoring. Anticholinergic poisoning may also cause prolonged QRS and QT intervals. In that case, sodium bicarbonate can be used to stabilize the myocyte membrane and prevent ventricular tachycardia. If a patient develops seizures, treat with benzodiazepines, NOT with phenytoin or fosphenytoin.

ORGANOPHOSPHATES

Etiology. Inhibits cholinesterase and has muscarinic and nicotinic effects. Patients will be farmers or gardeners.

Nicotinic effects are weakness and decreased respiratory drive. Muscarinic effects are as follows, otherwise known as DUMBELSS syndrome:

- Defecation
- Urinary incontinence
- Muscle weakness, miosis
- Bradycardia/bronchospasm
- Emesis
- Lacrimation
- Salivation
- Seizure

Diagnosis. Check RBC cholinesterase levels. Do not delay treatment while waiting for results.

Treatment. First step is for physician to put on protective clothing, as organophosphates are absorbed by the skin. Then, have patient remove clothing immediately. Start atropine immediately to treat the bradycardia. Start pralidoxime (2-PAM), which restores cholinesterase activity and reverses both the nicotinic and muscarinic effects.

ALCOHOL

A 35-year-old man is brought to the emergency department by his wife after he had a seizure. He is agitated and combative. He is yelling and trying to hit the nurses, and tells you that he is in France. He is also yelling at his mother, who is not in the room. His wife tells you that he drinks a liter of whiskey a day, though he has not had any in the last few days because he didn't have the money. His pulse is 130/min, blood pressure 160/90 mm Hg, and respirations 24/min. He is diaphoretic and extremely irritable. His temperature is 38° C (100.4° F). The rest of the exam is unremarkable.

Presentation. Alcoholics may present with any one of the following:

Mild withdrawal:

Symptoms are tremors, tachycardia, and anxiety. Seizures may be seen 6–12 hours after the last drink.

Delirium tremens (DT):
- Manifests 48–72 hours after the last drink but can last up to 10 days
- Mental confusion
- Autonomic hyperactivity
- Visual hallucinations
- Severe agitation
- Diaphoresis

Note

The diagnosis of all alcohol withdrawal–related syndromes is made clinically, not by lab values.

Alcoholic hallucinosis:

- May be confused with DT
- Starts 12–24 hours after last drink but can last days to weeks
- Paranoid psychosis without tremors and confusion
- Normal vital signs (no hypertension or tachycardia)
- No agitation
- Normal appearance except for auditory (most common), visual, or tactile hallucinations

Wernicke encephalopathy:

- Confusion, ataxia, and ophthalmoplegia (nystagmus)

Korsakoff psychosis:

- Amnesia and confabulations

Treatment. Alcohol withdrawal has a very high mortality rate (5%).

Benzodiazepines can be life-saving (important to taper dose slowly). Diazepam and chlordiazepoxide are common, due to their long half-life. There is no role for anticonvulsants.

Antipsychotics such as haloperidol should be avoided because they can lower the seizure threshold and cause prolonged QT interval.

Hydrate with isotonic fluids and electrolyte replacement.

Symptom-triggered therapy is recommended. A work-up for alternative diagnosis is also very important.

- Use only lorazepam or oxazepam for cirrhosis
- CT head to look for intracranial bleed
- Lumbar puncture to rule out meningitis if there is a fever
- Chest x-ray: look for aspiration pneumonia
- High doses of thiamine IV for Wernicke and Korsakoff. Treatment for alchoholic hallucinosis is benzodiazipines and haldoperidol (there is no risk of siezures, so it can be used here)

HEAD TRAUMA

A 20-year-old man is playing football when he is struck in the head and loses consciousness for a few minutes. He awakens and has some motor weakness of his left arm, which seems to slowly worsen over the course of the next hour as he is brought to the emergency department.

Definition. Any degree of traumatic brain injury resulting in a range of injury from scalp laceration to headache to loss of consciousness or focal neurologic deficits. The term does not imply a specific mechanism of injury. The injury can result in concussion, contusion, epidural hematoma, subdural hematoma, or traumatic subarachnoid hemorrhage. Cerebral contusion can progress to intraparenchymal hemorrhage.

Clinical Presentation. The presentation is often only suggestive of the degree of injury. The specific injury can only be determined by the use of CT scanning. All forms of head trauma can result in headache, amnesia, and loss of consciousness. The degree of amnesia is loosely associated with the degree of head trauma. That is to say, the worse the trauma, the more memory one loses. Memory loss starts from the time of the episode of injury and stretches both forward (anterograde), in which one doesn't remember events since the time of the injury, as well as backward (retrograde), in which one forgets past events. Retrograde amnesia starts from the time of the injury and moves further back in time depending on the severity of the injury. The more severe the injury, the further back in time you forget. Retrograde amnesia is more common. Recovery of memory starts with recollection of the most distant progressing to the most recent memories.

Loss of consciousness, although possible in any form of head trauma, is not always present, even with relatively severe forms of brain injury. You can have very severe intracranial bleeding (such as a subdural hematoma) without a loss of consciousness. This is particularly true of chronic subdural hematoma.

Concussion is generally not associated with focal neurologic findings, such as motor or sensory deficits. The presence of focal findings, starting in order of highest frequency, is most commonly associated with epidural and subdural hematomas and contusion.

Diagnosis. CT scanning of the head is the mainstay of diagnosis of brain injury. Contrast enhancement is not necessary because blood does not enhance with contrast. Hemorrhage should be visible instantly if present at the time of the initial presentation. When evaluating head CT scans, subdural hematomas are crescent-shaped and epidural hematomas are lens-shaped. Follow-up scanning is also accomplished with CT scanning when necessary. Skull x-rays are always the wrong answer when presented as one of the diagnostic choices. Normal x-rays do not exclude hemorrhage, and abnormal x-rays do not confirm the presence of a hemorrhage. Cervical spine x-rays should be obtained in head trauma if there are focal findings consistent with a cervical radiculopathy or if spinal tenderness is present. Even without these findings, you should have a very low threshold for obtaining cervical spine x-rays.

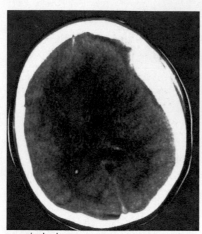

wyomingbrain.com

Figure 10-15. Subdural Hematoma

(venous in origin; may be acute or chronic and may or may not result in midline shift)

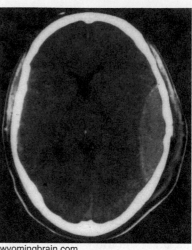

wyomingbrain.com

Figure 10-16. Epidural Hematoma

(usually arterial and associated with skull fractures)

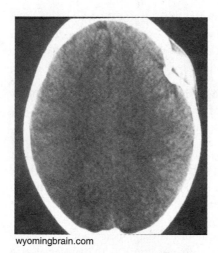

wyomingbrain.com

Figure 10-17. Depressed Skull Fracture

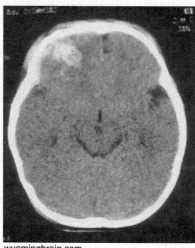

wyomingbrain.com

Figure 10-18. Cerebral Contusion

(petechial hemorrhage and/or edema, which may worsen over days)

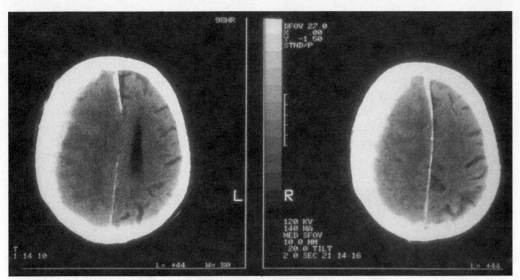

Dr. Conrad Fischer

Figure 10-19. CT Scan Demonstrating Subdural Hematoma with a Midline Shift

Treatment. Severe intracranial hemorrhage should be managed by lowering the intracranial pressure. This is accomplished acutely with hyperventilation to PCO2 of 30–35, which will cause vasoconstriction of cerebral vessels, leading to a decrease in intracranial pressure. It should be used in moderation and for limited amount of time.

Osmotic diuretics such as mannitol and elevation of the head of the bed are also helpful to reduce intracranial pressure. This is in preparation for surgical evacuation. Steroids are not effective, and when an answer choice in head trauma is a steroid, it is always wrong. Select simpler measures such as elevation of the head of the bed to 30 degrees and maintenance of systolic blood pressure to 110–160 mm Hg. This slight degree of hypertension assures that the cerebral perfusion pressure is adequate.

Cerebral perfusion pressure is best when mean arterial pressure ≥60 mm Hg above the intracranial pressure. Stress ulcer prophylaxis with PPI is used after all severe head trauma and after intubation.

SUBARACHNOID HEMORRHAGE

A 52-year-old woman is at her job in the office when she develops the sudden onset of a severe headache, stiff neck, photophobia, and loss of consciousness. She awakens within the hour that she arrived in the hospital. She is noted to have a severe headache, nuchal rigidity, photophobia, and a temperature of 38.5 C (101.3 F).

Definition. A subarachnoid hemorrhage (SAH) is the sudden onset of bleeding into the subarachnoid space.

Etiology. Aneurysm formation is the most common etiology. The aneurysms can be saccular or fusiform and are most commonly around the circle of Willis. There is an association with polycystic kidney disease, Ehlers-Danlos syndrome, and some other connective tissue diseases. SAH most commonly occurs spontaneously. Head trauma is rare as a cause of SAH.

Clinical Presentation. Sudden onset of severe headache is the hallmark of SAH. The sudden rise in intracranial pressure results in loss of consciousness in as many as 50% of patients. Focal neurologic symptoms occur in >30%, the most common from compression of the occulomotor cranial nerve. Sometimes the pressure of the bleed can dissect into the surrounding tissues and cause other neurologic defects. Nuchal rigidity, photophobia, headache, and papilledema occur because of meningeal irritation. Fever can occur 3–4 days after the initial hemorrhage. This can simulate meningitis because an SAH is a form of chemical meningitis from irritation by the blood. Seizures are also an extremely common finding. One-year mortality can be up to 50%, with half of the people dying upon immediate occurrence of the bleed.

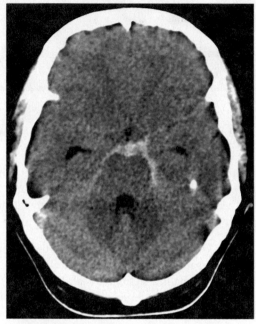

Copyright 2007 Gold Standard Multimedia Inc.

Figure 10-20. Subarachnoid Hemorrhage on CT Scan

Note

A spinal headache may occur after a lumbar puncture in some patients. This is treated with a blood patch.

Longer-term manifestations include the development of focal deficits, seizures, rebleeding, and hydrocephalus. Vasospasm after the bleed results in hypoperfusion to portions of the brain parenchyma and the development of stroke. Rebleeding occurs when the clot falls off of the original site of bleeding. Up to half of the people who rebleed will die. Hydrocephalus occurs when the blood cells clog up the arachnoid granulations through which CSF normally drains.

Diagnosis. The initial test is the CT scan, which is more sensitive than MRI for the diagnosis of SAH. The CT scan of the head is without the use of contrast and has a sensitivity of 90–95% within the first 24 hours after the onset of the bleed. The diagnostic sensitivity of the CT scan actually diminishes with time as the red cells within the CSF hemolyze and are resorbed and converted into the yellowish coloring described on CSF examination as *xanthochromia*.

If the initial CT scan is normal and an SAH is still suspected, *a lumbar puncture is done*. The lumbar puncture is the most sensitive diagnostic test. The absence of red cells on the lumbar puncture essentially excludes an SAH. Xanthochromia needs 4–6 hours to develop. Angiography is used to determine the specific anatomic site of the vascular defect and the site of the bleeding. EKG abnormalities, such as inverted or enlarged T-waves, are often associated with the development of an SAH and are not a cause for alarm.

Treatment. Initially, management consists of maintaining systolic blood pressure at 110-160 mm Hg. Pressure higher than this can provoke more bleeding. Pressure lower than this can provoke cerebral ischemia through hypoperfusion, given the increased intracranial pressure. Seizure prophylaxis is not necessary in these patients.

Nimodipine is a calcium-channel antagonist that can be used to lower the risk of spasm in the blood vessel and therefore, lower the risk of subsequent stroke. *Angiography* should be done to determine the anatomic site that will need catheter or surgical correction. It is important to perform this so that surgical correction (usually performed through embolization or clipping of the AVM) can occur before rebleeding develops. If hydrocephalus occurs, then shunting will be needed. Embolization is superior to surgical clipping.

BURNS

> A 32-year-old fireman is caught in a fire and is briefly trapped under a burning staircase. He is quickly extracted and brought to the emergency department. His respiratory rate is 14/min. He is fully alert and weighs 220 pounds. There is soot in his mouth and nose and on his face, and his sputum not carbonaceous. The nasal hairs are singed. He has no stridor or hoarseness, and the lungs are clear to auscultation. He has first-degree burns on his right leg and second- and third-degree burns on his right arm and chest.

Definition. Injuries due to burns can be divided into several types. The most common causes of death from fires are **smoke inhalation** and **carbon monoxide poisoning**. Thermal injury is most dangerous when it is respiratory related. Skin injury is labeled first degree when the skin is fully intact, even though it may be discolored. First-degree burns are not associated with blister formation and appear "sunburn-like." The skin may be red or gray, but capillary refill remains normal. **Second-degree** burns result in blister formation. **Third-degree** burns are deeper and destroy skin appendages such as sweat glands, hair follicles, and sometimes pain receptors. This leaves third-degree burns insensate. Pain perceived by third-degree-burn patients is from surrounding structures where pain receptors are intact.

Pathophysiology. Although not apparent at first, respiratory injury can be the most life-threatening injury. Soot in the mouth or nose, stridor, wheezing, altered mental status, burned nasal hairs, and burns involving closed spaces are all clues to impending pulmonary and laryngeal edema. Shock occurs not only from direct skin loss but also from the release of a host of mediators that result in **diffuse capillary leak** for the first 18-24 hours. Serious capillary leak occurs when the percentage of serious body surface area burn exceeds 20-25%.

Clinical Presentation. Altered mental status, dyspnea, headache, and chest pain are clues to severe carbon monoxide poisoning. Laryngeal edema can result in stridor, hoarseness, and dyspnea. Soot in the nose and mouth can imply impending airway compromise. Skin injury is estimated with the "Rule of Nines" to assess fluid resuscitation. The head and arms are 9% each. The chest, back, and legs are 18% each. Patchy burns can be estimated by using one hand's width as an estimate of 1% of body surface area burned. Circumferential burns are critical in the assessment because as they heal they tighten and cut off circulation, leading to limb compromise and the need for escharotomy.

Diagnosis. Besides the obvious burn, carboxyhemoglobin levels are essential in severe burns. Severe burns are defined as combined second- and third-degree burns >20% in adults or >10%

Note

The Rule of Nines differs between adults and children. Refer to Pediatrics for more information on the treatment and calculation of burns in children.

in the very old or very young or third-degree burns >5% of body surface area (BSA). Chest x-ray and bronchoscopy help determine the exact extent of respiratory injury when it is uncertain. Bronchoscopy can reveal severe thermal injury to the lungs even when the initial chest film is normal. Foley catheter placement helps determine the adequacy of fluid resuscitation.

Treatment. If the patient has signs of severe respiratory injury, as described above, the first step is to intubate the patient before more severe laryngeal edema can occur and make the intubation difficult. If the carboxyhemoglobin level is significantly elevated (>5-10%), 100% oxygen should be administered. Fluid resuscitation over the first 24 hours is based on a formula of 4 ml per % BSA burned per kg. Use Ringer's lactate as the preferred fluid. Use second- and third- degree burns in your calculation. Give half the fluid in the first 8 hours, with one-quarter in the second 8 hours, and one-quarter in the final 8 hours. This is known as the Parkland formula. Afterward, when the diffuse capillary leak improves, give enough fluid to maintain a urine output >0.5-1 mL per kg per hour.

Stress ulcer prophylaxis with H_2 blockers or PPIs should be given. Topical treatment with silver sulfadiazine is used to prevent infection. Do not break blisters and do not use steroids. Escharotomy is useful in circumferential burns. Skin grafting is done on the basis of the size and severity of the injury.

Heat Disorders

Definition. Heat disorders are divided into 2 main groups: exertional and nonexertional. Exertional disorders vary from mild heat cramps to more severe heat exhaustion to potentially lethal heat stroke. Nonexertional disorders are malignant hyperthermia and neuroleptic malignant syndrome.

- **Heat Cramps.** This is a mild disorder that can happen to any healthy person who develops fluid and electrolyte depletion. The patient develops painful muscular contractions lasting a few minutes with muscle tenderness present. The patient is able to sweat, and there are no neurologic abnormalities. The body temperature is normal. Treatment is rest, oral rehydration, and salt replacement.

- **Heat Exhaustion.** This is a more severe exertional heat disorder. The patient is weaker with more systemic symptoms. Body temperature may be slightly elevated. Mild neurologic symptoms such as headache, nausea, and anxiety may occur, but severe confusion is rare. Death is very unlikely, but the disorder can progress to heat stroke if not treated. The patient is still able to sweat and remove heat from the body. Treatment can be accomplished with oral fluid and electrolyte replacement, but with severe weakness, the patient may need IV hydration.

- **Heat Stroke.** This is a very severe and potentially life-threatening disorder. Most patients have lost the ability to remove heat from the body because of the impairment of the ability to sweat. Fifty percent of patients still retain some capacity to sweat, but in insufficient amounts to keep up with heat generation. Body temperature may become severely elevated (>41°C), resulting in confusion, disorientation, nausea, blurred vision, and seizures. Numerous laboratory abnormalities may occur such as hemoconcentration, rhabdomyolysis, and elevated BUN, creatinine, and white cell count. Anuria, DIC, and lactic acidosis may develop.

  Treatment of heat stroke is with IV fluid replacement and rapid cooling of the body (place in cool environment and spray with water, then fan to evaporate the fluid). Ice-water immersion can result in overcooling and hypothermia. Chlorpromazine and diazepam can be used to control shivering.

- **Malignant Hyperthermia.** This is a nonexertional heat disorder occurring as an idiosyncratic reaction to the use of anesthetic agents such as halothane or succinylcholine. Virtually any anesthetic may cause it. Rhabdomyolysis may develop. Treatment is with dantrolene.

- **Neuroleptic Malignant Syndrome.** This is an idiosyncratic reaction to a wide variety of phenothiazines or butyrophenones such as haloperidol. Muscular rigidity and rhabdomyolysis may occur as well. Treatment, besides stopping the drug, is with bromocriptine or dantrolene.

Hypothermia

Definition. A reduction of core body temperature below 35°C (normal 37°C). Core temperature is measured with a rectal probe or through the esophagus. Severe hypothermia is a core temperature below 30°C.

Etiology. Hypothermia often occurs in association with alcohol intoxication, particularly in the elderly.

Clinical Presentation. The most common symptoms of severe hypothermia are related to the central nervous system. Lethargy, confusion, and weakness may occur. Death is most commonly from **arrhythmia** (Osborne wave or J wave). This is from the effect of the cold on altering cardiac conduction.

Diagnosis. The EKG can show a wide variety of serious arrhythmias, including ventricular fibrillation or ventricular tachycardia. The most characteristic finding is an elevation of the J-point, known as Osborne waves. J-wave elevation may mimic ST-segment elevation.

Treatment. Most patients will respond well to common-sense treatment, such as a warm bed, bath, or heated blankets. Warmed IV fluids or warmed humidified oxygen can be used in very severe cases, although care must be taken because overly rapid rewarming can result in arrhythmias as well. When life-threatening arrhythmias occur, it is important to continue resuscitative efforts until the body temperature is >**35°C**. If the patient is cold but not shivering, active measures should be used:

Active external rewarming

- Only to truncal areas
- Warm blankets
- Heat lamps
- Hot-water bottles

Active internal rewarming

- Warm IVFs (45° C)
- Warm humidified oxygen (45° C)
- Warmed gastric lavage via NGT
- Warmed hemodialysis

Hypothermia is one of the few times in which a patient can be resuscitated from pulselessness beyond the usual 10 minutes of efforts.

Note

Hypothermia must be worked up for precipitant factors:

- Hypoglycemia (most common cause)
- Hypothyroidism
- Sepsis

RADIATION INJURIES

Ionizing radiation damages tissues primarily through destructive changes to DNA molecules. Ionizing radiation is lethal and can often cause cancer. Longer exposures give worse injury. **Nonionizing radiation** is less destructive to tissue and causes injury primarily as burns. Examples include infrared, ultraviolet, and microwave radiation.

Presentation. To give a sense of scale, mortality is almost zero with <2 Gy (or Sv) of exposure. This rises almost to 100% mortality with >10 Gy (or Sv). (10 Gy = 1,000 rad.)

Any cell can be damaged by ionizing radiation, but the more rapidly the cell divides, the more vulnerable it is to radiation. This is because more DNA damage can be done during the time of division.

Bone Marrow. As little as 2-3 Gy (200-300 rad) can depress the lymphocyte count. Neutrophils are the next most sensitive cell, and erythrocytes are the least sensitive. Long-term, leukemia is the earliest and most common cause of cancer from radiation exposure. Thrombocytopenia can result in death from bleeding. Overall, *infection* and *bleeding* from depressed bone marrow function are the most common causes of death in acute exposure.

Gonads. Two to 3 grays result in temporary aspermatogenesis. Four to 5 grays can make men permanently sterile. Testes are more sensitive than ovaries.

GI. Nausea and vomiting are the most common early symptoms of radiation exposure. This develops in 50% of cases with a 2 Gy (200 rad) exposure and in 100% of patients with >3 Gy exposure. In addition to nausea and vomiting, the rapidly reproducing intestinal lining ulcerates, leading to bleeding and infection later.

Other Sites. Other common sites of radiation injury are the skin, salivary glands, respiratory epithelium, and thyroid glands.

Treatment. The management of radiation injury is supportive only. There is no specific therapy to reverse radiation injury.

- Antiemetics. Given that nausea is such a common feature of radiation sickness, antiemetics are a mainstay of therapy.
- Blood products. Platelets and RBC transfusions are needed. WBC transfusions don't help.
- Colony-stimulating factors (G-CSF, GM-CSF). These will help restore marrow function.
- Antibiotics. Use as needed when infection develops.
- Bone marrow transplantations. These are occasionally useful.

ELECTRICAL INJURIES

Note

For USMLE purposes, anything ≤500–600 volts is considered low voltage and anything above that is considered high voltage.

Epidemiology. Lightning has an extremely high voltage, from 100,000 to 2 billion volts, but the duration of the contact is extremely small at <1 millisecond. Injury is a function not only of the amount of current, but the duration of the contact. High voltage (lightning) causes morbidity 5–10 × greater than low voltage.

Mechanism. Injury occurs because electrical injury is converted to heat. When resistance is high, there is more heat produced and therefore more injury. Dry skin is 1,000 times more resistant than wet skin, so more local injury is produced by dry skin. Nerves and blood vessels have low resistance. Wet skin conducts electricity along nerves and blood vessels to produce injury to parts of the body far from the point of contact with the electrical source. Hence, a relatively minor superficial wound can mask serious deep tissue damage.

Presentation. Local injury is the most common electrical injury. The conversion of electricity to heat results in first-, second-, or third-degree burns. Lightning may give a superficial "feathering" pattern on the skin as the energy is conducted over the outside of the body.

- Cardiopulmonary arrest. AC current can give ventricular fibrillation, and the DC current of lightning can result in asystole, although an arrhythmia is possible. Respiratory arrest can occur by injury to the medulla or paralysis of respiratory muscles.

- Neurologic effects. Central and peripheral nervous system injury can occur in 25-100% of electrocutions. Motor injury is more common than sensory. Lightning gives loss of consciousness in 75% of patients, and no patient ever remembers the strike. Neurologic injury can be delayed up to 3 years and may be as severe as spinal cord transection.

- Renal failure. Renal failure occurs from dehydration due to fluid sequestration into injured tissue. (They suck fluid out of the vasculature to form edema.) This dehydration combines with rhabdomyolysis from injury and tetanic contraction because injured muscle releases myoglobin.

- Cataracts. Cataracts develop in 5-30% of patients for unclear reasons.

Treatment. Pain management is imperative. Cardiopulmonary resuscitation primarily involves management of arrhythmias and ABCs. Provide fluid replacement to compensate for fluid sequestration into tissues and to prevent renal failure from rhabdomyolysis. Urine output is the best method for determining adequacy of hydration (the Rule of Nines is not used here because it can underestimate total body involvement). Lactated Ringer's (LR) solution is the fluid of choice because it causes no metabolic acidosis, as seen with normal saline.

Also provide local wound care—including debridement, fasciotomy, and amputation, if needed.

DROWNING

Risk/Mechanism. Alcohol and drug use are strongly associated with an increased risk of death by drowning. Muscular exhaustion, head and spinal trauma, or acute myocardial infarction are also predispositions to drowning and near drowning. Ten to twenty percent of drowning victims may have suffered dry drowning in that there is no water aspirated into the lungs. Dry drowning is secondary to laryngospasm.

Drowning from aspiration of water can be divided into 2 types:

- Freshwater, which is hypotonic, alters pulmonary surfactant, resulting in unstable alveoli, which then collapse. **The hypotonic freshwater is absorbed into the body, resulting in acute hypervolemia, hemodilution, and intravascular hemolysis.** At autopsy, the lungs may contain little water.

- With seawater, **the hypertonic water draws water out of the body into the lung, causing systemic hypovolemia and hemoconcentration.** The lungs become even more heavy and fluid-filled because the surfactant is essentially washed out.

Presentation. Only the presentation of near drowning is important to discuss because drowned victims are dead. The presentation can vary from coma to agitation. Cyanosis, coughing, and signs of pulmonary edema, such as tachypnea, tachycardia, and blood-tinged sputum, are common. Rales and rhonchi can be found on the exam. Hypothermia is also common.

Note

Tissue resistance: Bone > Fat > Tendons > Skin > Muscles > Blood > Nerves

Note

Near drowning is defined as survival after immersion, at least for some time. Morbidity is high and death may occur later. The exact definition is still the topic of much debate.

Drowning is defined as death within 24 hours after submersion in water.

Laboratory Findings. Arterial blood gases show hypoxia and hypercarbia, as well as metabolic acidosis from anaerobic metabolism. Hyperkalemia may be present if there is significant hemolysis. Renal insufficiency on the basis of hypoxia is a rare finding.

Treatment. The first task is to remove the patient from the water and do ABCs (airway/breathing/circulation) of resuscitation.

- Endotracheal intubation as needed
- Supplemental oxygen
- Positive pressure mechanical ventilation as needed

After removal from water, establishment of adequate airway is the most important initial step. Continuous positive airway pressure (CPAP) is the most effective treatment and gives the best correction of hypoxia and acidosis. Even if the patient appears comfort-able initially, continue observation for 24 hours because ARDS (acute respiratory distress syndrome) may develop as a late finding.

The following treatments **do not help and may be harmful**:

- *Abdominal thrusts.* These may lead to aspiration of gastric contents.
- *Prophylactic antibiotics.* Antibiotics are only indicated if pneumonia develops.
- *Steroids.* There are no benefits to administering steroids.

ANAPHYLAXIS

Definition. A syndrome of histaminergic release in which there are signs of severe injury such as urticaria, angioedema, hypotension, tachycardia, and respiratory compromise.

Etiology. As an idiosyncratic reaction, patients can potentially develop anaphylaxis from any food, medication, insect bite, or antigenic substance entering the body by oral or parenteral route. Although medications such as penicillin, phenytoin, contrast agents, and allopurinol are most often associated with anaphylaxis, patients can potentially be allergic to anything. Chocolate, peanuts, and strawberries are common, but patients can be allergic to any food. The same is true of insect stings. Although bees may be common, patients can conceivably be allergic to any insect's venom.

Clinical Presentation. Mild symptoms include a rash known as "hives." More severe symptoms include dyspnea, stridor, tachycardia, hypotension, and hemodynamic collapse.

Treatment. Mild allergies may respond to simply stopping the offending toxin and waiting. More severe symptoms require the use of an antihistamine, such as diphenhydramine. Severe symptoms of anaphylaxis with hemodynamic instability require epinephrine injections, IV fluids, antihistamines, and systemic corticosteroids.

VENOMOUS BITES AND STINGS

Cat and Dog Bites

Epidemiology. Dog bites are the most common bites in the United States.

Etiology/Presentation. Dog bites are usually ripping and tearing in nature, whereas, cat bites are usually in the form of a puncture wound. Infection is more likely in patients with a delay in treatment, extremes of age and extremity injuries. Infections are most often polymicrobial. Cat bites are highly associated with *Pasteurella multocida* and dog bites are associated with *Pasteurella, Eikenella*, b *hemolytic streptococci, Staph aureus*, and *Capnocytophaga canimorsus*.

Treatment. This includes exploration, debridement, irrigation, and proper wound care. If prophylactic antibiotics are indicated, the drug of choice is amoxicillin and clavulanate (a combination of clindamycin plus ciprofloxacin or trimethoprim/sulfamethoxazole or doxycycline can be used with penicillin allergy). Moxifloxacin may be used alone, as it has good aerobic and anaerobic activity.

Indications for antibiotic prophylaxis:

- For any cat bite
- Any bite on hand, face, or genitals
- Imunocompromised patients
- Asplenic patients (high risk of overwhelming sepsis from *Capnocytophaga canimorsus*)

Most wounds should be left unsutured except for facial wounds for cosmetic reasons. Never suture the hand.

Human Bites

Epidemiology. Human bites carry an infection rate of 15%, which is greater than cat and dog bites together.

Etiology. The most common organisms are anaerobic and aerobic bacteria, specifically, *Eikenella Corrodens*. Hepatitis B and HIV can also be transmitted through bites but is much less common.

Treatment. Clean and irrigate wound well. No place for cultures on fresh bites. If the bite is <12 hours old, close loosely. Give counseling for tetanus, hepatitis B, and prophylaxis. Initiate 5 to 7 day course of prophylactic antibiotics.

Rabies

Epidemiology. Carried by raccoons, rats, wild dogs, woodchucks, skunks, foxes. Nearly 100% fatal once the disease has been contracted. Bats are the most common cause.

Etiology/Clinical Presentation. Incubation period up to 1 year. Prodrome of 2 to 10 days including fevers and paresthesias at the bite site. Neurologic changes include aphasia, paralysis, hypersalivation, and myoclonus.

Diagnosis. Viral cultures from saliva, CSF, or serum

Note

All human and monkey bites should always receive prophylactic antibiotics.

Treatment. Ribavirin has been used in confirmed cases. Prophylaxis with human rabies immunoglobin (HR16), which gives immediate passive immunity, and human diploid cell vaccine (HDCV) should be given at 0, 3, 7, 14, and 28 days (5 shots total).

Snakebites

Epidemiology. Although 50,000 snakebites are reported per year worldwide, only about 8,000 of those are poisonous. There are <5–10 deaths per year, with rattlesnakes accounting for almost all fatalities.

Mechanism. Snake venom contains numerous potentially dangerous substances, such as hemolysis toxin, cardiotoxin, neurotoxin, and proteolytic enzymes, in addition to others. Some of these substances can result in neuromuscular blockade.

Factors that affect the severity of the bite:

- Body size. The smaller the body, the worse the effects; hence, bites tend to be worse in children.
- Location of bite. Trunk and face bites are worse than extremity bites.
- Exercising after bite. Muscular activity helps spread the venom through the lymphatics.
- Depth of injury. No poisoning occurs in 20-50% of bites because they are too superficial.

Treatment. Transport the patient immediately to the nearest medical facility.

1. Immobilize the patient. This will help to decrease the spread of venom through the lymphatics, which increases with muscular contraction.
2. Apply compression bandage. This will also help to decrease lymph flow. It should not be so tight as to decrease venous flow.
3. Antivenin. Be cautious of anaphylactic reactions that may occur to the horse serum.
4. Supportive. Hypotension is managed with fluids. Ventilatory support may be necessary.

Ineffective therapy includes incision and suction of the bites. Tourniquets and ice immersion do not help and might be harmful.

SPINAL CORD COMPRESSION

A 63-year-old African-American man is brought to the emergency department complaining of back pain that started gradually 3 days ago. The patient describes the pain as "band-like" around the abdomen, without radiation. His past medical history is significant for prostate cancer, diagnosed 3 years earlier, and treated with radiation.

Definition. An acute syndrome of back pain associated with compression of the spinal cord. It is considered a neurologic emergency.

Etiology. Commonly caused by cancer (lymphoma; multiple myeloma; carcinomas of prostate, lung, breast, kidney, or colon), herniated disk, epidural abscess, hematoma, or trauma. Acute cases are caused by trauma.

Clinical Presentation. Patients commonly present with insidious onset of mild sensory disturbance, lower extremity weakness, and/or sphincter or sexual dysfunction. Pain is the earliest symptom in the majority of patients (96%). Pain may be intensified by actions that increase intrathoracic and thus cerebral spinal fluid pressure. The diagnosis of acute spinal cord compression has to be suspected on the basis of the history and neurologic exam. The importance of having a high index of suspicion for the diagnosis is essential to instituting appropriate therapy early in the course of the disease. A history of cancer, fever, and bowel or bladder incontinence/retention are all points in the clinical history that strongly suggest the possibility of acute spinal cord compression. On neurologic exam, a dermatomal sensory level with bilateral lower extremity weakness, increased lower extremity muscle tone, and upper motor neuron signs below the level of compression are all consistent with the diagnosis of acute cord compression. The thoracic cord is the most common site of compression (70%) because the spinal cord is narrowest at that point. Symptoms may progress quickly.

Diagnosis. Plain x-rays are abnormal in 84 to 94% of all cases. The diagnostic test of choice is an MRI of the spine. When MRI of the spine is contraindicated, CT myelogram is the diagnostic test of choice.

Treatment. High-dose dexamethasone should be started immediately once the diagnosis is suspected. After the specific etiology is delineated more clearly by MRI, specific therapy may be initiated. For radiosensitive tumors, such as lymphoma or multiple myeloma, radiation therapy should be started as soon as possible. Surgical decompression is the treatment of choice for a herniated disk, epidural abscess, or hematoma. The prognosis depends mainly on the functional status of the patient at the time of presentation. Up to 80% of patients who are initially able to ambulate retain that ability after treatment. Only 5% of patients without antigravity leg strength are able to ambulate after treatment.

Note

Spinal Cord Compression

Acute: trauma

Subacute: most common cause—neoplams

Chronic: herniation

SYRINGOMYELIA

Syringomyelia is defined as cavitation of the spinal cord. It occurs as either communicating (with the CSF pathways) or noncommunicating. Communicating syringomyelia is usually associated with the congenital Arnold Chiari malformation, whereas the noncommunicating syringomyelia is typically secondary to trauma or tumors of the spinal cord.

In the cervical vertebrae of both gray and white matter, there is typically sensory dissociation with impaired pain and temperature and intact sensation to light touch. The loss of pain and temperature occurs in a cape-like distribution across the neck and arms. There is sparing of tactile sensation, position, and vibratory sense. Reflexes are lost.

As the lesion enlarges, there may be lower motor neuron manifestations at the level of the lesion with upper motor neuron signs below the lesion. Cavitation most commonly occurs at the level of the cervical cord. MRI is the most accurate diagnostic test. Treatment is surgical, but often unsatisfactory.

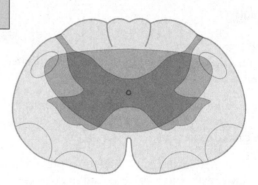

Note cavitation of spinal cord in shaded area

Figure 11-1. Syringomyelia

SUBACUTE COMBINED DEGENERATION

Subacute combined degeneration occurs with vitamin B_{12} deficiency. Patients will complain of distal paresthesias and weakness of the extremities followed by spastic paresis and ataxia. On exam there is a combined deficit of vibration and proprioception with pyramidal signs (plantar extension and hyperreflexia). Diagnosis is established by finding a low serum vitamin B_{12} and treatment is with vitamin B_{12} replacement.

ANTERIOR SPINAL ARTERY OCCLUSION

Anterior spinal artery occlusion presents with acute onset of flaccid paralysis that evolves into a spastic paresis over days to weeks. Additionally, there is loss of pain and temperature sensation with sparing of vibration and position sense as the posterior columns are supplied by the posterior spinal artery. Everything (motor, sensory, autonomic) is lost below the level of the infarction with the striking exception of retained vibration and position sense. Treatment is supportive.

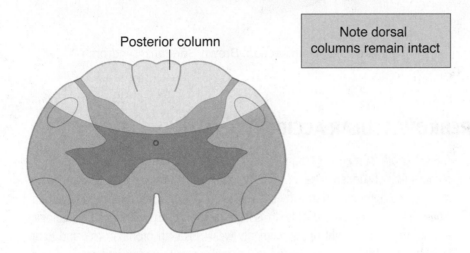

Posterior column

Note dorsal columns remain intact

Figure 11-2. Anterior Spinal Artery Occlusion

BROWN-SÉQUARD SYNDROME

Hemisection of the cord results in a lesion of each of the 3 main neural systems: the principal upper motoneuron pathway of the corticospinal tract, one or both dorsal columns, and the spinothalamic tract. The hallmark of a lesion to these 3 long tracts is presentation with 2 ipsilateral signs and 1 contralateral sign.

- Lesion of the corticospinal tract results in an ipsilateral spastic paresis below the level of the injury.
- Lesion to the fasciculus gracilis or cuneatus results in an ipsilateral loss of joint position sense, tactile discrimination, and vibratory sensations below the lesion.
- Lesion of the spinothalamic tract results in a contralateral loss of pain and temperature sensation starting 1 or 2 segments below the level of the lesion.

At the level of the lesion, there will be an ipsilateral loss of all sensation, including touch modalities as well as pain and temperature, and an ipsilateral flaccid paralysis in muscles supplied by the injured spinal cord segments.

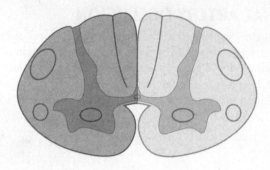

Figure 11-3. Hemisection: Brown-Séquard Syndrome

CEREBROVASCULAR ACCIDENT (CVA)

A 56-year-old woman is brought to the emergency department by her daughter complaining of sudden onset of right upper extremity weakness that began while she was watching television early this morning. The daughter became concerned when her mother was unable to talk in response to questions. Neurologic examination shows right upper extremity weakness with pronator drift and right facial nerve palsy. When questioned, the patient seems to understand what is being said but cannot clearly respond.

Definition. A sudden onset of a focal neurologic deficit.

Etiology. The principal mechanisms by which strokes occur are:
1. Large artery thrombosis
2. Small artery thrombosis (lacunar)
3. Embolic (cardiogenic or artery-to-artery)
4. Vascular dissection
5. Systemic hypertension
6. Bleeding

Clinical Presentation. Stroke should be considered in any patient who presents with acute onset of a focal neurologic deficit. The specific clinical syndrome is determined by the mechanism and vascular territory affected. The blood supply to the brain is divided into two major systems: the carotid (anterior) circulation, and the vertebrobasilar (posterior) circulation. The major blood vessels comprising the anterior circulation include the anterior cerebral artery (ACA) and middle cerebral artery (MCA).

Occlusion of the ACA presents with contralateral weakness and sensory loss in the leg more than in the upper extremity. Urinary incontinence, confusion, and behavioral disturbances are common. Lower extremity weakness exceeds upper extremity weakness.

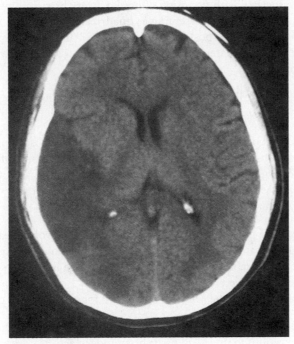

aic.cuhk.edu.hk/web8

Figure 11-4. CT Scan Demonstrating a Right MCA Infarction

Occlusion of the MCA presents with contralateral hemiplegia, hemisensory loss, and homonymous hemianopia with eyes deviated toward the cortical lesion. Dominant hemisphere involvement results in aphasia. Nondominant hemisphere involvement results in preserved speech, comprehension with confusion, and apraxia with spatial and constructional deficits.

The posterior circulation provides blood supply to the cerebellum, brain stem, occipital lobe of the cortex, and pons. The major blood vessels that comprise the posterior circulation are the posterior cerebral artery (PCA), basilar artery (BA), and vertebral arteries.

Table 11-1. Posterior Circulation Syndromes

	Ipsilateral	Contralateral
Weber	CN III	Hemiplegia
Benedikt	CN III	Ataxia
Wallenberg	Facial sensory loss	Body sensory loss

Occlusion of the PCA presents with contralateral homonymous hemianopia, visual hallucinations, and agnosias. Occlusion of the penetrating branches of this vessel can result in CN III palsy with contralateral hemiplegia (Weber syndrome) or CN III palsy with contralateral ataxia or athetosis (Benedikt syndrome).

Specific syndromes associated with occlusion of basilar artery branches include the "locked-in syndrome" (paramedian branches), presenting as quadriparesis with intact vertical eye movements; and Wallenberg syndrome (posterior inferior cerebellar artery), which presents as ipsilateral facial sensory loss, contralateral body sensory loss, vertigo, ataxia, dysarthria, dysphagia, and Horner syndrome.

Occlusion of the major cerebellar arteries produces vertigo, vomiting, nystagmus, and ipsilateral limb ataxia.

Diagnosis. The initial test of choice will always be a noncontrast CT scan of the head. This test is done to distinguish between hemorrhagic and ischemic stroke. Noncontrast CT is the most sensitive test for detecting blood in the brain. CT scans are often negative for ischemia within the first 48 hours after symptom onset. Diffusion-weighted MRI is the most accurate test for detecting cerebral ischemia.

The diagnostic workup of patients with acute ischemic stroke involves searching for embolic sources (echocardiogram, carotid duplex, and 24-hour Holter monitor). Also consider a workup for inherited hypercoagulability. Subarachnoid hemorrhage is associated with EKG abnormalities such as ischemia or inverted T-waves, called cerebral T-waves. A "bubble study" is done on the echocardiogram to detect the presence of a patent foramen ovale or other cardiac defect.

Treatment. Tissue plasminogen activator is given if the patient presents within 3 hours of symptom onset. Contraindications to the use of tissue plasminogen activator include stroke or serious head trauma within 3 months, hemorrhage (GI or genitourinary) within 21 days, surgery within 14 days, history of intracranial hemorrhage, BP >185/110 mm Hg, current use of anticoagulants, platelets <100,000/mm^3, or coagulopathy (PT >15 seconds). Patients who receive tissue plasminogen activator in an appropriate manner have better neurologic function 3 months after CVA as compared with patients who did not receive tissue plasminogen activator.

There is no clear benefit to the use of heparin with stroke. This is because of the increased risk of bleeding. Any benefit is offset by adverse events associated with treatment. For every stroke prevented, one intracranial hemorrhage is caused. Therefore, treatment with heparin in acute ischemic stroke is always wrong.

Antiplatelet therapy is most useful in secondary prevention of ischemic stroke. Aspirin is considered first-line treatment for secondary prevention of ischemic stroke. Aspirin is started 24 hours after TPA. When patients have a known allergy to aspirin or continue to have recurrent cerebrovascular events on aspirin alone, dipyridamole may be added or the patient may be switched to clopidogrel to enhance antiplatelet therapy. Ticlopidine is no longer used because the rates of thrombotic thrombocytopenic purpura and leukopenia are unacceptably high. For those with a recurrent stroke while on aspirin, the single best answer is to add dipyridamole or switch to clopidogrel. *Do not combine* aspirin and clopidogrel for a stroke. Combination of anti-platelet agents is used on coronary disease but not cerebral disease.

Subarachnoid hemorrhage is treated with nimodipine to reduce the risk of ischemic stroke. Early surgical intervention to clip off the aneurysm or embolize the vessel with a catheter should be done in good operative candidates. "Early" means within several days. Don't wait for the unrepaired aneurysm to rebleed. Unruptured aneurysms found incidentally should be repaired if they exceed 10 mm in size.

Carotid endarterectomy is recommended when an occlusion exceeds 70% of the arterial lumen and the lesion is *symptomatic.* Endarterectomy may benefit those who are asymptomatic if there is >60% stenosis in men age <60. The benefit of endoarterectomy is less certain in women because they have a lower risk of stroke. The more severe the disease, the greater the benefit. Carotid stenting is an alternative to endarterectomy.

Endarterectomy is simply not clear in asymptomatic carotid stenosis. The Step 2 exam does not engage in unanswerable, controversial issues.

Carotid angioplasty and stenting are not as good as endarterectomy for symptomatic patients with >70% stenosis. Angioplasty and stenting should be considered only for those who cannot undergo surgical endarterectomy.

SEIZURES AND EPILEPSY

A 29-year-old man is brought to the emergency department by ambulance after being found convulsing in his bedroom. The patient's mother says that during the episode her son was unable to respond to her frantic cries, and she describes jerking movements that became more frequent and then stopped after approximately 1 minute. The mother says that he seemed tired and lethargic for at least 20 minutes after the episode. She then called the ambulance to bring her son to the hospital.

Definition. A seizure is a paroxysmal event due to abnormally discharging central nervous system (CNS) neurons. Epilepsy is defined as a condition of recurrent seizures due to a chronic underlying process.

Etiology. Seizures are caused by "VITAMINS":

Vascular (stroke, bleed, arteriovenous malformation)
Infection (meningitis, abscess, encephalitis)
Trauma (especially penetrating)
Autoimmune (CNS vasculitis)
Metabolic (hyponatremia, hypocalcemia, hypomagnesemia, hypoglycemia, hypoxia, drug overdose/withdrawal)
Idiopathic
Neoplasm
pSychiatric

Clinical Presentation. A seizure is essentially a paroxysmal, involuntary event (associated with abnormal movement or change of consciousness or both). Characteristically, seizures are sudden in onset, with or without an aura. Patients often complain of disorientation, sleepiness, and aching muscles for minutes to hours after the event. Patients may also experience incontinence, tongue biting, and headache as a result of the seizure. It may be difficult at times to differentiate a seizure from syncope, and it is important to obtain a complete history from any individual who witnessed the event. Generally, patients with syncope will not complain of significant postictal symptoms. They will recover consciousness within several minutes of the event, and on physical exam will not have evidence of incontinence or tongue biting.

It is important to classify seizures according to their clinical features because this will determine what medications will be used for treatment. Seizures can be classified as **partial versus generalized** and **complex versus simple**.

Partial seizures occur within discrete portions of the brain. The patient will often complain of involuntary jerking of a finger or hand. When consciousness is maintained for the duration of the seizure, the seizure is termed a **simple partial seizure**. When there is a change in consciousness during the seizure, the seizure is termed a **complex partial seizure**. When a partial seizure progresses to a generalized seizure, it is called a partial seizure with secondary generalization. Typically, the seizure will begin focally and become generalized as the seizure activity involves both cerebral hemispheres.

Generalized seizures arise from both cerebral hemispheres spontaneously without any detectable focal onset. **Generalized tonic-clonic (grand mal)** seizures are characterized by tonic contraction of muscles throughout the body followed by intermittent relaxation of various muscle groups (clonic phase). **Absence seizures (petit mal)** are more common in children than adults; they are characterized by sudden, brief loss of consciousness without loss of postural tone. Characteristically, the EEG will show a generalized, symmetric 3-Hz spike-and-wave discharge pattern. Atonic seizures are characterized by sudden loss of postural tone lasting 1 to 2 seconds. Myoclonic seizures are characterized by sudden, brief muscle contraction.

Status epilepticus is defined as recurrent or continuous seizures (lasting at least 5–30 min).

Diagnosis. EEG is the test of choice for the diagnosis of epilepsy. The diagnosis of idiopathic seizures is made only after secondary precipitating factors have been ruled out. An abnormal EEG alone is not diagnostic of epilepsy. Approximately 2 to 18% of the population has an abnormal EEG. Always check serum electrolytes, glucose, toxicology, and arterial blood gas to rule out hypoxia as a cause of a patient's seizure. CT scan or MRI of the head is usually indicated to rule out a structural lesion as the cause of seizure. Think of any seizure as a symptom, much like shortness of breath or chest pain, which has an extensive differential diagnosis. The evaluation of any seizing patient is to rule out reversible causes of seizure.

Treatment. The treatment of seizures can be divided into the acute management of the acutely seizing patient (status epilepticus) and the chronic management of the epileptic patient.

The first step in the treatment of any acutely seizing patient is to secure the <u>a</u>irway, <u>b</u>reathing, and <u>c</u>irculation. Once an adequate airway is established, breathing is assured, and the patient is hemodynamically stable, the next step is to simultaneously evaluate and treat any precipitating causes of seizure. If a reversible cause is identified, treat aggressively. If the patient continues to seize, the following strategy is appropriate. The initial drug of choice is lorazepam or diazepam, both of which are benzodiazepines. These medications work by potentiating GABA receptor function. If the patient continues to seize, add phenytoin or fosphenytoin, which inhibits sodium-dependent action potentials. CNS side effects of phenytoin include diplopia, dizziness, and ataxia. Systemic side effects include gum hyperplasia, lymphadenopathy, hirsutism, and rash. If the patient continues to seize add phenobarbital. Side effects include sedation, ataxia, and rash. If, despite all of the above therapy, the patient continues to seize, add midazolam or propofol.

In patients with first-time seizure, anticonvulsant therapy should be started *only* if the patient has an abnormal neurologic exam, presented with status epilepticus, has a strong family history of seizure, or has an abnormal EEG. Otherwise, first-time seizures are generally not treated with long-term anticonvulsant therapy.

There is no superior drug in pregnancy. Valproic acid is clearly more dangerous in pregnancy.

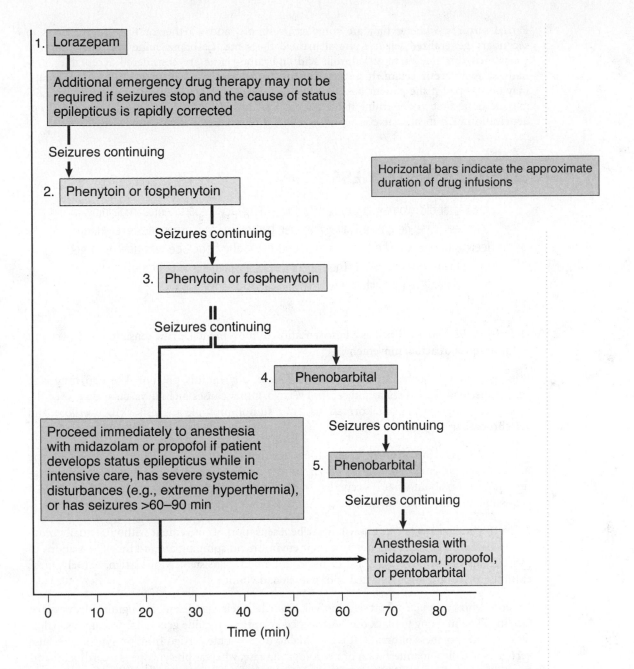

1. Lorazepam

Additional emergency drug therapy may not be required if seizures stop and the cause of status epilepticus is rapidly corrected

Seizures continuing

2. Phenytoin or fosphenytoin

Horizontal bars indicate the approximate duration of drug infusions

Seizures continuing

3. Phenytoin or fosphenytoin

Seizures continuing

4. Phenobarbital

Proceed immediately to anesthesia with midazolam or propofol if patient develops status epilepticus while in intensive care, has severe systemic disturbances (e.g., extreme hyperthermia), or has seizures >60–90 min

Seizures continuing

5. Phenobarbital

Seizures continuing

Anesthesia with midazolam, propofol, or pentobarbital

Time (min)

Figure 11-5. Development of Status Epilepticus

For primary generalized tonic-clonic seizures, valproic acid, phenytoin, lamotrigine, carbamazepine, or levetiracetam can be used. Lamotrigine works by decreasing glutamate release. Side effects include Stevens-Johnson syndrome. Absence seizures are treated with ethosuximide as first-line therapy. If ethosuximide is not an answer choice, valproic acid is an acceptable option. For myoclonic and atonic seizures, valproic acid is the treatment of choice. Overall, there is no single antiepileptic drug that's truly superior to the others—valproic acid, phenytoin, levetiracetam and carbamazepine are all nearly equal in efficacy.

Partial seizures, whether they are complex or simple, and whether or not they progress to secondary generalized seizures, are all treated the same. Carbamazepine and phenytoin are considered first-line therapy. Valproic acid and lamotrigine are considered acceptable alternatives, as is levetiracetam. It is very difficult to determine when to stop therapy. Therapy may be stopped if the patient has been free of seizures for 2–3 years. Sleep-deprivation EEG may be done first to determine if the patient is at low risk of a recurrence. A normal sleep-deprivation EEG means there is a lower likelihood of seizures.

VERTIGO AND DIZZINESS

A 53-year-old woman is brought to the emergency department complaining of dizziness. She describes walking to her bathroom and experiencing a sudden feeling of nausea. She then vomited and fell to the floor. She was unable to get up but was able to call 911. The patient describes a feeling of the room "spinning" around her, even though she realizes she was not moving.

Definition. Vertigo is defined as a false sensation of movement, i.e., the sensation of movement in the absence of actual movement.

Etiology. Vertigo may be caused by Ménière disease, labyrinthitis, positional vertigo, traumatic vertigo, perilymphatic fistula, and cervical vertigo. Other causes include vascular disease of the brain stem, arteriovenous malformations, brain tumor, multiple sclerosis, drug overdose, and vertebrobasilar migraine.

Clinical Presentation. With the dizzy patient, the first step in the evaluation is to determine the nature of the patient's complaints. "Dizziness" is a nonspecific term that provides no meaningful information about what is occurring to the patient. Simply by taking a complete history, it is possible to determine whether the patient is experiencing vertigo or presyncope.

Patients who experience vertigo will describe a sensation of movement without actually moving. Commonly, patients will describe their environment spinning around them. Sensations of tilting, swaying, or falling forward or backward are all consistent with vertigo. Acutely, these episodes are commonly associated with nausea and vomiting.

Patients who complain of presyncope will describe their symptoms as "lightheadedness" or "feeling like I'm going to black out." Associated symptoms include generalized weakness, palpitations, and shortness of breath. It is essential to differentiate vertigo from presyncope because vertigo is usually a manifestation of neurologic disease, whereas presyncope is a cardinal manifestation of cardiovascular disease.

Once you are convinced by the history that the patient is indeed experiencing an episode of vertigo, the next diagnostic question you have to answer is whether the vertigo is secondary to peripheral or central vestibular disease. This distinction is important because the management will differ between peripheral and central vertigo.

Several points on history and physical examination will distinguish central from peripheral vertigo.

Table 11-2. Vertigo

	Central Vertigo	Peripheral Vertigo
Onset	Gradual	Usually sudden
Tinnitus, hearing loss	Absent	Present
Neighborhood signs (diplopia, cortical blindness, dysarthria, extremity weakness/numbness)	Present	Absent
Nystagmus	Pure, vertical, does not suppress with fixation, and multidirectional	Mixed, horizontal, suppresses with fixation, and unidirectional

Once you have determined that the patient has peripheral vertigo, there is a wide differential diagnosis that should be considered.

Ménière disease is characterized by tinnitus, hearing loss, and episodic vertigo. Each episode lasts 1 to 8 hours. The symptoms wax and wane as the endolymphatic pressure rises and falls. The two most common causes of Ménière disease are syphilis and head trauma.

Benign paroxysmal positional vertigo is a cause of peripheral vertigo that characteristically is exacerbated by head movement or change in head position. Typically, episodes will occur in clusters that persist for several days. There will be a latency of several seconds after head movement before the onset of vertigo. The vertigo usually lasts 10 to 60 seconds.

Labyrinthitis presents with sudden onset of severe vertigo that lasts for several days with hearing loss and tinnitus. The disease frequently follows an upper respiratory tract infection.

Perilymphatic fistula is a form of peripheral vertigo related temporally to head trauma (blunt trauma to the ear, e.g., a slap to the ear) or extreme barotrauma during air flight, scuba diving, or vigorous Valsalva maneuver. Explosions deafen people.

Central vertigo is caused by any cerebellar or brain-stem tumor, bleed, or ischemia. Drug toxicity or overdoses are important causes of central vertigo. Also, in the young patient with unexplained central vertigo, consider multiple sclerosis.

Treatment. Symptomatic treatment for peripheral vertigo includes meclizine or, in severe cases, diazepam.

Ménière disease is treated with a low-salt diet and diuretics. In patients who fail medical therapy, you can consider surgical decompression.

Benign paroxysmal positional vertigo is treated with positional maneuvers that attempt to move the otolith out of the circular canals (e.g., Dix Hallpike and Barany maneuvers).

Vertigo secondary to *labyrinthitis* is treated symptomatically with meclizine and diazepam when the symptoms are severe. Steroids help labyrinthitis.

DISORDERS ASSOCIATED WITH HEADACHE

Headache

A 32-year-old woman comes to the office complaining of a headache that started 2 days ago. She locates her headache at the right side of her head and describes it as throbbing in quality. The headache is worsened by walking up stairs or around the block. She experiences nausea but denies vomiting. She also states that loud noise and bright light exacerbate her pain.

Definition. Headache is defined as pain located in the head, neck, or jaw.

Etiology. There are many causes of headache that can be divided into primary or secondary headache syndromes. Primary headache syndromes include migraine, cluster, and tension headache. Secondary causes of headache include intracranial hemorrhage, brain tumor, meningitis, temporal arteritis, and glaucoma. Migrane affects 15% of the general population.

Clinical Presentation. The single most important question that has to be answered in any patient who presents complaining of a headache is whether there exists a serious underlying cause for the symptoms. By taking a thorough history and performing an adequate physical examination, it is possible to make this differentiation. An essential point in the history is to determine whether this is the first episode of headache that the patient has experienced. A history of recurrent symptoms makes the diagnosis of a primary headache disorder more likely. A history of a first-time headache, especially when severe and rapidly peaking, speaks strongly for serious underlying pathology.

Headache with fever and nuchal rigidity suggests meningitis as the underlying cause. Conversely, a headache that is described as "the worst headache of my life" and/or "thunderclap" at onset, and is accompanied by nuchal rigidity *without* fever, suggests an intracranial hemorrhage as the underlying cause. Patients with brain tumors will present complaining of headache that is described as a deep, dull, aching pain that disturbs sleep. The history of vomiting that precedes the onset of headache by a number of weeks, or a history of headache induced by coughing, lifting, or bending, is typical of posterior fossa brain tumors. Patients with temporal arteritis complain of a unilateral pounding headache associated with visual changes, described as dull and boring with superimposed lancinating pain. Patients will also complain of polymyalgia rheumatica, jaw claudication, fever, weight loss, and scalp tenderness (difficulty combing hair or lying on a pillow). The scalp tenderness is from pain over the temporal artery. Temporal arteritis is a disorder of the elderly, generally presenting in patients age >50. Temporal arteritis gives an elevated sedimentation rate and is diagnosed with biopsy of the temporal artery. Do not wait for the biopsy results to initiate therapy with steroids. Patients with glaucoma will usually give a history of eye pain preceding the onset of the headache.

Once serious underlying pathology is excluded by history and physical examination, primary headache syndromes should be considered. The main primary headache syndromes are migraine, cluster, and tension headache.

Note

Any patient who presents with headache and the following should be considered to have a secondary headache syndrome:

- "Worst headache of my life"
- Worsening symptoms over days to weeks
- Abnormal neurologic exam
- Fever
- Vomiting preceding the headache
- Headache induced by coughing, bending, lifting; or onset age >55

Migraine headaches are defined as a benign and recurrent syndrome of headache, nausea/vomiting, and other varying neurologic dysfunctions. Patients will describe the headache as pulsatile, throbbing, unilateral, and aggravated by minor movement. Other associated features include photophobia, phonophobia, and the time to maximal pain (4 to 72 hours). Migraine is a likely diagnosis when a typical trigger can be identified. Typical triggers include alcohol, certain foods (such as chocolate, various cheeses, monosodium glutamate), hunger, or irregular sleep patterns.

- Migraine without aura is a migraine without a preceding focal neurologic deficit.
- Migraine with aura (classic migraine) is a migraine accompanied by a preceding aura that consists of motor, sensory, or visual symptoms. Focal neurologic symptoms usually occur during the headache rather than as a prodrome. The pathognomonic aura for classic migraine is the scintillating scotoma. Only 20% of migraine headaches are accompanied by an aura. Visual auras are also described as stars, sparks, and flashes of light. Migraine equivalent is defined as focal neurologic symptoms without the classic complaints of headache, nausea, and vomiting.
- Complicated migraine is migraine with severe neurologic deficits which persist after the resolution of pain.
- Basilar migraine is migraine associated with symptoms consistent with brain-stem involvement (vertigo, diplopia, ataxia, or dysarthria).

Tension-type headaches are described as tight, band-like headaches that occur bilaterally. Patients may also describe their headache as "vise-like," and these headaches may be associated with tightness of the posterior neck muscles. Patients will describe their pain as one that builds slowly, and the pain may persist for several days with or without fluctuations. Movement will not generally exacerbate the headache.

Cluster headaches, common in men, begin without warning and are typically described as excruciating, unilateral, periorbital, and peaking in intensity within 5 minutes of onset. They are rarely described as pulsatile in nature. The attacks last from 30 minutes to 3 hours and occur 1–3× day for a 4-to-8-week period. Symptoms associated with cluster headaches include rhinorrhea, reddening of the eye, lacrimation, nasal stuffiness, nausea, and sensitivity to alcohol. Horner syndrome is sometimes found. Emotion and food rarely will trigger a cluster headache.

Diagnosis. Patients with severe, sudden onset of a first-time headache accompanied by strong evidence for an underlying cause on history or physical examination should have a CT scan of the head to rule out any secondary causes.

Treatment. Always begin with an attempt to identify probable triggers for the patient and to modify lifestyle by avoiding those triggers. Most patients will require pharmacotherapy as well.

Pharmacologic treatment for migraine headaches can be divided into management of an acute episode and prophylaxis. Initially, for a mild migraine—which is defined as headache in the absence of nausea or vomiting—NSAIDs may be used.

Acutely, abortive therapy consists of sumatriptan, which acts as a serotonin receptor agonist. Dihydroergotamine is the alternative to the triptans. Ergotamine can be used in combination with caffeine. The triptans are contraindicated in patients with known cardiovascular disease, uncontrolled hypertension, or pregnancy. In addition to sumatriptan, there is almotriptan, naratriptan, zolmitriptan, and eletriptan. These medications can be given orally, intranasally, or even subcutaneously, depending on the severity of the headache. Alternatively, ergotamine can be given for acute abortive therapy. Dopamine antagonists such as metoclopramide can be given acutely as oral formulations to aid in the absorption of other abortive medications. When given parenterally, dopamine antagonists can provide relief acutely for migraine headaches.

Prophylactic treatment for migraine therapy should be initiated when patients have acute migraine headaches >3–4/month. The best prophylactic medication is a beta blocker. Propranolol, valproic acid, and topiramate are all considered first-line therapy for migraine prophylaxis. Verapamil and tricyclics can also be used. These medications take 2 to 6 weeks to have an effect and can be discontinued gradually over 6 months once clinical stabilization has occurred. Methysergide is not used because of the serious side effects associated with prolonged use (valvular and retroperitoneal fibrosis). SSRIs such as sertraline and fluoxetine can also be used for prophylaxis.

Table 11-3. Migraine Therapies

Abortive	Prophylactic
• NSAIDs, aspirin, acetaminophen • Triptans • Ergotamine derivatives	• Beta blockers • Calcium blockers • Tricyclics • SSRIs • Valproic acid • Topiramate

Opioid analgesics are not routinely recommended for the treatment of migraine headaches because of the possibility of developing addiction. They are used only in patients with severe, infrequent migraines that are unresponsive to other therapy. Other therapies for migraine headaches are acetaminophen and NSAIDs such as ibuprofen.

Treatment for tension headaches consists of relaxation. Patients should be encouraged to find activities that are relaxing for them. Initial pharmacotherapy consists of acetaminophen and NSAIDs. If the headache remains refractory to these medications, a muscle relaxant can be added to the regimen.

Cluster headaches are treated with a triptan or 100% oxygen. Prophylaxis of cluster headaches is best done with a calcium channel blocker. Prednisone and lithium are sometimes used.

Pseudotumor Cerebri

Definition. An idiopathic increase in intracranial pressure also known as benign intracranial hypertension.

Etiology. The disorder is 8 to 10 times more common in women. There is an association with obesity, chronic lung disease, Addison disease, oral contraceptives, tetracycline use, and vitamin A toxicity. Often there is no identified cause and the disorder resolves spontaneously after several months.

Clinical Presentation. Patients present with a headache, visual disturbances such as diplopia, and sixth cranial nerve (abducens) palsy. Clinical findings include diplopia, papilledema, and enlargement of the blind spot on visual field testing. The CT and MRI are normal, and evaluation of cerebrospinal fluid is normal beyond an increase in pressure.

Treatment. Treatment consists of weight loss, removing offending agents such as oral contraceptives, and the use of diuretics such as acetazolamide or furosemide. Steroids such as prednisone may help as well. In urgent cases, repeated lumbar punctures may help. If this is not effective and the disorder does not resolve, definitive treatment can be achieved with the placement of a surgical shunt between the ventricles and the peritoneum.

Trigeminal Neuralgia

Also known as tic douloureux, trigeminal neuralgia is an idiopathic pain syndrome resulting in sudden, severe, sharp pain starting near the side of the mouth and progressing to the ear, eye, or nostril. Attacks can be triggered by touch or movement such as talking or by eating. Trigeminal neuralgia can be so severe as to be nearly incapacitating. The pain lasts for a few seconds and disappears. Despite the pain, the sensory examination will be normal. Generally, trigeminal neuralgia is felt to be secondary to compression of the trigeminal nerve root by a blood vessel. Occasionally it can be a manifestation of multiple sclerosis or a posterior fossa tumor. With the exception of multiple sclerosis or the posterior fossa tumor, all imaging and neurologic testing will be normal.

Carbamazepine is the standard of care for treatment. In those not controlled with carbamazepine, phenytoin, baclofen, or gabapentin can be tried. In those not responding to any form of medical therapy, surgery or radio-frequency lesioning into the affected nerve may work.

GUILLAIN-BARRÉ SYNDROME (GBS)

A 46-year-old man is brought to your office complaining of "rubbery legs." The patient states that his symptoms began 2 days ago and that approximately 3 weeks ago, he experienced several episodes of diarrhea, which resolved spontaneously. On neurologic examination, bilateral lower-extremity weakness and a loss of reflexes are noted.

Definition. An acute, often severe polyradiculopathy whose underlying pathophysiology is an autoimmune destruction of myelin.

Etiology. Evidence suggests that GBS is caused by a misdirection of the immune response, where the body's immune system attacks self-antigens mistaken for foreign antigens (molecular mimicry).

Clinical Presentation. Most patients will present with rapidly developing weakness that typically begins in the lower extremities and moves upward. On physical examination the patient is noted to lack reflexes in the muscle groups affected. The progression of the symptoms will develop over the course of hours to days. The legs are usually more affected than the arms and face. Fever, constitutional symptoms, or bladder dysfunction are rare and should raise the possibilities of alternate diagnoses.

In addition to the motor weakness, patients will typically complain of sensory disturbances that can take the form of pain or tingling dysesthesia. Sensory changes are due to loss of large sensory fibers, producing loss of reflexes and proprioception. Autonomic instability (profuse sweating, postural hypotension, labile blood pressure, cardiac dysrhythmias) occurs in severe GBS, requiring patient treatment in an intensive care unit.

Approximately 75% of patients who present with GBS will have a history of an infection 1 to 3 weeks preceding the onset of symptoms. The infection is typically in the respiratory or GI systems (*Campylobacter jejuni*), although GBS may be preceded by infections with human herpesvirus, cytomegalovirus, or the Epstein-Barr virus. The only association between immunizations and GBS occurred in 1976 with the introduction of the swine influenza vaccine. More recent formulations of influenza vaccine are associated with one case of GBS per million patients immunized. GBS occurs more frequently in patients with HIV, systemic lupus erythematous, and lymphoma.

Diagnosis. Diagnosis lies principally in recognizing the typical pattern of weakness with the absence of reflexes, fever, and constitutional symptoms. A lumbar puncture for protein and cell count is always the best initial test. The characteristic finding is an elevated protein without an associate rise in the cell count on CSF. These changes in the cerebral spinal fluid do not occur until 48 hours after the onset of symptoms. The most accurate test for the diagnosis is electromyography (EMG). EMG is used to detect evidence of demyelination of the peripheral nerves.

Treatment. Treatment should be initiated as quickly as possible because available therapy becomes ineffective approximately 2 weeks after the onset of symptoms.

IV immunoglobulin and plasmapheresis are equally effective treatments. There is no benefit to combination therapy. Glucocorticoids are not effective in the treatment of acute GBS. Also, it is extremely important to monitor the vital capacity in patients with GBS and initiate early respiratory support to prevent death from respiratory failure.

MYASTHENIA GRAVIS

A 35-year-old woman comes to the clinic complaining of double vision that seems to worsen near the end of the day. She also complains of difficulty chewing meat and other hard foods. She notices that her symptoms improve following a good night's sleep. On neurologic examination, you note a snarling appearance when the patient is asked to smile, and a nasal tone is heard in her voice. You also note a weakness in the upper extremities when the patient is asked to clench her fist around your finger repeatedly.

Definition. Myasthenia gravis (MG) is a disease of the neuromuscular junction characterized by weakness and fatigability.

Etiology. In myasthenia gravis, an autoimmune process characterized by acetylcholine-receptor antibodies leads to a decreased number of active and functional acetylcholine receptors at the postsynaptic membrane.

Clinical Presentation. The major features in a patient's history that help to diagnose myasthenia gravis are muscle weakness and fatigability. Initially, patients will complain of diplopia, ptosis, and difficulty swallowing. Speech may have a "mushy" or nasal quality and facial weakness may manifest as a "snarling" appearance when smiling. As the disease progresses, weakness may become generalized, involving proximal muscles in an asymmetric pattern. Deep tendon reflexes are intact. Pupillary responses are normal. There are no sensory abnormalities. Very severe disease may affect the muscles of respiration.

Eaton-Lambert myasthenic syndrome is characterized by *increasing* muscle strength on repetitive contraction. This syndrome is seen in association with malignancy, especially small-cell carcinoma of the lung.

Botulism may cause a myasthenic-like illness, but the pupils are usually dilated and repetitive nerve stimulation (on EMG) shows an incremental increase in muscular fiber contraction (opposite of myasthenia gravis).

Diagnosis. The best initial test for the diagnosis of myasthenia gravis is the acetylcholine-receptor antibody test. In generalized myasthenia gravis, 80–90% of patients will have a positive test. In the presence of fatigable muscle weakness, a positive antibody test is specific and virtually diagnostic. Antibodies are present in only 70% of those with disease limited to the eyes.

The edrophonium (Tensilon) test is sensitive but not specific for the diagnosis. Additionally, patients may experience nausea, diarrhea, fasciculations, syncope (rare), or bradycardia during the test, which are cholinergic symptoms.

Imaging studies of the chest such as x-rays and CT scan should be performed to detect a thymoma. Thymoma is found in 10–15% of patients. Thymic hyperplasia is found in 65%.

The most accurate test for the diagnosis of myasthenia gravis is electromyography (EMG). The characteristic finding is a decremental decrease in muscle fiber contraction on repetitive nerve stimulation.

Treatment. Anticholinesterase (usually pyridostigmine or neostigmine) medications are useful for the symptomatic treatment of myasthenia gravis. Pyridostigmine is longer lasting. If treatment with anticholinesterase medications is unsuccessful in providing symptomatic relief, the physician should consider immunosuppressive therapy.

There are numerous medications used for immunosuppressive therapy. These interventions primarily differ in the onset of therapeutic benefit. They are used if thymectomy is not effective.

Glucocorticoids are effective in improving weakness but take 1 to 3 months for you to observe a clinical benefit. Steroids are the initial immunosuppressive of choice. If patients fail steroid therapy, azathioprine is the most widely used medication used in combination with steroids. The benefits of azathioprine therapy may take >3–6 months to peak. Cyclosporine and cyclophosphamide are alternatives to azothiaprine but are more toxic.

Plasmapheresis and IV immunoglobulin are immunosuppressive therapies noted for their ability to rapidly improve weakness in myasthenia gravis. They are therefore reserved for patients in acute myasthenic crisis. These therapies are used when respiratory involvement occurs or when patients go to the operating room.

Thymectomy is indicated in postpubertal patients and in those age <60 with generalized myasthenia gravis before initiation of immunosuppressive therapy. Thymectomy is performed in those not controlled with anticholinesterase medications to prevent the use of potentially toxic medication such as systemic steroids. Thymectomies are also performed when a thymoma is present to prevent the spread of malignant thymic disease.

Aminoglycoside antibiotics may exacerbate myasthenia gravis and should be avoided. In fact, many medications may worse myasthenia gravis.

Mycophenolate is a newer immunosuppressive drug with less adverse effects than steroids or cyclophosphamide.

AMYOTROPHIC LATERAL SCLEROSIS

Amyotrophic lateral sclerosis (ALS) is an idiopathic disorder of both upper and lower motor neurons. ALS has a unique presentation of muscle weakness combined with signs of upper motor neuron loss, cranial nerve palsies, respiratory involvement, and lower motor neuron destruction, while at the same time preserving bowel, bladder sensory, cognitive, and sexual function. The cranial nerve, or bulbar, palsies result in dysphagia, difficulty chewing, decreased gag reflex, dysarthria (difficulty in articulating words), and difficulty in handling saliva. Since there is often respiratory muscle involvement, recurrent aspiration pneumonia is the most common cause of death. A weak cough is also characteristic, and this only worsens the respiratory problem.

There is no pain from abnormal sensory neuropathy because this is entirely a motor neuron disease. On the other hand, the upper motor neuron involvement gives significant spasticity that can lead to pain. Mentation, bowel, bladder, and sexual function remain intact for the same reason. In other words, a fully mentally alert patient loses nearly all motor control while still being able to think and perceive. The patient becomes fully aware of being trapped in a body that does not function. Head ptosis occurs because the extensor muscles of the neck become too weak to keep the head up.

Upper motor neuron manifestations are weakness with spasticity and hyperreflexia. Lower motor neuron manifestations are weakness with muscle wasting, atrophy, and fasciculations; this includes tongue atrophy. The combination of upper and lower motor neuron weakness is the unique presentation of ALS. The most accurate confirmatory test is the electromyogram, which will show diffuse axonal disease. CPK levels are sometimes mildly elevated, and the cerebrospinal fluid and MRI scans are normal.

The only treatment that may slow down the progression of the disease is riluzole, which is thought to work by inhibiting glutamate release. Death typically results in 3–5 years. Spasticity is treated with baclofen and tizanidine.

Many of the exam questions regarding ALS will be ethical questions on issues of the withholding of care. Since ALS has no impact on cognitive function, the patient is felt to retain the capacity to make medical decisions. This means the patient has the right to refuse potentially lifesaving therapy such as antibiotics, nasogastric tube placement, tracheostomy, or the use of mechanical ventilation. The patient should not be allowed to commit suicide nor should the physician assist with the suicide. Withholding intubation or antibiotics is not considered assisting a suicide. Every adult patient with the capacity to understand the implications of their choice is allowed to refuse any therapy they do not want.

MULTIPLE SCLEROSIS

A 32-year-old woman comes to the emergency department complaining of numbness and tingling in her right hand. Her symptoms began several days ago and have worsened over the last several hours. She states that 3 years ago she had an episode of "seeing double" that lasted 2 days and resolved on its own. Physical examination is significant for hyperreactive reflexes bilaterally in her lower extremities. Increased spasticity is also noted in her lower extremities.

Definition. An autoimmune inflammatory disease of the CNS white matter characterized by a relapsing or progressive course.

Etiology. The cause of multiple sclerosis (MS) is thought to be multifactorial. There is evidence that genetic susceptibility plays an important role. The disease occurs primarily in female populations of Northern European descent and of child-bearing age, respectively. This implies a role for some sort of environmental trigger (infectious, dietary, climatic). Pathologically, focal areas of demyelination are characteristic of the disease.

Clinical Presentation. Commonly, patients will present complaining of weakness, numbness, tingling, or unsteadiness of a limb. Urinary urgency or retention, blurry vision, and double vision are all common initial manifestations of the disease. Symptoms may persist for several weeks or may resolve spontaneously over a few days.

There are several forms of the disease that may change the course of management and are therefore important to recognize. Most patients will have a months-long to years-long disease-free period after their first exacerbation.

- **Relapsing remitting disease:** progression is characterized by relapses of active disease with incomplete recovery during the periods of remission
- **Secondary progressive disease:** progression becomes more aggressive so that a consistent worsening of function occurs
- **Primary progressive disease:** symptoms are progressive from the onset of disease with the early onset of disability (least common form)

It is important to understand when the diagnosis of multiple sclerosis should be suspected. Classically, the diagnosis is made clinically when a young patient (usually age <55) presents with a history of multiple neurologic complaints that cannot be explained by the presence of one CNS lesion. In other words, suspect the diagnosis when a patient presents with multiple neurologic deficits **separated by time and space (anatomy)**.

A number of triggers are known to exacerbate the disease. Infections or trauma may acutely worsen the disease. Pregnancy, especially the 2 to 3 months following birth, may also exacerbate symptoms. However, there are generally fewer attacks during the pregnancy. Uncomplicated MS typically has no adverse effects on the outcome of the pregnancy.

Diagnosis. To diagnose MS you have to rely on clinical criteria supplemented with radiologic and laboratory confirmations. The advent of MRI scanning of the brain has dramatically changed the methods by which multiple sclerosis is diagnosed.

MRI of the brain is the most accurate test to diagnose MS, reaching a sensitivity of 85 to 95% in symptomatic persons. Increased T2 and decreased T1 intensity represent the increased water content of demyelinated plaques in the cerebrum and spine. Enhancement of lesions with gadolinium indicates active MS lesions that may enhance for up to 2 to 6 weeks after an exacerbation. MS is an unusual disease in that the best initial test for the diagnosis is also the most sensitive one, namely MRI of the brain and spine.

Evoked response potentials detect slow or abnormal conduction in response to visual, auditory, or somatosensory stimuli. The limitation of this test for the diagnosis of MS is that many other neurologic diseases can give an abnormal result. The test is not specific for the diagnosis of MS. As a result, evoked potentials are rarely used to make the diagnosis.

Cerebrospinal fluid (CSF) analysis usually reveals a mild pleocytosis (usually <50 cells/μL) and a total protein that is mildly elevated. A protein level exceeding 100 mg/dL is unusual and should be considered as evidence against the diagnosis of MS. An elevated IgG index (oligoclonal bands) is found in 70 to 90% of patients with MS. The finding is nonspecific, and as a result, CSF for oligoclonal banding is recommended only when the MRI is nonconfirmatory but clinical suspicion for MS remains high.

Treatment. The treatment of multiple sclerosis can be divided into disease-modifying therapy, treatment of complications, and treatment for symptomatic relief during an acute exacerbation. The specific agents used depend on progression of the disease at the time of diagnosis.

In relapsing-remitting disease, there are 3 disease-modifying agents that have been shown to reduce the number of clinical exacerbations and the number of MRI lesions:

- Interferon-β1a
- Interferon-β1b
- Glatiramer acetate

More importantly, these medications seem to delay the onset of significant disability. Glatiramer is also known as copolymer I.

In secondary progressive disease, interferon-β1b and mitoxantrone have been shown to reduce the number of exacerbations, decrease MRI activity, and delay onset of disability. In patients who receive mitoxantrone, dose-related cardiotoxicity is a concern; mitoxantrone should be given only to patients with a normal ejection fraction. Mitoxantrone is not a first-line agent to prevent disease progression because of its cardiotoxicity. In patients with relapsing-remitting disease or secondary progressive disease who cannot tolerate treatment with IFN-β1b, IFN-β1a, or glatiramer acetate, you can consider treatment with methotrexate, mitoxantrone, cyclophosphamide, IV immunoglobulin, or azathioprine. ACTH is no longer used.

No approved disease-modifying therapy exists at this time for primary progressive disease.

Mitoxantrone, cyclophosphamide, and natalizumab are not used for a first episode of disease. Natalizumab is associated with progressive multifocal leukoencephalopathy (PML).

The length and intensity of an acute exacerbation is shortened by the administration of glucocorticoids. Typically, an acute exacerbation is treated with 3 days of intense IV steroids followed by a course of oral medication tapered over 4 weeks. In patients with severe disease who are unresponsive to steroid therapy, plasma exchange can be used as an alternative treatment.

For patients with spasticity, baclofen is the most effective medication. Tizanidine and diazepam are useful for nocturnal spasticity but are limited in their use for daytime symptoms because they cause intense somnolence. Pain secondary to trigeminal neuralgia and dysesthesias responds well to carbamazepine, gabapentin, phenytoin, pregabalin, or tricyclic antidepressants. Bladder hyperactivity is treated with oxybutynin, whereas urinary retention is treated with bethanechol. Fatigue may be treated with amantadine or fluoxetine. Erectile dysfunction can be treated with sildenafil acetate.

All disease-modifying therapies are relatively contraindicated in pregnancy. Interferon and glatiramer should both be stopped for a pregnancy.

Fingolimod is an oral disease-modifying medication that decreases rates of MRI progression. It prevents lymphocytes from proliferating outside of lymph nodes. Cardiac toxicity can be severe.

Dalfampridine is an oral disease-modifying medication that increases walking speed. It is a unique potassium channel blocker for which the precise mechanism of action (for improved walking speed) is not clearly known.

DEMENTIA

> A 67-year-old woman is brought to the clinic complaining of forgetfulness. She states that recently she has been forgetting common phone numbers and the name of her mailman, whom she has known for 25 years. Her past medical history is significant for hypertension, coronary artery disease, and high cholesterol. Her physical examination is unremarkable.

Definition. Cognitive function is measured by various mental functions, including memory, concentration, language, praxis, visuospatial functioning, and executive functions. "Dementia" refers to loss of memory with impairment of any other cognitive function sufficient to interfere with social or occupational functioning.

Etiology. There are >100 identifiable causes of dementia in the elderly. Among the many **reversible causes** of dementia, you should consider hypothyroidism, vitamin B_{12} deficiency, hepatic or uremic encephalopathy, CNS vasculitis, syphilis, brain abscess, brain tumor (primary or metastatic), medications (especially anticholinergics), obstructive sleep apnea, central sleep apnea, trauma, subdural hematoma, normal pressure hydrocephalus (NPH), and depression. **Irreversible causes** of dementia include progressive multifocal leukoencephalopathy, Alzheimer disease, dementia with Lewy bodies, frontotemporal degeneration including Pick disease, vascular dementia including multi-infarct dementia and Binswanger disease, and Creutzfeldt-Jakob disease (CJD). Alzheimer disease accounts for 60 to 80% of all causes.

The prevalence of dementia is 1–5% between ages 65–69, rising to 45% by age 100. Only 5% of Alzheimer disease is inherited.

Clinical Presentation. The most common cause of dementia is Alzheimer disease. Typically, patients will present with problems in memory and visuospatial abilities that generally occur early in the course of the disease. Social graces can be retained despite significant loss of cognitive decline. Hallucinations and personality changes typically occur late in the course of the disease.

Mild cognitive impairment refers to memory loss without dysfunction of other cognitive domains. These patients have a higher risk of developing Alzheimer disease later in life but do not have Alzheimer disease. The rate of progression is 15–20% per year.

Alzheimer disease is, by definition, the loss of memory as well as other cognitive disturbances, such as aphasia, agnosia (the failure to identify entities despite intact sensory function), apraxia, or the loss of the ability to make plans and execute them. There is no single diagnostic test for Alzheimer disease.

Patients with frontotemporal dementias such as Pick disease will typically present with personality changes early in the course of their disease, with relative sparing of their visuospatial function. Social, interpersonal, and emotional abnormalities precede memory impairment. Frontotemporal dementia is often noted primarily by the family because the patient lacks insight into their condition. There is no proven therapy for this condition.

Dementia with Lewy bodies (DLB) can be confused with delirium and is characterized by fluctuating cognitive impairment.

Dementia secondary to Parkinson disease should be accompanied by clinical findings consistent with that disease. Recurrent visual hallucinations are also characteristic.

Dementia secondary to CJD is characterized by a shorter (weeks to months), more aggressive course than Alzheimer disease. Patients with CJD will present with dementia and myoclonus. Variant CJD is bovine spongiform encephalopathy (BSE). BSE is from the ingestion of prions from affected cattle. The diagnosis of CJD is by rapidly progressive dementia, myoclonus, ataxia, and the presence of 14-3-3 protein in the CSF. EEG may also help diagnose. These criteria can eliminate the need for brain biopsy.

Vascular dementia is divided into multi-infarct dementia, which typically has a stepwise progression associated with discrete cerebrovascular events, and Binswanger disease, involving the subcortical white matter, which presents with a slowly progressive course.

Normal pressure hydrocephalus will present with prominent gait abnormalities early in the course of the disease that usually precede the onset of cognitive impairment. There will also be associated urinary incontinence.

Diagnosis. All patients with cognitive impairment should be assessed with a Mini Mental Status Examination (MMSE) to identify the areas of cognitive impairment.

Initially, the workup should focus on ruling out reversible causes of the dementia. If a reversible cause is identified, it should be treated, with the hope that cognitive function can be recovered. Laboratory studies should include a complete blood count (CBC), electrolytes, calcium, creatinine, liver function studies, glucose, thyroid-stimulating hormone (TSH), vitamin B_{12}, RPR, and HIV.

Brain imaging is most useful for patients who have a focal neurologic exam, seizures, gait abnormalities, and an acute or subacute onset of their symptoms. EEG and CSF evaluation are not necessary except for NPH-opening pressure. No CSF marker is proven beneficial with the exception of 14-3-3 protein in CJD.

Treatment. Treatment of dementia revolves around insuring that the family and the patient have the proper medical and emotional support to cope with the disease. Caregivers are at an increased risk for depression and anxiety. Their concerns and frustrations should be addressed at frequent intervals.

Raising the level of acetylcholine in CSF benefits patients with Alzheimer disease. Pharmacotherapy with donepezil has been shown to improve cognitive function in mild to moderate dementia. Other anticholinesterase inhibitors (rivastigmine, galantamine) appear to have similar efficacy.

Memantine is a disease-modifying drug used in advanced disease either alone or with a cholinesterase inhibitor. Memantine seems to be neuroprotective and reduces the rate of progression of disease.

HUNTINGTON DISEASE

A 34-year-old man comes to the clinic for an evaluation of strange spontaneous movements that have been occurring lately. Recently, while sitting at a family dinner, the patient experienced uncontrolled grimacing with grunting. His father died at the age of 41 from "dementia."

Definition. A genetic degenerative brain disorder.

Etiology. Huntington disease is caused by the presence of the HD gene located on chromosome 4p. The gene contains a CAG trinucleotide repeat expansion that codes for a protein called *huntingtin*. The HD mutation leads to abnormal cleavage of the huntingtin protein, interfering with nuclear mechanisms, and causing cell death. The disease is inherited in an autosomal dominant fashion. Successive generations tend to have the disease occuring at an earlier age. This is called *anticipation*.

Clinical Presentation. The clinical hallmarks of the disease include chorea and behavioral disturbance. Onset is usually in the fourth or fifth decade and can begin with either chorea or behavioral change. The personality changes consist of irritability, anger, paranoia, or signs of depression. Antisocial behavior may develop. The chorea may begin as fidgeting that progresses to sudden movements of the trunk or limbs. Gait is poorly coordinated and has a choreic quality. Memory is usually preserved until late in the disease but lack of judgment, disinhibition, and inattention are early manifestations. There is frequently an associated depression. Dementia becomes severe later in the disease.

Diagnosis. Diagnosis is made by genetically testing for the presence of the CAG trinucleotide DNA repeat expansion. There is a 50% chance of passing it on to children. CT scanning shows cerebral atrophy. Atrophy of the caudate nucleus is severe later.

Treatment. Tetrabenazine helps the movement disorder of Huntington disease but will not reverse or cure the underlying disease process. Death occurs 15–20 years after the diagnosis. Haloperidol or clozapine can be used to control behavioral changes.

PARKINSON DISEASE

A 56-year-old man is brought to the office by his wife for evaluation of a resting tremor that she noticed recently. She also states that her husband has been moving "very slowly" as of late. When questioned, the patient states that he feels fine and does not know why his wife is dragging him from doctor to doctor. His past medical history is significant for mild hypertension that has been treated with a thiazide diuretic.

Physical examination is significant for a resting tremor noted in his right hand. When walking, the patient is stooped forward, taking small steps. You note cogwheel rigidity in his right upper extremity with a positive Myerson sign.

Definition. Parkinson disease is defined as a neurologic syndrome resulting from the deficiency of the neurotransmitter dopamine as a consequence of degenerative, vascular, or inflammatory changes in the basal ganglia.

Etiology. There are numerous causes of Parkinsonism. Many drugs can cause Parkinsonism, including neuroleptic agents (haloperidol, chlorpromazine), antiemetics (metoclopramide), alpha-methyldopa, and reserpine. Poisoning from MPTP, carbon monoxide, cyanide, and manganese are also causes of Parkinsonism. Any structural lesion around the basal ganglia (trauma, tumor, abscess, infarct) can produce clinical Parkinson disease. Patients who have survived an episode of encephalitis can develop *postencephalitic Parkinsonism.*

Clinical Presentation. The cardinal manifestations of Parkinson disease are bradykinesia (manifested by slow movements, mask facies, reduction of automatic movements), cogwheel rigidity, postural instability, and resting tremor. A useful mnemonic is to think of Mr. Parkinson as a fine **BRIT**ish gentleman.

> **B**radykinesia
>
> **R**igidity (cogwheel)
>
> **I**nstability (postural)
>
> **T**remor (resting)

There are a number of "Parkinson plus" syndromes, which are characterized by their relative lack of response to therapy with levodopa/carbidopa.

> Parkinsonism + vertical gaze palsy = supranuclear palsy
>
> Parkinsonism + prominent ataxia = olivopontocerebellar atrophy
>
> Parkinsonism + prominent orthostatic hypotension = Shy-Drager syndrome (now called *multiple-system atrophy*)

Several other diseases can imitate Parkinsonism. Severe depression can cause a paucity of spontaneous movement that can mimic Parkinsonism. Essential tremor can be mistaken for the tremor of Parkinson disease, but the lack of other neurologic symptoms and a positive family history of tremor and its amelioration with alcohol distinguish the two entities. A normal pressure hydrocephalus can present with ataxia and gait disturbances, which can also be mistaken for Parkinson disease. The presence of dementia and urinary incontinence with dilated ventricles on a CT scan of the head can help identify this disorder. Huntington disease can present with akinesia and chorea. The positive family history and dementia usually suggest the correct diagnosis.

Diagnosis. The diagnosis of Parkinson disease is a clinical one. It is important to identify any secondary causes of a patient's Parkinsonism that are potentially reversible. There is no diagnostic test of choice that can identify patients with Parkinson disease.

Treatment. There are many medications available for the treatment of Parkinson disease. The underlying pathophysiology that causes Parkinson disease is the imbalance of dopaminergic (too little) and cholinergic (too much) tone on the basal ganglia. Thus, medical treatment revolves around increasing dopaminergic tone or decreasing cholinergic tone on the basal ganglia.

Not surprisingly, the medications available for the medical treatment of Parkinson disease directly stimulate dopamine receptors (carbidopa/levodopa, dopamine agonists), indirectly increase the amount of dopamine available (COMT inhibitors, selegiline, amantadine), or block acetylcholine stimulation of the basal ganglia (benztropine, trihexyphenidyl).

Direct-acting dopamine agonists such as pramipexole or ropinirole can be used alone as initial therapy or in combination with small doses of levodopa/carbidopa. Two other dopamine agonists are bromocriptine and cabergoline. All of them are less efficacious than levodopa. Dopamine agonists do, however, have less dyskinetic side effects. Bromocriptine and pergolide are ergot derivatives and can cause cardiac toxicity.

The first step when considering what medication to start with is evaluating the patient's functional status. Patients with an intact functional status are managed differently from patients with a compromised functional status.

Patients with intact functional status (less bradykinesia) are not generally given carbidopa/levodopa as initial therapy. Such patients are started on anticholinergic medication when they are age <60. This is particularly true for those in whom tremor is the predominant symptom. When age >60, the treatment of choice is amantadine. The reason why anticholinergics are relatively contraindicated in elderly patients is because the side effects (dry mouth, urinary retention, constipation, confusion/hallucinations) occur more frequently and severely. Anticholinergics such as benztropine and trihexyphenidyl are used mostly to relieve tremor and rigidity. Avoid with BPH and glaucoma.

For patients with compromised functional status (more significant bradykinesia), the best initial therapy is carbidopa/levodopa. Carbidopa inhibits extracerebral dopa-decarboxylase, allowing more of the levodopa to reach the central nervous system, where it is needed. Levodopa is the precursor to dopamine. Carbidopa protects the levodopa from breakdown in the periphery, ensuring its secure delivery to the central nervous system. There are several late complications to carbidopa/levodopa therapy: Dyskinesia (abnormal movements), akathisia (restlessness), and "on-off" phenomena are all disconcerting to the patient. All of these late side effects are termed "response fluctuations" and can be managed by using a sustained release form of carbidopa/levodopa, adding a dopamine agonist, selegiline, or a COMT inhibitor, or restricting the main protein meal to the night. COMT inhibitors are tolcapone and entacapone. They are always used in conjunction with levodopa to help reduce the dose or modify response fluctuations. COMT inhibitors have no effect alone; they decrease the metabolism of the levodopa. They are an adjunct to the use of levodopa to reduce adverse effects.

Selegiline was once thought to slow the progression of the disease. Selegiline can be used in those with a declining or fluctuating response to levodopa. Selegiline offers mild symptomatic benefit in early disease. Rasagiline is a newer version.

Surgery should only be considered for patients who cannot tolerate or respond adequately to medical therapy. The procedures usually performed are pallidotomy or thalamotomy. The placement of deep brain stimulators is also effective when placed in the globus pallidus or subthalamic nuclei. Surgical therapy is a last resort.

BENIGN ESSENTIAL TREMOR

This is an idiopathic disorder consisting of an isolated tremor of the hands, head, or both. The lower extremities tend to be spared. Essential tremor can be worsened by the use of caffeine or beta agonists. Examination reveals no other abnormalities. Although the level of disability tends to be limited, there can be interference with manual skills such as the ability to write. It is characteristic of this disorder that there is an improvement with the use of alcohol. The patient will describe shaky hands, which improve with 2–3 drinks.

There is no specific diagnostic test for this disorder. Treatment is propranolol. If propranolol is ineffective, alternate medications are primidone, alprazolam, and clozapine. If no medical therapy is effective, thalamotomy is indicated.

RESTLESS LEG SYNDROME

Restless leg syndrome (RLS) is an idiopathic condition resulting in a sensation of creeping and crawling dysesthesia within the legs, leading to involuntary movements during sleep. Often the condition is brought to attention because of multiple bruises sustained by the sleep partner. The condition can be familial and is exacerbated by sleep deprivation, caffeine, and pregnancy. There is also an association with uremia, iron deficiency, and peripheral neuropathy.

There is no specific diagnostic test for this disorder. Treatment is a dopamine agonist such as pramipexole or ropinirole, although some patients may need levodopa/carbidopa. Other therapies are narcotics and benzodiazepines.

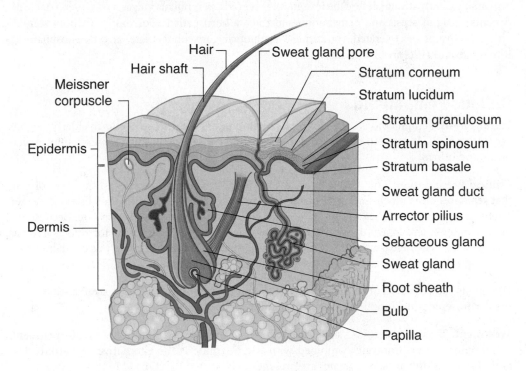

Figure 12-1. Skin

BULLOUS/BLISTERING DISEASES

Pemphigus Vulgaris

Pathogenesis. Pemphigus vulgaris is an *autoimmune* disease of unclear etiology in which the body essentially becomes allergic to its own skin. Antibodies are produced against antigens in the intercellular spaces of the epidermal cells. They attack the *"glue" that holds the epidermal cells together*. "Pemphix" is from the Greek word for bubble, which is what a bulla looks like before it is broken. Pemphigus vulgaris is most often idiopathic, but ACE inhibitors or penicillamine can occasionally cause it.

Clinical Presentation. Vulgaris occurs in patients age 30s and 40s, whereas bullous pemphigoid occurs in those age 70s and 80s. Pemphigus vulgaris is a much more serious and potentially life-threatening disease than pemphigoid. Vulgaris occurs prominently in the mouth and often starts there. The oral lesions are erosions, not bullae. The bullae are very thin and flaccid and break easily. This leads to the loss of large volumes of skin surface area, so it acts like a burn. This is because the bullae occur from destruction *within* the epidermis, making them thinner and more fragile. The presence of the *Nikolsky sign* (the easy removal of skin by just a little pressure from the examiner's finger, pulling the skin off like a sheet) is seen in pemphigus vulgaris, staphylococcal scalded skin syndrome, and toxic epidermal necrolysis.

The lesions of pemphigus vulgaris are *painful,* not pruritic.

Diagnosis. The most accurate diagnostic test is to *biopsy* the skin and to use immunofluorescent stains. These stains will detect intercellular deposits of *IgG and C3* in the epidermis.

Treatment. Treatment is with systemic glucocorticoids, such as prednisone. Topical steroids will not be sufficiently strong. Before the invention of steroids, pemphigus vulgaris was often fatal, with patients dying of sepsis and dehydration—just like a burn patient. For those in whom steroids are ineffective or not tolerated, you can use azathioprine, mycophenolate, or cyclophosphamide. Rituximab and *IVIG* are also effective.

Bullous Pemphigoid

Pathogenesis. Pemphigoid is 2× as common as pemphigus vulgaris and occurs in elderly persons age 70s and 80s. It can also be drug induced with sulfa drugs, including furosemide, penicillamine, and others.

Clinical Presentation. The defect occurs at the *dermo-epidermal junction*, so the layer of skin that separates off is much thicker. Because the fracture of the skin causing the blisters is deeper, the bullae are thicker walled and much less likely to rupture. Oral lesions are rare. Because the bullae are tense and intact, the skin is better protected. There is no dressing for skin as good as skin itself. Hence, there is much less fluid loss, and infection is much less likely as compared with pemphigus vulgaris. Mortality is much less likely in bullous pemphigoid.

Diagnosis. The most accurate diagnostic test is a biopsy with immunofluorescent antibodies at the dermo-epidermal junction (basement membrane).

Treatment. Systemic steroids, such as prednisone, are the standard means of treatment. Tetracycline or erythromycin combined with nicotinamide is the alternative to steroids. Use *topical* steroids only if *no oral lesions* are present.

Porphyria Cutanea Tarda

Pathogenesis. Porphyria cutanea tarda is a disorder of porphyrin metabolism. Deficiency of the enzyme uroporphyrinogen decarboxylase results in an abnormally high *accumulation of porphyrins*, which then leads to a photosensitivity reaction. The test question should give a history of HIV, alcoholism, liver disease, chronic hepatitis C, or a woman taking oral contraceptives. The liver disease may be from any cause but is most likely to involve chronic infectious hepatitis or hemochromatosis because porphyria cutanea tarda is associated with increased liver iron stores. Diabetes is found in 25% of patients.

Clinical Presentation. Fragile, *nonhealing blisters* are seen on the *sun-exposed* parts of the body, such as the backs of the hands and the face. This leads to hyperpigmentation of the skin in general and hypertrichosis of the face.

Diagnosis. The diagnostic test is a level of **urinary uroporphyrins**. Uroporphyrins are elevated 2–5× above the coproporphyrins in this disease.

Treatment. The best initial step in management is to *stop drinking* alcohol (although it is unlikely to be effective) and to *discontinue all estrogen use.* Combine treatment with barrier sun protection, such as clothing, because most sunscreens do not seem to block the wavelength of light causing the dermal reaction. The most effective therapy to use if this is insufficient is phlebotomy to remove iron. Deferoxamine is used to remove iron if phlebotomy is not possible. Also, the antimalarial drug chloroquine increases the excretion of porphyrins.

DRUG ERUPTIONS/HYPERSENSITIVITY

Urticaria

Pathogenesis. Acute urticaria is a hypersensitivity reaction most often mediated by *IgE and mast cell activation*, resulting in evanescent *wheals and hives*. It is a type of localized, cutaneous anaphylaxis, but without the hypotension and hemodynamic instability. The most common causes of acute urticaria are allergic reactions to medications, insect bites, and foods, and occasionally, the result of emotions. The most common medications are aspirin, NSAIDs, morphine, codeine, penicillins, phenytoin, and quinolones. ACE inhibitors are also associated with urticaria, as well as angioedema. The most common foods are peanuts, shellfish, tomatoes, and strawberries. Contact with latex in any form can also cause urticaria.

Clinical Presentation. Acute urticaria lasts <6 weeks in duration and two-thirds of cases are self-limited. Chronic urticaria lasts >6 weeks in duration and is associated with pressure on the skin, cold, or vibration. Pressure on the skin resulting in localized urticaria is also known as *dermatographism*. In acute cases, the onset of the wheals and hives is usually within 30 minutes and lasts for <24 hours. Itching is prominent. In patients with chronic urticaria lasting >6 weeks, you should investigate the etiology.

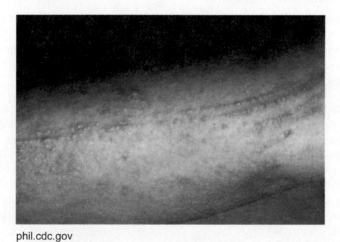

phil.cdc.gov

Figure 12-2. Contact Dermatitis Due to Poison Ivy

Treatment. Urticaria is treated with H_1 antihistamines. Severe, acute urticaria is treated with older medications, such as diphenhydramine (Benadryl®), hydroxyzine (Atarax®), or cyproheptadine. If it is life-threatening, use H_2 antihistamines when H_1 antihistamines fail and add systemic steroids. Chronic therapy is with newer, nonsedating antihistamines, such loratadine, desloratadine, fexofenadine, or cetirizine. Astemizole and terfenadine should never be used and are no longer marketed; they cause potentially fatal rhythm disturbances particularly when combined with other medications, such as macrolide antibiotics, because of their effect on the hepatic P450 system.

Note

For urticaria:

- Answer "**terfenadine**" or "astemizole" only when the test question asks what will kill the patient or which is the most dangerous medication.

- Answer "**desensitization**" when the trigger cannot be avoided, e.g., a beesting in a farmer. Beta-blocker medications must be stopped prior to desensitization because they inhibit epinephrine, which may be used if there is an anaphylactic reaction.

Morbilliform Rashes

Pathogenesis. A morbilliform rash is a milder version of a hypersensitivity reaction compared with urticaria. This is the "typical" type of drug reaction and is *lymphocyte mediated*.

Clinical Presentation. The rash resembles measles and is usually secondary to medications that the patient is allergic to, such as penicillin, sulfa drugs, allopurinol, or phenytoin. It is a generalized, maculopapular eruption that *blanches* with pressure. The reaction can appear a few days after the exposure and may begin even after the medication has been stopped.

Treatment. Antihistamines are effective, and steroids are rarely necessary.

Erythema Multiforme

Although erythema multiforme (EM) may be caused by the same types of medications that cause urticaria and morbilliform rashes (penicillins, phenytoin, NSAIDs, and sulfa drugs), the *most common cause* of EM is a *reaction to infection*. The majority of cases follow infection with herpes simplex or *Mycoplasma*.

Clinical Presentation. The most characteristic feature of EM is *target-like lesions* that occur especially on the *palms and soles*. These lesions can also be described as "iris-like." Bullae are not uniformly found. EM of this type usually does not involve mucous membranes.

Treatment is with antihistamines and by treating the underlying infection.

Stevens-Johnson Syndrome

Pathogenesis. Stevens-Johnson syndrome (SJS) is sometimes called **erythema multiforme major**. It is sometimes difficult to distinguish SJS from toxic epidermal necrolysis (TEN) and, in fact, the two diseases may be considered a spectrum of severity of the same disorder. All of these disorders may arise as a hypersensitivity response to the same set of medications, such as penicillins, sulfa drugs, NSAIDs, phenytoin, and phenobarbital.

Clinical Presentation. SJS usually involves <10 to 15% of the total body surface area, and the overall mortality rate is <5 to 10%. There is mucous-membrane involvement in 90% of cases, most often of the oral cavity and the conjunctivae, although there may be extensive involvement of the respiratory tract.

Treatment. These patients should be treated with early admission to a burn unit, withdrawal of the offending drug, and supportive care. Respiratory-tract involvement may be so severe as to require mechanical ventilation. Death occurs from a combination of infection, dehydration, and malnutrition.

There is *no* proven benefit for steroids. The best initial therapy for severe disease is IV immunoglobulins. Other therapies of unclear value are cyclophosphamide, cyclosporine, and thalidomide.

Toxic Epidermal Necrolysis

Pathogenesis. Toxic epidermal necrolysis (TEN) is the *most serious* version of a cutaneous *hypersensitivity reaction*. Mortality may be as high as 40 to 50%.

Clinical Presentation. Much more of the body surface area (BSA) is involved and may range from 30 to 100%. The Nikolsky sign is present, and the skin easily sloughs off. TEN has certain features similar to staphylococcal scalded skin syndrome; however, TEN is *drug induced* as opposed to being caused by a toxin coming from an organism.

Diagnosis. The diagnosis is usually clinical. The most accurate diagnostic test is a skin biopsy, which will reveal full thickness epidermal necrosis. A skin biopsy is usually not necessary.

Treatment. Sepsis is the most common cause of death, but *prophylactic* systemic antibiotics are *not* indicated. Systemic steroids are *not* effective and may, in fact, decrease survival.

Fixed Drug Reaction

Pathogenesis. This is a *localized* allergic drug reaction that recurs at precisely the *same anatomic site* on the skin with repeated drug exposure. It is not known why the reactions are anatomically localized and do not become generalized morbilliform rashes. The most commonly implicated drugs include aspirin, NSAIDs, tetracycline, and barbiturates.

Clinical Presentation. Fixed drug reactions are generally round, sharply demarcated lesions that leave a hyperpigmented spot at the site after they resolve.

Treatment. In addition to discontinuation of the offending drug, the reactions can be treated with topical steroids.

Erythema Nodosum

Pathogenesis. Erythema nodosum (EN) is a localized inflammatory condition of the skin or panniculitis. It is secondary to recent infections or inflammatory conditions. It is also associated with pregnancy. The most common causes of EN are recent streptococcal infections, coccidioidomycoses, histoplasmosis, sarcoidosis, inflammatory bowel disease, syphilis, TB, and hepatitis. Enteric infections such as *Yersinia* also cause the disorder.

Clinical Presentation. Erythema nodosum consists of multiple painful, red, raised nodules on the anterior surface of the lower extremities. They are extremely tender to palpation. They do not ulcerate, and they generally last about 6 weeks.

Diagnosis. ASLO titers can help determine who has recently had a streptococcal infection if there is no other etiology apparent from the history.

Treatment. Therapy consists of treating the underlying disease, as well as the use of analgesics and NSAIDs. Potassium iodide solution can be used in those who do not respond to symptomatic therapy. Erythema nodosum is usually a self-limiting condition.

> **Clinical Pearl**
>
> Always do a chest x-ray on a patient with EN, to exclude sarcoidosis.
>
> A biopsy of EN lesions will show nonspecific inflammation.

INFECTIONS

Fungal Infections

Tinea pedis, cruris, corporis, versicolor, capitis, and onychomycosis

All of the superficial fungal infections of the body share a number of common characteristics leading to the same answer on the test for similar questions for each of these diseases. "Superficial fungal infections" refer to those infections limited to the skin, nails, and hair. Remember, though, that these answers would not be valid for more deep-seated, life-threatening infections, such as fungal endocarditis, meningitis, or abscesses.

Clinical Presentation and Diagnosis. All superficial fungal infections of the skin, hair, and nails are primarily diagnosed by their *visual appearance* and confirmed by a potassium hydroxide *(KOH) test* of the skin. The leading edge of the lesion on the skin or nails is scraped with a scalpel to remove some of the epithelial cells or some of the nail and hair. KOH has the ability to dissolve the epithelial cells and collagen of the nail, but does not have the ability to melt away the fungus. Hence, a KOH preparation gives an immediate diagnostic answer by revealing fungal hyphae. This is particularly characteristic in tinea versicolor, where the *Malassezia furfur (Pityrosporum orbiculare)* organism appears in a "spaghetti and meatballs" pattern.

The most accurate test is to culture the fungus. This is usually not clinically practical because molds that grow on the skin (dermatophytes) take up to 6 weeks to grow even on specialized fungal media. A specific species usually does not need to be isolated in most cases, unless it is an infection of the hair or nails. In the case of nail and hair infections, oral therapy is necessary, and it is important to be precise because there are fewer medications that can be used to effectively treat onychomycosis. Tinea tonsurans is the cause of >90% of cases of tinea capitis.

Treatment. For onychomycosis (nail infection) or hair infection (tinea capitis), the medications with the greatest efficacy are oral terbinafine or itraconazole. These medications are used for at least 6 weeks for fingernails and 12 weeks for toenails. Terbinafine is potentially hepatotoxic, and it is important to periodically check liver function tests. Griseofulvin must be used for 6 to 12 months in the treatment of fingernails and has much less antifungal efficacy than terbinafine. Griseofulvin is no longer recommended in the treatment of oncomycosis of the toenails. In the treatment of tinea capitis, griseofulvin is recommended for 6 to 8 weeks.

All of the other fungal infections of the skin that don't involve the hair or nails may be treated with any of the following *topical medications:* ketoconazole, clotrimazole, econazole, terbinafine, miconazole, sertaconazole, sulconazole, tolnaftate, or naftifine. There is no clear difference in efficacy or adverse effects between them when used topically. Ketoconazole has more adverse effects when used systemically, such as hepatotoxicity and gynecomastia. This is why ketoconazole is not a good choice for onychomycosis. There is no topical form of fluconazole. Fluconazole is also less efficacious for dermatophytes of the nails when used systemically.

Antifungal medications generally should not be used in combination with topical steroids, unless a diagnosis has been confirmed. Steroids in a cream can relieve redness and itching and give the appearance of improvement even in impetigo and contact dermatitis.

Tinea versicolor

Definition. Skin infection characterized by multiple macules (usually asymptomatic), varying in color from white to brown.

Etiology. Pityrosporum orbiculare (Malassezia furfur).

Clinical Presentation. Tan, brown, or white scaling macular lesions that tend to coalesce; found on chest, neck, abdomen, or face. Lesions do not tan.

Diagnosis. Skin scrapings examined with 10% KOH under a microscope. The classic description is of "spaghetti and meatballs," which refers to the hyphae and spores that can be seen in the KOH prep.

Treatment. Topical selenium sulfide, clotrimazole, ketoconazole, or oral itraconazole. The need for local or systemic therapy is decided on the basis of the amount of surface area involved.

Note

Drug of choice for oral antifungal treatment:

- Tinea capitis and onchomycosis
  - Terbinafine or itraconazole

Clinical Correlate

Tinea versicolor has some additional features that are important in its management. It presents with lesions of different colors from tan to pink (hence the name *versi*color). The lesions often do not tan, and they present with pale areas in the middle of a normal tan. This can be distinguished from vitiligo by the fact that vitiligo has *no* pigmentation, whereas tinea versicolor presents with *altered* pigmentation. The organism may also be contagious. A KOH preparation and fungal culture are used in the same manner as for the other dermatophytes. The main therapeutic difference is the use of topical selenium sulfide every 2 to 3 weeks versus oral therapy with itraconazole or fluconazole. This is not because of antifungal resistance; it is because tinea versicolor is much more likely to involve large amounts of body surface area so it is difficult to cover this volume of skin with an ordinary topical cream or lotion.

Candidiasis

Definition. A yeast infection usually involving skin and mucous membranes, but it can also be systemic.

Etiology. *Candida albicans.* Usually spreads in patients with decreased host defenses. Patients with any of the following have an increased susceptibility: systemic antibacterial therapy, obesity, diabetes mellitus, corticosteroid or antimetabolite therapy, pregnancy, debilitating disease and blood dyscrasias, or HIV.

Clinical Presentation

- *Intertriginous infection:* Well-demarcated, erythematous, itchy, exudative patches, usually rimmed with small red-based pustules that occur in the groin, gluteal folds (diaper rash), axilla, umbilicus, and inframammary areas.
- Vulvovaginitis: White or yellowish discharge with inflammation of the vaginal wall and vulva. Common in pregnant women and patients with diabetes mellitus.
- Oral candidiasis (thrush): White patches of exudates on tongue or buccal mucosa
- Candidal paronychia: Painful red swelling around the nail

Diagnosis. Potassium hydroxide on slide to visualize fungal forms. Culture is definitive.

Treatment

- Topical nystatin, clotrimazole, miconazole, ciclopirox, econazole, or terconazole
- Systemic amphotericin in serious invasive infections. Fluconazole in less serious infections. *Candida paronychia* requires systemic therapy.

Bacterial Infections

Antistaphylococcal antibiotics

The most common bacterial organisms to cause skin infections of any kind are *Staphylococcus* and *Streptococcus.* Antibiotics used to treat *Staphylococcus* are dicloxacillin, cephalexin (Keflex®), or cefadroxil (Duricef®). Cefadroxil, cefazolin, or cephalexin are the preferred agents. If a patient is allergic to penicillin, but the reaction is only a rash, then cephalosporins can be safely used. There is far less than 5% cross-reaction between penicillins and cephalosporins. The IV equivalents of oral dicloxacillin include oxacillin and nafcillin. The IV equivalent of cefadroxil is cefazolin.

If the penicillin reaction is anaphylaxis then cephalosporins cannot be used. The alternative antibiotics that will treat the skin are macrolides, such as erythromycin, azithromycin, clarithromycin, or the newer fluoroquinolones (levofloxacin or moxifloxacin). Ciprofloxacin will not adequately cover the skin. Vancomycin is only for IV use for skin infections, and oral vancomycin is not absorbed. Oral therapy for MRSA is with clindamycin, TMP/SMX, or doxycycline. The ultimate form of oral MRSA therapy is linezolid.

Impetigo

Definition. A superficial, pustular skin infection, seen mainly in children (ecthyma is an ulcerative form of impetigo), with oozing, crusting, and draining of the lesions. It is a superficial bacterial infection of the skin largely limited to the epidermis and not spreading below the dermal-epidermal junction.

Etiology. Group A beta-hemolytic *Streptococcus* and *S. aureus* (*bullous impetigo*).

Clinical Presentation. Because it is limited to the epidermis, the purulent material is easily able to express itself through the surface; therefore, the patient history will describe the infection with words such as "weeping," "oozing," "honey colored," or "draining." Impetigo occurs more often in warm, humid conditions, particularly when there is poverty and crowding of children. This is because it is both contagious and autoinoculable. More common on arms, legs, and face. May follow trauma to skin. Begins as maculopapules and rapidly progresses to vesicular pustular lesions or bullae. The crusts are described as having a golden or yellow appearance and if untreated can progress to lymphangitis, furunculosis, or cellulitis, and acute glomerulonephritis. Impetigo may cause glomerulonephritis, but it will not cause rheumatic fever.

Note

Group A *streptococci* and *S. aureus* are the most common causes of impetigo.

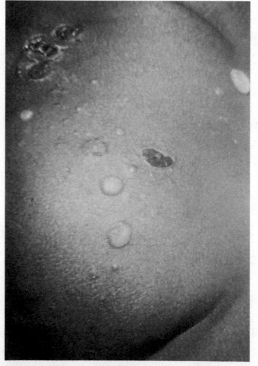

phil.cdc.gov

Figure 12-3. Bullous Impetigo of the Buttocks

Treatment

- Oral first-generation cephalosporin or semisynthetic penicillin, e.g., oxacillin, cloxacillin, dicloxacillin (for severe or widespread cases)
- Topical mupirocin, bacitracin, or retapamulin for mild cases of impetigo
- Penicillin-allergic patients can be treated with macrolides such as clarithromycin or azithromycin.
- TMP/SMZ, clindamycin, or doxycycline for MRSA

Erysipelas

Pathogenesis. Erysipelas is a bacterial infection of a deeper layer of the skin than impetigo. Erysipelas involves both the dermis and epidermis and is most commonly caused by group A Streptococcus (pyogenes).

Clinical Presentation. Because it involves lymphatic channels in the dermis, erysipelas is more likely to result in fever, chills, and bacteremia. It often involves the face, giving a bright red, angry, swollen appearance. Usually bilateral, shiny red, indurated edematous tender lesions on the face, arms, and legs. These lesions are often sharply demarcated from the surrounding normal skin. Differentiate from herpes, contact dermatitis, and angioneurotic edema.

Treatment. Semisynthetic penicillin or first-generation cephalosporin if you cannot distinguish it from cellulitis; penicillin (if *Streptococcus* is certain).

Cellulitis

Pathogenesis. Cellulitis is a bacterial infection of the dermis and subcutaneous tissues with Staphylococcus and Streptococcus.

Clinical Presentation. Cellulitis is characterized by redness, swelling, and warmth and tenderness of the skin. Because it is *below the dermal-epidermal junction*, there is no oozing, crusting, weeping, or draining.

Treatment. Cellulitis is treated with the antibiotics prescribed for erysipelas on the basis of the severity of the disease. If there is fever, hypotension, or signs of sepsis or if oral therapy has not been effective, then the patient should receive IV therapy. Oxacillin, nafcillin, or cefazolin is the best therapy. Treatment is generally empiric because injecting and aspirating sterile saline for a specific microbiologic diagnosis has only a 20% sensitivity. Oral therapy for MRSA is with clindamycin, TMP/SMX, or doxycycline.

Folliculitis, furuncles, and carbuncles

Pathogenesis. Folliculitis, furuncles, and carbuncles represent *3 degrees of severity* of staphylococcal infections occurring around a hair follicle. Occasionally, folliculitis can be the result of those who contract *Pseudomonas* in a whirlpool or from a hot tub.

Clinical Presentation. As folliculitis worsens from a simple superficial infection around a hair follicle, it becomes a small collection of infected material known as a furuncle. When several furuncles become confluent into a single lesion, the lesion becomes known as a carbuncle, which is essentially a localized skin abscess. Folliculitis is rarely tender, but furuncles and carbuncles are often extremely tender.

Treatment. Folliculitis mainly can be treated with warm compresses locally without the need for antibiotics. If antibiotics are required, mupirocin is the best choice. Furuncles and carbuncles

Note

Retapamulin is a topical antibacterial more active against staph and strep than mupirocin or bacitracin are.

require treatment with systemic antistaphylococcal antibiotics, and in the case of carbuncles, should be administered intravenously. Treatment with dicloxacillin, cephalexin, or cefadroxyl is acceptable. A large furuncle or carbuncle will also require surgical drainage.

Necrotizing fasciitis

Pathogenesis. Necrotizing fasciitis is an extremely severe, life-threatening infection of the skin. It starts as a cellulitis that dissects into the fascial planes of the skin. *Streptococcus* and *Clostridium* are the most common organisms because they are able to produce a toxin that further worsens the damage to the fascia. Diabetes increases the risk of developing fasciitis.

Clinical Presentation. The features that distinguish necrotizing fasciitis from simple cellulitis are a *very high fever*, a portal of entry into the skin, pain out of proportion to the superficial appearance, the presence of *bullae*, and *palpable crepitus*.

Diagnosis. Laboratory evidence of necrotizing fasciitis is an elevated creatine phosphokinase and an x-ray, CT scan, or MRI that show *air in the tissue or necrosis*. All of these laboratory methods of establishing a diagnosis lack both sensitivity and specificity. Surgical debridement is the best way to confirm the diagnosis and is also the mainstay of therapy.

Treatment. Surgery is the mainstay of therapy. The best empiric antibiotics are the beta-lactam/ beta-lactamase combination medications, such as ampicillin/sulbactam (Unasyn®), ticarcillin/ clavulanate (Timentin®), or piperacillin/tazobactam (Zosyn®). If there is a definite diagnosis of group A *Streptococcus (pyogenes)*, then treat with clindamycin and penicillin. Without adequate therapy, necrotizing fasciitis has an 80% mortality rate.

Paronychia

Paronychia is an infection loculated under the skin surrounding a *nail*. It is generally treated with a small incision to allow drainage and with antistaphylococcal antibiotics. The antistaphylococcal antibiotics are dicloxacillin, cefadroxil, or cephalexin orally, or oxacillin, nafcillin, or cefazolin intravenously.

Viral Infections

Herpes simplex

Pathogenesis. Herpes simplex infections of the genitals are characterized by multiple, painful vesicles.

Clinical Presentation. The vesicles are usually obvious by examination, and antibiotic therapy should be initiated immediately without waiting for results of the tests.

Diagnosis. This is done with active lesions only. In the event that the diagnosis is not clear or the lesions have become confluent into an ulcer, the best initial test is a Tzanck smear. The Tzanck smear is somewhat nonspecific in that it will determine only that the infection is in the herpes-virus family. Tzanck smears detect *multinucleated giant cells* and are similar in technique to a Pap smear. A scraping of the lesion is immediately placed on a slide and sprayed with fixative. Tzanck smears have 75% sensitivity in diagnosing facial herpetic lesions, but only 40% sensitivity in diagnosing genital lesions.

The most accurate diagnostic test is a viral culture, which will grow in 24 to 48 hours. Serology is *not* a useful test for diagnosing herpes infections.

Treatment. Immediate therapy is with oral acyclovir, famciclovir, or valacyclovir. Topical acyclovir has extremely little efficacy; it will slightly improve resolution in primary lesions and will do absolutely nothing for recurrent herpes simplex lesions. Topical penciclovir has some use for oral herpetic lesions, but it must be applied every 2 hours. The treatment of acyclovir-resistant herpes is with foscarnet.

Herpes zoster/varicella

Pathogenesis. Chickenpox is primarily a disease of children. Complications of varicella are pneumonia, hepatitis, and dissemination. Episodes of dermatomal herpes zoster, also known as shingles, occur more frequently in the elderly and in those with defects of the lymphocytic portion of the immune system (i.e., leukemia, lymphoma, HIV, or those on steroids).

Clinical Presentation. The vesicles are 2 to 3 mm in size at all stages of development and are on an erythematous base.

Diagnosis. Although the Tzanck prep and viral culture are the best initial and most accurate diagnostic tests, they are generally not necessary because little else will produce a band of vesicles in a dermatomal distribution besides herpes zoster.

Treatment. Chickenpox is generally not treated with antivirals. If the child is immunocompromised or the primary infection occurs in an adult, then acyclovir, valacyclovir, or famciclovir should be given.

Steroid use is still not clearly beneficial, although the best evidence for efficacy is in elderly patients with severe pain. The rapid administration of acyclovir still has the best efficacy for decreasing the risk of postherpetic neuralgia.

Other treatments for managing the pain are gabapentin, tricyclic antidepressants, and topical capsaicin. The most effective analgesic specific for postherpetic neuralgia is gabapentin. Nonimmune adults exposed to chickenpox should receive varicella zoster immunoglobulin within 96 hours of the exposure in order for it to be effective.

Molluscum contagiosum

Definition. Skin-colored, waxy, umbilicated papules.

Etiology. Poxvirus.

Clinical Presentation. Small papules that appear anywhere on the skin (genital and pubic area), usually by venereal contact, and are asymptomatic. The lesions have a central umbilication. They can be transmitted by skin-to-skin contact or sexually. Commonly seen in children; frequency is increased severalfold in patients infected with HIV.

Diagnosis

- Mainly on appearance; lab testing is rarely, if ever, necessary.
- Giemsa stain: large cells with inclusion bodies

Treatment. Freezing, curettage, electrocautery, or cantharidin.

PARASITIC INFECTIONS

Scabies

Pathogenesis. Scabies involves vesicular eruptions resulting from the females of the *Sarcoptes scabiei (hominis)* burrowing into the skin.

Definition. A parasitic skin infection characterized by superficial burrows, intense pruritus, and secondary infections.

Etiology. Itch mite, *Sarcoptes scabiei*. Transmitted by skin-to-skin contact.

Clinical Presentation. Scabies primarily involves the web spaces of the hands and feet. It also produces pruritic lesions around the penis, breasts, and axillary folds. Itching can be extreme. Because *Sarcoptes scabiei* is quite small, all that can be seen with the naked eye are the burrows and excoriations around small pruritic vesicles. Scabies often spares the head. Immunocompromised patients, such as those with HIV, are particularly vulnerable to an extremely exuberant form of scabies with severe crusting and malodorousness, known as Norwegian scabies.

Diagnosis. The diagnosis in all cases is confirmed by scraping out the organism after mineral oil is applied to a burrow; however, skin scrapings are usually not necessary and are not routinely done.

Treatment. Scabies can be successfully treated with permethrin. Lindane (Kwell) has equal efficacy, but also greater toxicity. Lindane should not be used in pregnant women. Ivermectin is a suitable alternative and is given as oral therapy if the disease is extensive. Treat Norwegian scabies with a combination of permethrin and ivermectin.

Pediculosis

Definition. Skin infestation by lice.

Etiology

- Head: *Pediculus humanus capitis*
- Body: *Pediculus humanus corporis*
- Pubic area: *Phthirus pubis* ("crab louse")

Clinical Findings. Itching, excoriations, erythematous macules and papules, and sometimes secondary bacterial infection.

Diagnosis. Direct examination of the pubic area, axillae, scalp, and other hair-bearing surfaces for the organism (louse or nits).

Treatment. Permethrin, lindane (Kwell).

TOXIN-MEDIATED DISEASES

Toxic Shock Syndrome

Pathogenesis. This disorder is a systemic reaction to a toxin produced from *Staphylococcus* attached to a foreign body. The majority of cases now are not from a menstrual source, such as a tampon or vaginal packing. Nasal packing, retained sutures, or any other form of surgical material retained in the body can promote the growth of the type of staphylococci that produces the toxin.

Clinical Presentation/Diagnosis. Because there is no single specific test, cases are matters of definition. The definition of a case of toxic shock syndrome is the presence of 3 or more or of the following findings: fever >102°F, a systolic blood pressure <90 mm Hg, a desquamative rash, vomiting, involvement of the mucous membranes of the eyes, mouth, or genitals, elevated bilirubin, or platelets <100,000. In addition, toxic shock is a systemic disease that also raises the creatinine, creatine phosphokinase (CPK), and liver function tests; lowers the platelet count; and can cause central nervous system dysfunction, such as confusion. Hypocalcemia is common, usually because of a diffuse capillary leak syndrome that drops the albumin level. Streptococcal toxic shock syndrome is essentially the same.

Treatment. In addition to removing the source of the infection, treatment is with vigorous fluid resuscitation, pressors (such as dopamine), and antibiotics. Empiric treatment is with clindamycin plus vancomycin until cultures return. In confirmed cases of methicillin sensitive strains, treatment should be with clindamycin plus an antistaphylococcal medication (oxacillin, nafcillin). In methicillin resistant strains (MRSA), either vancomycin or linezolid can be used.

Staphylococcal Scalded Skin Syndrome

Pathogenesis. Staphylococcal scalded skin syndrome (SSSS) is transmitted through physical contact with surroundings. It most commonly occurs in infants and young children and in the immunocompromised.

Clinical Presentation. SSSS is mediated by a toxin from *Staphylococcus*. The major presentation is the loss of the superficial layers of the epidermis in sheets. Nikolsky sign is present. It is markedly different from toxic shock syndrome in that there is normal blood pressure and no involvement of the liver, kidney, bone marrow, or central nervous system.

Treatment. Patients should be managed in a burn unit and given oxacillin or other antistaphylococcal antibiotics. Vancomycin can be added because of the possibility of MRSA.

BENIGN AND PRECANCEROUS LESIONS

The predominant method of distinguishing between benign and malignant lesions is by the shape and color of the lesion. Benign lesions, such as the junctional or intradermal nevus, do not grow in size and have smooth, regular borders with a diameter usually <1 cm. In addition, they are homogenous in color, and this remains constant. Biopsy is the most accurate method of making a diagnosis, and benign lesions need to be removed only for cosmetic purposes.

Note

Differential Diagnosis

SSSS:

- From an infection
- Splits off only the superficial granular layer of skin

TEN:

- From drug toxicity
- Full-thickness split of skin

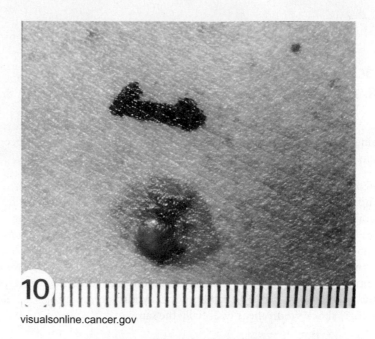

visualsonline.cancer.gov

Figure 12-4. Dysplastic Nevus

Seborrheic Keratosis

Pathogenesis. This is a benign condition with hyperpigmented lesions occurring in the elderly. Seborrheic keratosis has no malignant potential and no relation to either actinic keratosis or seborrheic dermatitis.

Clinical Presentation. The lesions have a "stuck on" appearance and are most common on the face shoulders, chest, and back.

Treatment. They are removed only for cosmetic purposes with liquid nitrogen or curettage.

Actinic Keratosis

Pathogenesis. Actinic keratosis presents with precancerous lesions occurring on sun-exposed areas of the body in older persons. The lesions occur more often in those with light skin color. They contain chromosomal abnormalities, and although only 1:1,000 lesions progresses to squamous cell cancer, an individual patient may have dozens of them. Hence, the rate of transformation to squamous cell cancer is 0.25% per patient.

Clinical Presentation. Although the lesions are usually asymptomatic, they can be tender to the touch and lighter in color.

Treatment. Therapy is universally with sunscreen to prevent progression and recurrence. In addition, the lesions should be removed with cryotherapy, topical 5 fluorouracil (5-FU), imiquimod, topical retinoic-acid derivatives, or even curettage.

MALIGNANT DISEASES

Melanoma

Pathogenesis. Superficial spreading melanoma is the most common type of malignancy, accounting for two-thirds of cases. The rate of occurrence of melanoma is rising faster than any other cancer in the United States.

Clinical Presentation. Malignant lesions grow in size, have irregular borders, are uneven in shape, and have inconsistent coloring. Lentigo maligna melanoma arises on sun-exposed body parts in the elderly. Acral-lentiginous melanoma arises on the palms, soles of feet, and nail beds.

Diagnosis. Biopsy diagnosis is best performed with a full-thickness sample because tumor thickness is by far the most important prognostic factor.

Table 12-1. Ten-Year Survival Rates for Melanoma

Lesion Size (mm)	Survival Rate
<0.76	96%
0.76–1.69	81%
1.7–3.6	57%
>3.6	31%

Treatment. Melanoma is removed by excision. Huge 5-cm margins are not routinely indicated. The size of the margin is determined by the thickness of the tumor. Melanoma in situ needs only a 0.5-cm margin, with a 1.0-cm margin for those lesions <1 mm in thickness. Lesions 1- to 2-mm depth get 2-cm margins, and those >2 mm in depth get 2- to 3-cm margins. There is no definitive chemotherapy for any form of skin cancer. Interferon seems to reduce recurrence rates.

Squamous Cell Carcinoma

Pathogenesis. Develops on sun-exposed skin surfaces in elderly patients.

Clinical Presentation. It is particularly common on the lip, where the carcinogenic potential of tobacco is multiplicative. Ulceration of the lesion is common. Metastases are rare (3–7%).

Diagnosis. Biopsy.

Treatment. Surgical removal. Radiotherapy can be used for lesions that cannot be treated surgically.

Basal Cell Carcinoma

Pathogenesis. Sixty-five to eighty percent of all skin cancers are basal cell. (10–25% percent are squamous cell.)

Clinical Presentation. Shiny or "pearly" appearance. Rate of metastases is <0.1%.

Diagnosis. Confirmed by shave or punch biopsy.

Treatment. Surgical removal. Mohs microsurgery has the greatest cure rate. In this technique, instant frozen sections are done to determine when enough tissue has been removed to give a clean margin. 5-FU can be used in treatment of superficial lesions.

Kaposi Sarcoma

Pathogenesis. Human herpes virus 8 is the causative organism.

Clinical Presentation. These are purplish lesions found on the skin, predominantly of patients with HIV and CD4 counts $<100/\text{mm}^3$.

Treatment. Antiretroviral therapy to raise the CD4 count. When that does not occur, the specific chemotherapy for Kaposi sarcoma is liposomal doxorubicin hydrochloride or vinblastine.

SCALING DISORDERS (ECZEMA)/PAPULOSQUAMOUS DERMATITIS

Psoriasis

Pathogenesis. The etiology of psoriasis is unknown.

Clinical Presentation. Silvery scales develop on the extensor surfaces. It can be local or enormously extensive. Nail pitting is a common accompaniment. The Koebner phenomenon is the development of lesions with epidermal injury.

Treatment. Salicylic acid is used to remove heaped-up collections of scaly material so that the other therapies can make contact. If the disease is relatively localized, topical steroids are used. Severe disease also needs coal tar or anthralin derivatives. To avoid the long-term use of steroids, which can cause skin atrophy, and to avoid coal tars, which are messy to use, substitute topical vitamin D and vitamin A derivatives. The vitamin D derivative most frequently used is calcipotriene. Tazarotene is a topical vitamin A derivative.

All patients should use emollients such as Eucerin®, Lubriderm®, Aquaphor®, Vaseline®, or mineral oil. When >30% of the body surface area is involved, it is difficult to routinely use topical therapy to control disease. Ultraviolet light in that case is the most rapid way to control extensive disease. The most severe, widespread, and progressive forms of the disease can be controlled with methotrexate; however, it has the highest toxicity and may cause liver fibrosis.

The newest therapy is immunomodulatory biologic agents, such as alefacept, efalizumab, etanercept, and infliximab. These are monoclonal antibodies that target defects in the immune system, such as tumor necrosis factor.

Atopic Dermatitis

Pathogenesis. Atopic dermatitis is an extraordinarily pruritic disorder characterized by high IgE levels.

Clinical Presentation. Red, itchy plaques appear on the flexor surfaces. In children, lesions are common on the cheeks and scalp. Adults present with lichenification.

Treatment. Preventive therapy is achieved by keeping the skin moist with emollients, avoiding hot water and drying soaps, and using only cotton clothes because these patients are extremely sensitive to drying.

Active disease is managed with topical steroids, antihistamines, coal tars, and phototherapy. Antistaphylococcal antibiotics are used if there is impetiginization of the skin. Topical immunosuppressants, such as tacrolimus and pimecrolimus, can be used to decrease dependence on steroid use. Every effort must be made to avoid scratching. The topical tricyclic doxepin can be used to help stop pruritus.

Seborrheic Dermatitis

Pathogenesis. An oversecretion of sebaceous material and a hypersensitivity reaction to a superficial fungal organism, *Pityrosporum ovale*, underlie seborrheic dermatitis.

Clinical Presentation. These patients present with "dandruff," which may also occur on the face. Scaly, greasy, flaky skin is found on a red base on the scalp, eyebrows, and in the nasolabial fold.

Treatment. Therapy consists of low-potency topical steroids, such as hydrocortisone, or topical antifungals in the form of shampoos, such as ketoconazole or sulfide. Zinc pyrithione is also used as a shampoo.

Stasis Dermatitis

Pathogenesis. Stasis dermatitis is a hyperpigmentation built up from hemosiderin in the tissue. It occurs over a long period, from venous incompetence of the lower extremities leading to the microscopic extravasation of blood in the dermis.

Treatment. There is no way to reverse this problem. Prevention of progression is with elevation of the legs and lower-extremity support hose.

Contact Dermatitis

Pathogenesis. Contact dermatitis is a hypersensitivity reaction to soaps, detergents, latex, sunscreens, or neomycin over the area of contact. Jewelry is a frequent cause, as is contact with the metal nickel from belt buckles and wristwatches.

Clinical Presentation. It can occur as linear, streaked vesicles, particularly when it is from poison ivy.

Diagnosis. A definitive diagnosis can be determined with patch testing.

Treatment. Identify the causative agent and treat with antihistamines and topical steroids.

Pityriasis Rosea

Pathogenesis. Pityriasis rosea is a pruritic eruption that begins with a "herald patch" 70 to 80% of the time. It is mild, self-limited, and usually resolves in 8 weeks without scarring.

Clinical Presentation. It is erythematous, salmon colored, and looks like secondary syphilis, except that it spares the palms and soles and has a herald patch. The lesions on the back appear in a pattern like a Christmas tree (if the observer is especially imaginative).

Diagnosis. The VDRL/RPR is negative. This is a clinical diagnosis.

Treatment. Very itchy lesions may be treated with topical steroids.

DECUBITUS (PRESSURE) ULCERS

Pathogenesis. Decubitus ulcers are chronic sores that occur in the pressure areas of the body, where bone is closer to the skin. It is often associated with patients who are immobilized or bedridden.

Clinical Presentation. Stage I lesions consist of nonblanchable redness. Stage II lesions result in destruction of the superficial epidermis or partial destruction of the dermis. Stage III lesions have destroyed the full thickness of the skin, but not the fascia, and stage IV lesions show destruction all the way to the bone.

Diagnosis. Never culture a swab of the superficial ulcer or drainage from the ulcer. It will be impossible to determine whether it is a genuine infection or simply colonization. A definitive microbiologic diagnosis is often obtained only in the operating room after debridement.

Treatment. The major theme of management is to relieve pressure. If the lesions are definitely infected, then antibiotics are useful.

HAIR

Alopecia Areata

Pathogenesis. This is an autoimmune disease in which antibodies attack the hair follicles and destroy hair production.

Treatment. The majority will resolve spontaneously over time. Immediate therapy is with localized steroid injection into the area of hair loss.

Telogen Effluvium

Pathogenesis. This is the loss of hair in response to an overwhelming physiologic stress, such as cancer or malnutrition.

Treatment. The management is to correct the underlying stress or disease.

ACNE

Pathogenesis. The contributing organism is *Propionibacterium acnes*. Pustules and cysts occur, which rupture and release free fatty acids, which in turn causes further irritation. Acne is more common in girls, but boys have more severe disease.

Clinical Presentation. There are both closed comedones, which are white, and open comedones, which are black. The discharge, although purulent, is odorless.

Treatment. Mild disease is treated with topical antibiotics, such as clindamycin, erythromycin, or sulfacetamide. In addition, the bacteriostatic agent benzoyl peroxide is used. Topical retinoids are applied if the attempts to control the load of bacteria locally are ineffective.

Moderate disease treatment combines benzoyl peroxide with the retinoids tazarotene, tretinoin, and adapalene. Severe cystic acne is treated with oral antibiotics, such as minocycline, tetracycline, clindamycin, and oral isotretinoin. Oral retinoic-acid derivatives are a strong teratogen.

Radiology/Imaging

This concise section should help you understand when to order each of the different types of tests in radiology. A description of what is found on each type of test is provided. For example, What does a sonogram show, and what doesn't it show? When does one use a CT scan or an MRI? When is contrast the best answer in a test question?

CHEST X-RAY

The most basic radiologic examination is a chest x-ray. Standard x-rays are based on the degree of density of tissue and how much x-ray energy each type of tissue will absorb. The closer a bone structure is in density, the greater the energy it will absorb. Therefore, because bones block the most amount of x-ray energy, they will come out white on the film. Conversely, air absorbs or blocks the least amount of energy and thus will appear darkest.

Chest x-rays are *not* routine screening tests. There is no routine screening of the general population for cancer or tuberculosis. You can do a chest x-ray if the PPD skin test is positive, but this is not the same thing as just doing a general screening.

Most x-rays are posterior-anterior (PA) films. The x-ray plate is placed in front of the chest, and the patient is leaning forward against the plate. The x-ray beam is directed from posterior to anterior. The patient must be able to stand for a PA film to be performed.

Anterior-posterior (AP) films are less accurate but must be done in patients who are too ill or unstable to stand up. All patients with central venous lines or chest tubes, or unstable patients, such as those in the intensive care unit, undergo AP films. The single greatest difference on AP films is that the heart size is artificially enlarged on them because the heart is more anterior in the chest and will therefore cast a wider shadow. On a normal PA film, the heart should be <50% of the total transthoracic diameter. This is increased to >50% on an AP film. (This phenomenon is no different than holding your hand in a light shined against a wall. The farther your hand is away from the wall, the larger your hand's shadow will appear.)

Technical Aspects of Normal Film Quality

When examining a chest x-ray, first assess the film for its technical quality. If the patient's body is abnormally rotated, then the film will be less accurate. You can determine this by seeing if the trachea and the spinous apophysis are midway between the clavicles.

Chest x-rays should be performed when the patient is holding in a full inhalation. There should be at least 10 ribs visible, counting from top to bottom.

An underexposed film will have the structures appearing too white. An overexposed film will have the blood vessels appearing too dark, preventing one from accurately assessing the blood vessels.

Note that on a PA film, the right hemidiaphragm is typically higher than is the left hemidiaphragm. This is because the liver is underneath the right hemidiaphragm, pushing it up.

Expiratory Films

Expiratory films are used when one is looking for a pneumothorax. The lungs will appear smaller because less air will remain in the lungs on expiration. Because a pneumothorax is air outside the lungs in the pleural space, this air will appear relatively larger. The volume of air in the pleural space does not decrease on exhalation.

Lateral Chest X-ray

Lateral chest x-rays will determine whether a structure in the chest is more anterior or posterior. For example, they can determine whether a mass that is visible in the center of the mediastinum on a PA film is posterior, making it more likely to be a neurally derived tumor attached to the spinal cord or an anterior mass. Anterior mediastinal masses are from the thymus, thyroid, lymph nodes, or a teratoma.

Lateral x-rays also have a greater sensitivity for the detection of small pleural effusions. On a PA film, you need at least 100 to 200 mL of fluid present to even begin to see an effusion. Each hemithorax can contain 3 liters of fluid if it is filled to capacity. A lateral chest x-ray can detect as little as 50 mL. These figures represent the amount of fluid needed to barely begin seeing "blunting," or obliteration, of the costophrenic angle.

On a lateral x-ray, the right hemidiaphragm is the one crossing the heart shadow.

Note

The right hemidiaphragm will appear higher on a lateral x-ray and a PA film because the liver pushes it upward.

Decubitus Films

Decubitus films help detect the presence of a pleural effusion. These are taken with the patient lying on his or her side and are employed when blunting or obscuration of the costophrenic angle is seen on a PA or lateral x-ray. Effusions will move and form a layer on the side of the chest wall. Infiltrates from alveolar disease do not move with gravity. You cannot determine if an effusion is infected just from its appearance on an x-ray.

APPEARANCES OF COMMON DISORDERS ON CHEST X-RAY

COPD/Emphysema

The most common appearance of COPD on a chest x-ray is related to hyperinflation of the lung. This leads to a darkening of the lung fields because more air is present. This trapped air also flattens the diaphragm and gives the impression of an elongated or tubular-shaped heart because it has been stretched down. There is an increased anterior/posterior diameter, or "barrel chest." Further, bullae are large, air-filled cavities that can give thin, white lines on a chest x-ray as the walls of the cavities press up against each other.

Pneumonia

Lobar pneumonia causes a whitening of each individual lobe of the lung because of the greater density of the lung. The "silhouette" sign is present, which is when the border between the affected lobe and the surrounding denser structure is obscured. (The density of the lung increases because of alveolar infiltration to the point where it takes on the density of the nearby heart or diaphragm; hence, one can no longer tell where the lung ends and the denser structure nearby begins). Lower lobe pneumonia gives a silhouette over each half of the diaphragm. Right middle-lobe pneumonia obscures the right heart border and will not pass the minor or horizontal fissure seen on a PA chest x-ray. Upper-lobe infiltration will not pass the major fissure, and this is more easily seen on a lateral x-ray. You cannot determine a specific microbiologic etiology from the x-ray alone.

Diseases of the lung outside the airspace but in the interstitial membrane give a fine, lacy appearance visible in most, if not all, of the lobes. Examples of disorders that give interstitial infiltrates are *Pneumocystis* pneumonia, *Mycoplasma*, viruses, chlamydia, and sometimes *Legionella*. Noninfectious etiologies of an interstitial infiltrate are pulmonary fibrosis secondary to silicosis, asbestosis, mercury poisoning, berylliosis, byssinosis (from cotton), or simply idiopathic pulmonary fibrosis. As the long-standing disorders become worse and more chronic, a greater degree of fibrosis occurs. This leads to greater thickening of the membrane. The terms that are used for this more chronic, thicker appearance are *reticular-nodular* and, later, *honeycombing*.

Congestive Heart Failure

The majority of pulmonary vascular flow is normally at the base of the lungs because of gravity. When there is fluid overload, the blood vessels toward the apices become fuller. This is known as pulmonary vascular congestion, or "cephalization" of flow. The term *cephalization* is used because more flow is moving toward the head. The other findings associated with CHF are cardiomegaly, effusions, and Kerley B lines.

Kerley B lines are the least important. They are small, horizontal lines at the bases that represent fluid in the interlobular septa. Each lung has several lobes. When fluid builds up outside the lobes, this is known as a pleural effusion. When fluid builds up within each lobe, in between the lobules, this is known as a Kerley B line. This type of subtle radiologic finding is less important in the evaluation of congestive heart failure since the advent of the widespread use of echocardiography.

Position of Lines and Tubes

Chest x-rays are routinely used to determine the appropriate position of central venous lines and both endotracheal and chest tubes. The proper position of the tip of an endotracheal tube is 1 to 2 cm above the carina. It is important to keep some space above the carina so that when the head moves forward, the tube does not push into the carina, which is extremely uncomfortable and will provoke coughing. The tip of central venous lines is at the junction of the superior vena cava and the right atrium, at the point where the right mainstem bronchus is seen. The tip of the line should not be fully inside the atrium because this can irritate the heart and may provoke an arrhythmia.

Note

Interstitial Syndromes of the Lung include:

- **S**arcoidosis
- **H**istiocytosis X
- **I**PF (interstitial pulmonary fibrosis)
- **T**umor
- **F**ailure
- **A**sbestosis
- **C**ollagen disorders
- **E**nvironmental
- **D**ust
- **D**rugs

Air under the Diaphragm

When there is perforation of an abdominal hollow organ, such as the duodenum, air is released and is visible under the diaphragm. The proper film to detect this is a chest x-ray taken in the upright position. This will allow the air to collect under the diaphragm, which should be easily visible. Abdominal x-rays do not always visualize the top of the diaphragm because of differences in body size. Chest x-rays always visualize the top of the diaphragm.

Imaging Tools for Lung Parenchyma

High resolution CT scan provides greater detail than a chest x-ray or CT scan because of 1 mm cut. This has a sensitivity of 95% and a specificity of close to 100% for lung parenchymal disease. High resolution CT scan is indicated in the following conditions:

- Symptomatic patients with a normal chest x-ray
- Detecting metastatic lesions, solitary nodules, bullae, bronchiectasis, and diffuse parenchymal disease (i.e., idiopathic lung diseases)
- To determine the type of lung biopsy required and site of biopsy

ABDOMINAL X-RAYS

Compared with chest x-rays, standard abdominal films without barium contrast provide far less information. Abdominal x-rays are beneficial only in the detection of an abdominal obstruction, such as an ileus or a volvulus; they do *not* reliably detect mass lesions, polyps, cancer, ascites, or inflammatory bowel disease. Mass lesions in all abdominal organs are best detected with CT scan or MRI of the abdomen. Polyps are best detected by colonoscopy. Ascites are visualized by sonography (U/S) or CT scanning. Inflammatory bowel disease, diverticulosis, and cancer are best detected by either endoscopy or barium studies of the bowel. Although 80 to 90% of kidney stones (nephrolithiasis) can be seen on abdominal films, they are also best detected by sonography or CT scanning. Only 10 to 15% of gallstones can be detected on an abdominal film because most of them do not calcify. Pancreatic calcifications can be detected in 30 to 50% of patients with chronic pancreatitis.

Sonography (U/S)

Sonography is used for evaluation of abdominal and pelvic pathology. Sonograms should be employed first for evaluation of the biliary tract because of their accuracy in evaluating dilation and obstruction of the ducts. The majority of cholelithiasis should be detected with sonography because cholesterol gallstones should be easily visible by sonography. The majority of nephrolithiasis is visible by sonography, although there is less accuracy in detecting stones in the ureters because they become retroperitoneal structures.

Sonography is useful in the evaluation of masses in the liver, spleen, pancreas, and pelvis, as well as for evaluating the presence of ascites. Despite this accuracy, CT scanning tends to have a greater sensitivity and specificity for the abdomen and pelvis. Sonography is particularly valuable in the evaluation of pregnant patients because it avoids radiation exposure to the fetus. Although less accurate, sonography is also practical in patients who have an absolute contraindication to the use of IV contrast. A total of 1:10,000 patients have a life-threatening reaction to the use of iodinated contrast agents.

There is very little utility of sonography in the evaluation of thoracic structures because the ribs block the sound waves. Also, sonography in the evaluation of intracranial structures, such as the brain, is not recommended because the skull blocks the sound waves.

Endoscopic U/S involves introducing a sonographic device into the abdomen at the end of an endoscope. Endoscopic U/S is extremely accurate in evaluating pancreatic pathology that is not easily visualized on CT scanning, such as a gastrinoma. Pancreatic lesions can also be effectively evaluated in this way.

Endoscopic Retrograde Cholangiopancreatography

Endoscopic retrograde cholangiopancreatography (ERCP) is an endoscopically introduced contrast procedure designed to visualize the biliary tract and pancreatic structures. ERCP is for therapy. The endoscope is introduced into the small bowel, and a catheter is placed through the sphincter of Oddi. Contrast is injected through the catheter. This allows extremely accurate visualization of the pancreatic ductal and biliary systems. ERCP is excellent for detecting strictures, stones, and neoplastic causes of obstruction. The other advantages of ERCP are the ability to perform therapy with the removal of these stones, to dilate strictures, and to perform biopsies. The scope does not routinely go up the sphincter of Oddi because it is too large to pass. MRCP is an MRI alternative to ERCP. It is less invasive than ERCP but does not allow an intervention.

The most common complication of ERCP is acute pancreatitis (around 10% in some series). Most of the time the pancreatitis is mild.

Barium Studies

Barium studies of the large bowel are never as accurate for colonic pathology as is endoscopy. In addition, you cannot biopsy with barium studies or perform therapeutic procedures, such as cautery or epinephrine injection for bleeding. The upper GI series is never as accurate as is upper endoscopy for the same reasons.

However, barium studies of the esophagus are a good test to start with for the evaluation of esophageal pathology. Barium esophagram is particularly good for the detection of strictures, rings, and webs, or Zenker diverticulum. Barium is not as accurate as an upper endoscopy for the detection of esophageal cancer because a biopsy is required. (Endoscopy is far superior for the detection and therapy of esophageal varices as well.) Barium is not as accurate as manometry for the confirmation of the diagnoses of achalasia or muscular disorders, such as diffuse esophageal spasm and nutcracker esophagus.

Capsule Endoscopy

The ileum and jejunum are the hardest parts of the bowel to visualize by radiologic studies or endoscopy. In the past, a "push enteroscopy" was performed by introducing an extremely long, thin scope into the small bowel. Capsule endoscopy is a new technology that allows direct visualization of the small bowel by swallowing a camera that electronically relays thousands of photographic images from the small bowel to a receiver outside the body. The drawback of this procedure is that it is not possible to perform therapeutic interventions in this way. If a patient has GI bleeding that is serious and both upper and lower endoscopy do not reveal the source, then answer "capsule endoscopy" on the exam.

Note

MRCP: diagnosis

ERCP: treatment

Clinical Pearl

Capsule endoscopy is not a screening test to detect colon cancer. Perform capsule endoscopy to evaluate obscure small bowel GI bleeding.

HIDA Scanning

This is a nuclear medicine scan useful only in the detection of acute cholecystitis. HIDA scanning is most useful in patients in whom the diagnosis of cholecystitis is not clear. An abnormal or positive test is the lack of visualization of the gallbladder. This is because the neck of the gallbladder or cystic duct becomes too edematous to allow the passage of the nuclear material. A normal scan will visualize the gallbladder. An abnormal scan will not visualize or fill the gallbladder.

Virtual Colonoscopy

This procedure uses CT scan or MRI to provide a computer-simulated bidimensional or tridimensional image of the air-filled, distended colon.

PET SCANNING

Positron emission tomography (PET) scans are useful in the detection of cancer. They are particularly useful in determining whether lesions that are visible on a CT scan of the chest are malignant or benign. Cancer is typically associated with the increased uptake of fluoro-deoxyglucose. PET scanning is used after chemotherapy to assess for the presence of residual cancer in some patients and can also be used to determine whether a patient is an operative candidate to remove a primary cancer. If the PET scan does not reveal malignancy, then the resection of certain primary cancers, such as lung cancer, is more likely to be successful.

Remember that slow-growing cancers (e.g., broncheoalveolar) may have a negative PET scan. Be careful when evaluating pulmonary nodules with PET scanning.

CENTRAL NERVOUS SYSTEM VISUALIZATION

In general, the most accurate test for evaluating the central nervous system is magnetic resonance imaging (MRI). The MRI is superior for the detection of stroke, cancer, multiple sclerosis, and infections and in the evaluation of the posterior fossa, such as the cerebellum and brainstem.

The CT scan does not visualize the brainstem well. For example, a stroke is visible on an MRI in >90% of cases within the first 24 hours after its onset, whereas the CT scan needs 3 to 4 days before >90% are visible. This is because the MRI is based on the water content of tissues rather than on the calcium content or simple density of tissue. Within a few hours after the onset of a stroke, the cells begin to swell and increase their water content. This is immediately visible on an MRI, whereas for a CT scan to detect an abnormality, the cells must die to decrease the density of visible cells.

The single exception in which a CT scan is superior to an MRI is in the detection of blood. As soon as bleeding occurs, it is visible on a CT scan. Therefore, the two cases in which a CT scan is a better study are to evaluate head trauma and to exclude hemorrhagic stroke. When a patient arrives within 3 hours of the onset of the symptoms of a stroke, a CT scan is first performed to exclude hemorrhage. This is to see if a patient is eligible for the use of thrombolytic therapy within these first 3 hours.

A CT scan is also used first for the detection of subarachnoid hemorrhage. On the first day after the stroke's onset, the CT scan has 95% sensitivity. The sensitivity diminishes by about 5% per day as the blood is hemolyzed and removed.

Clinical Pearl

Always check the patient's glucose before doing a PET scan. If the glucose is elevated, the PET scan can be falsely negative.

Contrast on a scan of the head is indicated primarily for the detection of cancers and infection. When an abscess or neoplastic process is present, there is some disruption of the blood-brain barrier, causing some extravasation of the contrast, which is visible as a contrast, or "ring"-enhancing lesion around the mass.

BONE IMAGING

An x-ray is certainly the first study to implement when evaluating trauma and fracture. Unfortunately, the bone scan has much less specificity and does not reliably distinguish between bone infection and infection of the overlying soft tissue. The MRI is both 90 to 95% sensitive and 90 to 95% specific.

Osteomyelitis

When there is the suspicion of osteomyelitis, then an x-ray is done first. Although plain x-rays lack sensitivity for the first 1 to 2 weeks, the specificity for osteomyelitis is excellent. More than 50% of the calcium content of bone must be lost for osteomyelitis to be visible. The earliest finding of osteomyelitis on an x-ray is elevation of the periosteum. If the film returns normal and there is still suspicion of osteomyelitis, then the best test is an MRI. The MRI and technetium nuclear bone scan have the same sensitivity (90–95%); however, the MRI's specificity is far greater (90–95%). Both studies should become abnormal within 2 days of the onset of osteomyelitis. Therefore, a negative bone scan is very useful if it is normal; it means that there is no osteomyelitis. If it is abnormal, you may still need to perform an MRI.

RETINAL DISEASES

Diabetic Retinopathy

Pathogenesis. The etiology of diabetic retinopathy is based on damage to the endothelial lining of the small blood vessels of the eye. This is identical in pathogenesis to the damage that diabetes causes to all blood vessels in the body, such as in the heart, kidney, brain, and peripheral nervous system. The endothelial lining of the retinal vessels becomes damaged, leading to progressive occlusion on a microscopic level. The occlusion leads to obstruction and increased pressure.

The earliest form of this adverse effect on the retina is called **nonproliferative** (or **background**) retinopathy. Nonproliferative retinopathy is characterized by dilation of veins, microaneurysms, retinal edema, and retinal hemorrhages. Hemorrhages into the retina are not as damaging as intravitreal hemorrhages because they do not obstruct sight.

Proliferative retinopathy is a more advanced form of the disease and is markedly more serious, meaning it progresses more rapidly to blindness. As the microvascular damage to the vessels worsens, these vessels secrete increased amounts of an angiogenesis factor. The vessels are not providing sufficient nutrition to the retina. The vessels themselves exert an increased effort to have more of them produced in an effort to deliver more nutrition and oxygen to the retina. Unfortunately, this "neovascularization," or new blood vessel formation, leads to the optic nerve getting covered with abnormal new vessel formation. In addition, hemorrhages protrude into the vitreous chamber. Vitreal hemorrhages are much more serious than microaneurysms or intraretinal hemorrhages because they are much more sight threatening.

The whole point of therapy for diabetic retinopathy is to first prevent the patient from ever progressing to the proliferative phase and, second, to slow down the disease's progress with laser photocoagulation, if it occurs.

Clinical Presentation. The clinical presentation of diabetic retinopathy is highly variable. There may be very advanced disease occurring with no symptoms. Vision may decrease slowly or rapidly. Vitreal hemorrhages may develop suddenly, and patients will complain of "floaters" in their vision.

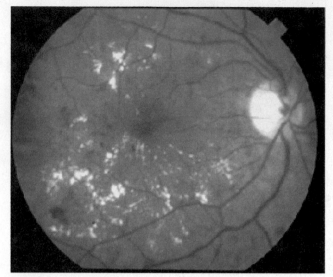

Retina-Vitreous Surgeons of Central New York

Figure 14-1. Features of Diabetic Retinopathy

Diagnosis. Screening for the presence of retinopathy should be performed on an annual basis by an ophthalmologist. This is how candidates for fluorescein angiography and laser photocoagulation are found. Fluorescein helps identify which vessels should undergo laser photocoagulation. The laser selectively destroys focal areas of the retina and diminishes the production of the angiogenesis factor, which causes the proliferative retinopathy.

Treatment of both stages of diabetic retinopathy involves the attempt to have tight control of glucose, blood pressure, and lipid levels. Proliferative retinopathy additionally involves immediate treatment with laser photocoagulation. Aspirin, clopidogrel, and other platelet-inhibiting medications have shown no benefit. The more tightly the glucose is controlled within the normal range, the slower the progression of the retinopathy. Blood pressure should be controlled to a level of <130/80 mm Hg.

Diabetes is considered by the National Cholesterol Education Program (NCEP) to be the equivalent to coronary artery disease in terms of its effect on cardiac mortality and on LDL targets. Even if there is no evidence of coronary artery disease, the target LDL in a diabetic patient is <100 mg/dL. If the patient is diabetic *and* has evidence of coronary disease, then the target LDL can be as low as <70 mg/dL. Glucose control is the most effective of these methods of retarding progression of the disease.

Retinal Detachment

A 71-year-old woman presents to the physician with blurry vision in her left eye since that morning. She says it was as if "a curtain came down." She has had floaters in the periphery of her left eye over the past few weeks but has had no pain or erythema. She has a history of stage I hypertension but is otherwise healthy.

Pathogenesis. Retinal detachment is usually spontaneous, but it may result from trauma. The term rhegmatogenous, which is used to describe the detachment, is from the Greek word for "tear." The two most common predisposing factors are myopia and surgical extraction of cataracts. Traction on the retina can also occur from proliferative retinopathy from diabetes, retinal vein occlusion, and age-related macular degeneration.

Clinical Presentation. The most common presentation is blurry vision developing in one eye without pain or redness. The patient may complain of seeing "floaters," as well as flashes at the periphery of vision. Sometimes it is described as a "curtain coming down," as the retina falls off the sclera behind it.

Diagnosis is made by ophthalmologic examination.

Treatment. Various methods of trying to reattach the retina are employed. Patients should lean their heads back to promote the chance that the retina will fall back into place. The retina can be mechanically reattached to the sclera surgically, by laser photocoagulation, cryotherapy, or by the injection of expansile gas into the vitreal cavity. The gas will press the retina back into place. A "buckle," or belt, can be placed around the sclera to push the sclera forward so that it can come into contact with the retina. If all of these methods fail to reattach the retina, then the vitreous can be removed and the retina can be surgically attached to the sclera. The majority (80%) of uncomplicated rhegmatogenous retinal detachments can be cured with one operation, with 15% needing a second operation.

Age-Related Macular Degeneration

Pathogenesis. Age-related macular degeneration (ARMD) is the most common cause of legal blindness in older persons in the Western world. The etiology is unknown. ARMD is characterized by the formation of deposits of extracellular material collecting into yellowish deposits seen on ophthalmoscopy. These deposits are known as "drusen." They are small, granular, subretinal deposits that are age related.

Clinical Presentation. There are 2 types of ARMD. The first is a *dry,* or atrophic, form characterized by slowly progressive visual loss in the elderly. Diagnosis is confirmed by finding clearly visible drusen on dilated eye exam.

The second type of ARMD is the *wet,* or exudative, form of the disease, characterized by the abnormal growth of vessels from the choroidal circulation into the subretinal space. These vessels leak, leading to collections of subretinal fluid and a localized, exudative retinal detachment.

Dry-type ARMD leads to visual loss of a slow, gradual nature. Wet type can present with the rapid distortion of vision over weeks to months. Fluorescein angiography will help confirm the diagnosis of exudative ARMD.

Treatment. There is no clear evidence that any therapy will stop the progression of dry-type ARMD. There is some evidence that zinc, antioxidant vitamins such as vitamins C and E, and beta-carotene may retard the progression of the disease. Wet-type ARMD is treated with VEGF inhibitors ranibizumab and bevacizumab.

Central Retinal Artery Occlusion

Pathogenesis. The etiology of the disorder can be from carotid artery embolic disease, temporal arteritis, cardiac thrombi or myxoma, or any of the usual causes of thrombophilia, such as factor V Leiden mutation.

Clinical Presentation. There is a sudden, painless, unilateral loss of vision. There is no redness of the eye. Ophthalmoscopy reveals a pale retina, with overall diminished perfusion and a "cherry-red" spot at the fovea. There is also "box-car" segmentation of the blood in the veins.

Diagnosis. These patients should undergo evaluation with carotid artery imaging, echocardiography, and evaluation for thrombophilia.

Treatment. Central retinal artery occlusion is managed in much the same way as for a stroke (cardiovascular accident [CVA]) or a transient ischemia attack (TIA). It includes laying the patient flat and supplying oxygen and ocular massage in an attempt to unobstruct the vessel. Other potential therapies are acetazolamide and thrombolytics. Anterior chamber paracentesis has been used to try to decompress the pressure in the eye and dislodge the embolus.

Central Retinal Vein Occlusion

Pathogenesis. Patients with retinal vein occlusion are at particularly high risk for developing glaucoma. These patients should be monitored for the possible use of laser photocoagulation. Younger patients should be investigated for inherited causes of thrombophilia, such as factor V mutation, protein C deficiency, and antiphospholipid syndromes.

Clinical Presentation. These patients have a clinical presentation similar to those with retinal artery occlusion. There is the sudden loss of vision without pain, redness, or abnormality in pupillary dilation. Ocular examination by funduscopy reveals disk swelling, venous dilation, tortuosity, and retinal hemorrhages.

Diagnosis. Retinal hemorrhages are the main way of distinguishing venous obstruction from arterial obstruction. You can't have a hemorrhage in the retina if you don't have blood getting into the eye.

Treatment. There is no specific therapy for retinal vein obstruction.

GLAUCOMA

Pathogenesis. The precise etiology of the majority of glaucoma is not clearly known. Acute angle-closure glaucoma can be precipitated by the use of anticholinergic medications, such as ipratropium bromide or tricyclic antidepressants; however, the majority of people with narrow angles in their anterior chambers never develop glaucoma.

In those with open-angle glaucoma, the precise etiology of the decrease in the outward flow of aqueous fluid has never been elucidated. Hence, the precise cause of the increase in intraocular pressure is not known.

Open-Angle Glaucoma

This disorder accounts for >90% of cases of glaucoma. Patients are asymptomatic for a long time, and this is the reason why it is important to screen older patients.

Diagnosis. The first clue to the diagnosis is a cup-to-disk ratio of >0.3, which should be confirmed by repeated measurements of an elevation in intraocular pressure as determined by tonometry.

Treatment of glaucoma is based on decreasing the production of aqueous humor while increasing its drainage. Medications that decrease the production of aqueous humor are beta-blockers (timolol, betaxolol, levobunolol), alpha-adrenergic agonists (apraclonidine, brimonidine), and carbonic anhydrase inhibitors (dorzolamide and brinzolamide).

Medications that increase the outflow of the humor are prostaglandin analogs, such as topical latanoprost, travoprost, and bimatoprost. The prostaglandin analogs can lead to a change in the color of the eyes and a darkening of the eyelid. Pilocarpine is a miotic agent that constricts the pupil to allow greater outflow of the aqueous humor.

Surgery is performed if maximal medical therapy is ineffective in controlling intraocular pressure. Laser trabeculoplasty or surgical trabeculectomy are the most commonly performed procedures.

Closed-Angle Glaucoma

Pathogenesis. This disorder is often an ophthalmologic emergency precipitated by the use of medications that have anticholinergic properties.

Clinical Presentation. It presents with an eye that is red, painful, hard to palpation, and associated with a fixed midpoint pupil. The cornea has a hazy cloudiness, and there is marked diminishment of visual acuity.

Treatment of acute angle-closure glaucoma is an ophthalmologic emergency. IV acetazolamide, urea, and osmotic diuretics, such as mannitol or glycerol, are used acutely. Pilocarpine can be used to open the canal of Schlemm, and beta-blockers are used to decrease humor production. If these medical therapies are ineffective, laser trabeculoplasty can be performed.

CATARACTS

Pathogenesis. Cataracts are opacifications of the lens. They are slowly progressive, with a blurring of vision occurring over months to years. Glare from the headlights of cars is particularly a problem when driving at night. Color perception is reduced in general. The etiology of cataracts is unknown, although there is an association with cigarette smoking.

Clinical Presentations. Mature cataracts can be easily seen on physical examination. Earlier-stage disease is seen with a slit lamp.

Treatment. There is no medical therapy for cataracts. Surgical removal with the placement of an intraocular lens is the standard of care.

CONJUNCTIVAL DISEASES

Conjunctivitis

Pathogenesis. Conjunctivitis can occur from any infectious agent, including bacteria, viruses, and fungi.

Clinical Presentation. Bacterial conjunctivitis is more often unilateral and presents with a marked purulent discharge from the eye. This is most symptomatic in the morning, when the patient's eye has developed a significant crust overnight, sometimes making it hard to open the eye. There is less itching compared with viral conjunctivitis. Although the eye can be red, there is a normally reactive pupil, as well as normal ocular pressure and no impairment of visual acuity.

Viral conjunctivitis is more often bilateral in nature, with much more severe ocular itching and enlarged preauricular adenopathy. The eyes are also red, but again, the pupil reacts normally and there is no photophobia.

Treatment of bacterial conjunctivitis is with topical antibiotics, such as erythromycin ointment, sulfacetamide drops, or topical fluoroquinolones. There is no specific microbiologic treatment for viral conjunctivitis. It is treated symptomatically with topical antihistamine/decongestants.

Subconjunctival Hemorrhage

Subconjunctival hemorrhage is more dangerous in its appearance than in its actual damage to vision or even the eye itself. The most common cause is trauma, particularly in the presence of thrombocytopenia. The collection of the hematoma stops at the limbus, which is the anatomic connection between the conjunctiva and the cornea. Because this prevents the blood from covering the cornea, there is no impairment of vision. There is no intraocular or intravitreal damage and hence no impairment of vision. No specific therapy for subconjunctival hemorrhage is necessary.

KERATITIS

Pathogenesis. Keratitis refers to any infection or inflammation of the cornea. Usually, keratitis happens as a result of trauma to the cornea with the inoculation of bacterial or fungal elements into the cornea.

Herpes Simplex Keratitis

Clinical Presentation. Herpes simplex keratitis is characterized by severe pain in the eye and a sensation that something is caught under the eyelid.

Diagnosis. The diagnosis is based on finding a characteristic dendritic pattern over the cornea on fluorescein staining of the eye with examination under a blue light.

Treatment. Therapy for herpes simplex keratitis is with oral acyclovir, famciclovir, or valacyclovir and topical trifluridin 1% solution or idoxuridine. It is most important for the general physician to *never* use oral or topical steroids in an attempt to relieve inflammation. This can markedly worsen the growth of the virus and essentially acts as fertilizer for the virus.

PERIORBITAL CELLULITIS

Pathogenesis. Cellulitis is caused by *Staphylococcus aureus* or *Streptococcus* invading the dermis and subcutaneous tissues surrounding the eye.

Treatment. Antistaphylococcal penicillins, such as oxacillin or nafcillin, should be administered. If there is an allergic reaction to penicillins, such as a rash, then first-generation cephalosporins can be used (i.e., cefazolin).

UVEITIS

Pathogenesis. The uveal tract refers to the iris, ciliary body, and choroid. When these structures are inflamed, the condition is called uveitis. The etiology of uveitis is from a large number of systemic inflammatory conditions, such as psoriasis, sarcoidosis, syphilis, Reiter syndrome, or inflammatory bowel disease.

Clinical Presentation. Uveitis leads to a painful, red eye with marked photophobia. One of the clues to the diagnosis is that pain occurs even when shining a light in the unaffected eye. This is because of the consensual light reflex in which the affected pupil will constrict even when light is shined in the normal eye.

Diagnosis. A specific diagnosis is made by slit lamp examination. Inflammation of the iris, ciliary body, and choroid is visible. Inflammatory cells may accumulate on the inside of the cornea after they precipitate out of the aqueous humor, rather like an accumulating snowfall. These focal collections are called keratic precipitates.

Treatment. The basic management, despite the varied underlying conditions, is to treat with topical or, sometimes, systemic steroids.

Index

Nultinucleated giant cells, 382
Nutcracker esophagus, 73

O

Obstructive sleep apnea (OSA), 304
Occlusion, of central retinal vessels, 402–403
Octreotide, 13
Onychomycosis, 378–379
Open-angle glaucoma, 402–403
Ophthalmology
  cataracts, 403
  conjunctival diseases, 403–404
  glaucoma, 403–404
  keratitis, 404
  periorbital cellulitis, 404
  retinal diseases, 399–402, 402
  uveitis, 405
Ophthalmopathy, in Graves disease, 20
Opiate toxicity, 328
Opioid analgesics, for migraine headaches, 360
Opportunistic infections, in AIDS, 225–227
Oral hypoglycemic drugs, 30–32
Organophosphate poisoning, 333
Orthostasis, in gastrointestinal bleeding, 93–94
Osmotic fragility test, 170
Osteoarthritis, 47, 62–64
  acromegaly and, 12
Osteodystrophy, in end-stage renal disease, 250
Osteomyelitis, 214–215
  imaging studies in, 402
Osteoporosis, prevention of, 6
Otitis media, 192
Outpatient setting, asthma patients in, 286
Oxacillin, 185
Oxalate crystals, acute renal failure and, 240
Oxygen delivery, gas exchange disturbances and, 278
Oxygen therapy
  home, in COPD, 291
  supplemental
    in asthma, 285
    in COPD, 290
Oxytocin, pituitary gland storage of, 9

P

Pancreatic B-cell tumor, 36
Pancreatic pseudocyst, 95
Pancreatitis
  acute, 94–95
  chronic, 87–88
  epigastric pain in, 75
  severe necrotizing, 95
Papillary carcinoma, of thyroid, 24
Papillary necrosis, acute renal failure and, 241–242
Pap smear, 2
Papulosquamous dermatitis, 388–389

Parapneumonic effusions, 280
Parasitic infections, of skin, 384
Parathyroid glands, diseases of, 24–28
Parkinson disease, 370–372
  dementia secondary to, 368
Parkland formula, 340
Paronychia, 382
Paroxysmal nocturnal hemoglobinuria (PNH), 171–172
Paroxysmal supraventricular tachycardia, 149–150
Partial seizures, 356
Partial thromboplastin time (PTT), 182–184
Patent foramen ovale, thromboembolism in, 298
Pediculosis, 384
Pegvisomant, 13
Pelvic inflammatory disease (PID), 208
Pemphigus vulgaris, 374–375
Penicillins
  allergic cross-reactivity and, 186
  for bacterial infections of skin, 385
  gram-negative bacilli and, 186–187
  gram-positive cocci and, 185
  skin reactions to, 379, 380
Pentamidine, 241
Peptic ulcer disease, 77–79
Percutaneous coronary intervention (PCI), 109, 113–115
Pericardial disease, 142–145
Pericardial effusion, 143
Pericarditis
  acute, 142–143, 225–226
  acute coronary syndrome and, 119
  chest pain and, 103
  constrictive, 144–145
Perilymphatic fistula, 357
Perinephric abscess, 213–214
Periorbital Cellulitis, 404
Peritonitis, spontaneous bacterial, 96
Petechial hemorrhage, in septicemia/endocarditis, 222
Petit mal (absence) seizures, 354
PET (positron emission tomography), 396
Peutz-Jeghers syndrome, 92
Pharyngitis, 193–194
Phenytoin therapy, 361
Pheochromocytoma, 43–44
  secondary hypertension in, 268
Philadelphia chromosome, 173
Phlebotomy, for hemochromatosis, 98
Phosphatidyl inositol glycan A (PIG-A), 171
Photosensitivity rash/recation
  in porphyria cutanea tarda, 378
  in SLE, 55
Physical examination, in cardiovascular disease, 100
Pick disease, 379
Pigments, acute renal failure and, 238–239
Pill esophagitis, 74
Pituitary apoplexy, 13
Pituitary gland, 9
  action of, 11

Staphylococcal scalded skin syndrome (SSSS), 385
Staphylococcus/Staphylococcus aureus infection
  antibiotics for, 382
  brain abscess and, 191
  infectious diarrhea and, 84
  meningitis and, 188
  methicillin-resistant. See Methicillin-resistant Staphylococcus
    aureus (MRSA)
  scalded skin syndrome, 385
  septic arthritis and, 66
  toxic shock syndrome and, 233, 385
Stasis dermatitis, 389
Statins, 117
Status epilepticus, 354
  development of, 355
ST elevation myocardial infarction (STEMI), 113–118
Steroids, for inflammatory bowel disease, 82–83
Stevens-Johnson syndrme, 376
Streptococcal bacteria
  gram-positive, 185
  in postinfectious glomerulonephritis, 247
Streptococcus bovis, 90
Stroke, 353–356
  hypopituitarism and, 14
ST segment
  depression, in ischemic heart disease, 108
  elevation, in acute pericarditis, 142–143
Subacute combined spinal cord degeneration, 348
Subacute (de Quervain) thyroiditis, 22
Subarachnoid hemorrhage (SAH), 337–338
  CT sensitivity in, 400
  in cerebrovascular accident, 356–357
Subconjunctival Hemorrhage, 404
Subdural hematoma, 337–338, 337–339
Sudden cardiac death, 119
Sugar-water test, 171
Sulfasalazine, in RA management, 52, 53
Sulfonylureas
  for diabetes mellitus, 31, 32
  overdose of, 332
Supplemental oxygen therapy
  in asthma, 285
  in COPD, 290
Supraventricular arrhythmias, 148–153
Supraventricular tachycardia (SVT), 317–320
Surgery. See also Transplantation; specific procedures
  in necrotizing fasciitis, 386
  in ST elevation myocardial infarction, 117
  mitral valve replacement, 133
Swan-Ganz catheterization, in ARDS, 303
Symptom-triggered therapy, in alcohol withdrawal management, 334
Syndrome of inappropriate secretion of ADH (SIADH), 17–18, 253
Synovial fluid analysis, 48
Syphilis, 208–209
Syringomyelia, 348
Systemic lupus erythematosus (SLE), 47, 54–55
  antinuclear antibodies in, 49

  glomerulonephritis and, 247
  malar rash in, 54, 55
Systemic sclerosis (SSc), 47, 56–58
  progressive, esophageal involvement in, 72–73
Systolic dysfunction, in congestive heart failure, 121, 126
  medical devices for, 128

T

Tabes dorsalis, in syphilis, 405
Tachycardia
  supraventricular, 317–320
  with pulses, management algorithm for, 316
Tegaserod, 87
Telangiectasias, in CREST syndrome, 57
Telogen effluvium, 390
Temporal arteritis (TA), 68, 358
Tension-type headache, 359
Terbinafine, 378
Terfenadine, 375
Testicular diseases, 45
Tetanus, 230
Thalassemia, 164
Theophylline, for COPD, 290
Thiamine, for toxic ingestion, 324
Thiazides, for congestive heart failure, 126
Thiazolidinediones, 31, 32
Third-degree (complete) atrioventricular block, 148
Thoracocentesis, 281
Thrombocythemia, essential, 176
Thrombocytopenia, heparin-induced, 184
Thromboembolic disease, 299–305. See also Deep vein thrombosis
    (DVT)
  acute coronary syndrome and, 119
Thrombolytics
  contraindicated, in STEMI, 115–116
  for pulmonary thromboembolism, 300
  for ST elevation myocardial infarction, 115–116
Thrombotic thrombocytopenic purpura (TTP), 245–246
Thymectomy, 363
Thymoma, 363
Thyroid gland, 18–19
  diseases of, 18–23
  neoplasia of, 23
Thyroiditis, 22
Thyroid-reactive iodine uptake (RAIU), 19–20
Thyroid stimulating hormone (TSH) test, 18–19
Thyroid stimulating immunoglobulin (TSI), 18–19, 21
Thyroid storm, 21
Thyrotopin (TSH), 14
Thyrotropin-releasing hormone (TRH), 11
Tic douloureux, 361
Tigecycline, 186
Tinea capitis, 378–379
Tinea corporis, 379–380
Tinea cruris, 379–380
Tinea pedis, 377–378